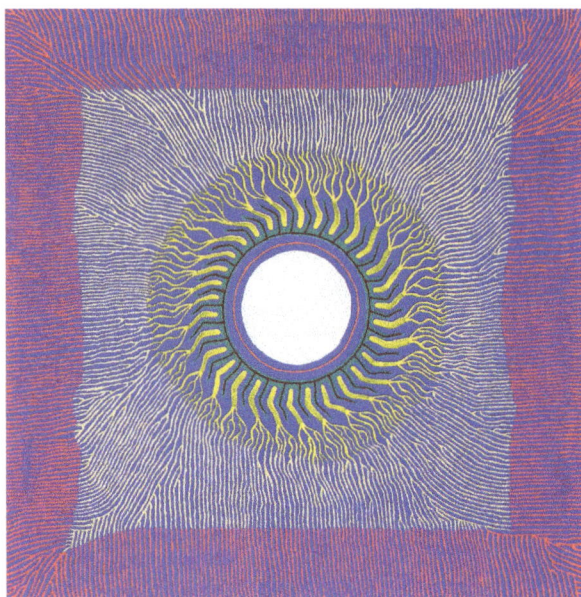

Mother Earth

Paul Dutton, the artist: Kali (Dingo Totem), Mukwarra (Moiety), Barkindji (mob) - Baaka (of the river - Darling). Striving for Mother Earth. Sharing for Humanity. Separated Stolen Generation, lived Sydney, reunited when 19 years old. Connected to my family, country and Spirits. Long-held belief in Just Justice and Social Inclusion is way forward to unite.

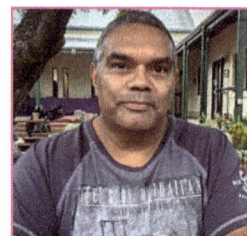

Mother Earth provides the story of all living things to which the rhythm of being flows. All existence flows from Mother Earth's spirit, one living being to another, from our creatures to our plants, air, water and beyond to the multitude of planetary universes and their Mother Earth's of spirit.

Humanity must learn to re-connect that gift for our own existence and future. We are individuals but communal beings, to live, heal, work, walk and breathe it must be done in unity to reach our 'meaning of life'.

ISBN 978-0-9876161-2-8
© 2017 Croakey.org

Suggested citation

Finlay, S.M., Williams, M., McInerney, M., Sweet, M., Ward, M., (Eds), 2016: #JustJustice: Tackling the over-incarceration of Aboriginal and Torres Strait Islander peoples (2nd edition). NSW.

#JustJustice

Tackling the over-incarceration of Aboriginal and Torres Strait Islander peoples

SECOND EDITION

#JUSTJUSTICE

Acknowledgements

We acknowledge the Traditional Owners upon whose country these articles were written and published, as well as Aboriginal and Torres Strait Islander people across Australia whose lives and families continue to be affected by punitive, unjust and culturally unsafe policing and justice systems, as well as a lack of accessible and culturally safe health, legal and community services. We acknowledge the enormous contributions made by many Aboriginal and Torres Strait Islander people and organisations in working for #JustJustice. This publication includes diverse styles and terminology, respecting that contributors have used differing terminology.

We caution Aboriginal and Torres Strait Islander readers that this publication may contain images and references to deceased persons, as well as to traumatic events.

NOTE: This book is published in both hard copy and e-book format. The hyperlinks (in red text) are of course not functional in the print version, and we apologise for any inconvenience. We encourage you to locate the online, hyperlinked articles if seeking further information from the links. Minor editorial changes have been made in the e-version of this book.

This book has been made possible through the generosity of more than 300 donors to the crowdfunding campaign that concluded on 7 June, 2015, and the generosity of two premium sponsors, Jesuit Social Services and Frank Meany of One Vision. In December 2016, Western Sydney University provided a $5,000 grant to enable this second edition of #JustJustice to be produced with some additional stories, and for dissemination strategies. See the full list of donors on page 243.

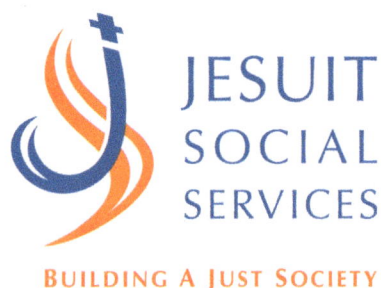

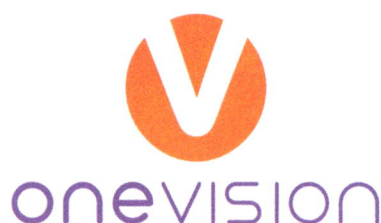

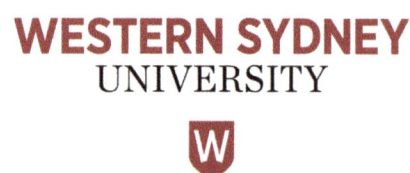

JESUIT SOCIAL SERVICES

BUILDING A JUST SOCIETY

onevision

WESTERN SYDNEY UNIVERSITY

We also acknowledge the dozens of contributing authors and organisations, as listed on page 247.

The #JustJustice team is:

Summer May Finlay • Dr Megan Williams • Marie McInerney • Melissa Sweet • Mitchell Ward

We also thank Luke Pearson, founder of IndigenousX, for social media consultancy for the crowdfunding project.

We thank Professor Tom Calma AO and Mr Mick Gooda for their support in launching the project. We also thank and acknowledge Sandy Davies and the Geraldton Regional Aboriginal Medical Service for inviting Croakey to attend the "PRISON HEALTH - From the Inside Out" conference, in Geraldton in 2015, and covering flight and accommodation costs for Marie McInerney.

Warm thanks to Karen Wyld and Sally Fitzpatrick for their generous help with the final editing.

Read more about the project and the team on page 241.

The #JustJustice articles were first published at Croakey.org, a social journalism project for public health.

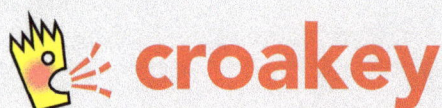

croakey

Foreword

In Aboriginal and Torres Strait Islander affairs we are continually exposed to the horrendous statistics of the disadvantage Aboriginal and Torres Strait Islander people experience across the board and of the mainstream media who portray us as a failed peoples. Government Ministers are notorious in talking about failed experiments, cultural museums, lifestyle choices, the high expenditure on Indigenous affairs and our burden on society – all of which generally portrays a negative and deficit viewpoint about Aboriginal and Torres Strait Islander people.

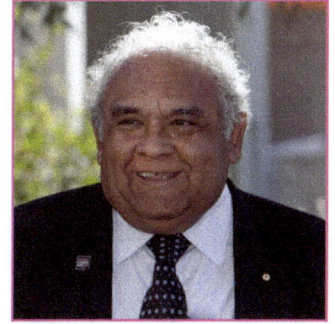

Ministers and senior bureaucrats rarely reflect on their role or accept, as numerous independent reports have highlighted, that they are often the key contributors to the state of Indigenous affairs. Their *imposed* policies and programs that have not been developed in consultation or collaboration with affected persons, their regular restructuring of programs and short-sighted funding arrangements and their lack of engagement with Indigenous peoples' peak body have significantly contributed to the state of Aboriginal and Torres Strait Islander peoples' advancement.

The blame game has to stop and we must all be active and willing partners in determining the strategies and pathways that must be taken if we are to realise positive and sustainable changes. The first step is to respect and value the contribution of Aboriginal and Torres Strait Islander peoples in the journey. Secondly, we need to develop long term generational plans and strategies and fund them appropriately. Thirdly, they must enjoy multi-party support and they must survive political and ministerial terms to give confidence to the community and to the bureaucrats who are administering the programs. Finally, research and best practices, both domestically and internationally, must influence the way forward.

The fantastic collection of ideas recorded in this very important book addresses many of the principles I have cited. When considered in conjunction with Chapter 2 of the Aboriginal and Torres Strait Islander Social Justice Report 2009 and the Senate's Legal and Constitutional Affairs References Committee's 2013 Report titled "Value of a justice reinvestment approach to criminal justice in Australia", we will understand that solutions are within our grasp if politicians have the courage and willingness to embrace them.

The unacceptable over-representation of Aboriginal and Torres Strait Islander peoples in juvenile and adult corrections centres in all jurisdictions has given rise to a collaborative social journalism project, #JustJustice, to agitate for change through sharing stories that promote public awareness and action.

This book highlights and recognises the foundational work of the many human rights and social justice advocates, be they individuals, communities and organisations, who have the vision and courage required to make a difference and it is now time for politicians and policy makers to join us to address this national crisis. One very important solution would be to implement a justice reinvestment approach.

I urge you to read the stories and join us in the fight for a fair and just Australia.

Professor Tom Calma AO

Justice Reinvestment advocate
Chancellor, University of Canberra
Read more here.

Contents

Introduction/overview

By Karen Wyld

More than 90 articles profiling solutions to the over-incarceration of Aboriginal and Torres Strait Islander people have been published as part of the crowdfunded #JustJustice campaign.

This book compiles those articles, providing a significant intervention into public and policy debate about the over-incarceration of Aboriginal and Torres Strait Islander people.

By privileging the voices of Aboriginal and Torres Strait Islander people from across the country, and taking a strengths-based, solutions-focused approach, this book reveals the depth of knowledge, social and cultural capital, and leadership among Aboriginal and Torres Strait Islander communities.

The stories and voices in this book demand a strong response, and that must include action from governments, policymakers and service providers, including those working in the health sector.

This book also demands a response from all Australians, that we individually and collectively acknowledge the true history of the colonisation of this country, in order to enable healing and justice.

As these stories show, one of the longstanding strategies of colonisation has been to criminalise, institutionalise and incarcerate Aboriginal and Torres Strait Islander people; we must acknowledge this history in order to stop repeating it.

This book also demands a response from the mainstream media, to move beyond colonial constructions and representations that problematise and pathologise Aboriginal and Torres Strait Islander people.

Enact your watchdog roles; hold governments to account; and maintain a strong spotlight on not only the problems caused by "tough on crime" rhetoric and "law and order" policies, but also on the solutions to over-incarceration.

As the stories in this book show over and over again, communities have the solutions. The media must help governments to do a better job of listening and responding appropriately.

The #JustJustice series was published at the social journalism for health project, Croakey.org, between April 2015 and November 2016. It highlights the complex correlations between the criminal justice system and the health and wellbeing of Aboriginal and Torres Strait Islander peoples.

Within this book are stories of people's lives and aspirations, and their ongoing efforts to achieve fairer treatment within the justice sector for Aboriginal and Torres Strait Islander people.

This book provides an honest account of the over-incarceration of Aboriginal and Torres Strait Islander people, and the complex circumstances that might lead people to being brought before the criminal justice system.

Drawing on personal stories, the generational effects of crime and incarceration become painfully obvious. Aboriginal and Torres Strait Islander contributors have generously shared their stories, in the hope that real change can occur for their families and communities.

These stories are balanced with evidenced-based accounts of the impact of the justice system on the health and wellbeing of Aboriginal and Torres Strait Islander people, families and communities.

This book also exposes the unacceptably high number of Aboriginal and Torres Strait Islander people with health conditions, such as foetal alcohol spectrum disorder and hearing loss, who have become trapped in a cycle of incarceration, often for minor offences.

More than anything, this book brings together community members, professionals, policy makers, and health practitioners to share their expertise.

Collectively, they present politicians, policy makers, health and justice sectors, and the wider community with road-maps to move forward.

The #JustJustice campaign kicked off on 9 April 2015 with a call for action from Mick Gooda, who at that time was Australia's Aboriginal and Torres Strait Islander Social Justice Commissioner.

Mick Gooda stated that:

> *Tackling the over-incarceration of Aboriginal and Torres Strait Islander peoples will require leadership and action at multiple levels.*
>
> *The evidence from around the world tells us that putting people in jail for minor crimes does not create safer communities. But it does create a cycle of incarceration that is tearing apart families and communities.*
>
> *I am supporting the #JustJustice campaign because we need to encourage a public debate that is focused on ensuring effective, evidence-based solutions to over-incarceration.*

During the 2015 – 2016 #JustJustice campaign, research evidencing over-incarceration and inequitable treatment of Aboriginal and Torres Strait Islander people was reinforced by a number of incidents that gained widespread public attention (see timeline on page 10).

In chapter one, **Cultural solutions**, the positive influences of culture, family and community are highlighted. Leadership, and the role of Elders and mentors to help young people to avoid destructive cycles, are shown as vital elements.

People on the ground collectively call on government and policy makers to see first-hand the successful initiatives that communities have developed to address complex health and social issues.

" *We are the people that know our own problems and we're the only ones who can solve them. If you give us the means to do it, it will happen.*

Clinton Walker, Ngarluma and Yindjibarndi man from the Pilbara region in Western Australia.

Stories from the heart is the theme of chapter two. People shared personal stories of family violence, recollections of friends who have been trapped in cycles of crime, and the impact of incarceration on communities. They've also provided solutions to reducing both crime rates and incarceration, such as through investing in community initiatives and social infrastructure.

" *What the young people around here need are more activities and programs to keep them out of trouble. They need to be put in touch with culture, not drugs and alcohol.*

Michaela Crowe, Yinggarda woman from Carnarvon in Western Australia.

Chapter three, **Landmarks in advocacy**, explores the benefits of using evidence-based advocacy to generate stronger accountability and drive change. The Blueprint For Change, released in November 2015, provided a twelve-principle plan to close the gap within imprisonment rates and to cut disproportionate rates of violence experienced by Aboriginal and Torres Strait Islander people; particularly women and children. This leading document was developed by Change the Record, a coalition of Aboriginal and Torres Strait Islander organisations, as well as allies within the human rights and legal sectors.

" *In 1992, Federal and State Governments agreed to report annually on their progress in implementing the recommendations of the Royal Commission.*

Not only have governments generally failed to provide these annual reports, they have also failed to implement most of the recommendations. Amnesty International review of the implementation of Royal Commission into Aboriginal Deaths in Custody.

Indigenous leadership is the focus of chapter four. Throughout Australia, there are many people speaking up, mentoring young people, and actively contributing to change. Strong leadership does exist but they require more support and accountability from funding bodies, policy makers and non-indigenous organisations.

" *The progress we have made can be the springboard for us to address current challenges and tackle unfinished business. This is not just a job for Aboriginal and Torres Strait Islander families and communities alone. It needs the engagement of all Australians. We have the opportunity to collectively address the truth of Australia's history and the impact on Aboriginal and Torres Strait Islanders.*

Richard Weston, CEO Healing Foundation.

Cultural solutions, respect, collaboration and setting achievable justice targets are key themes in chapter five, **Community-driven innovation – Justice reinvestment**.

" *Justice Reinvestment is a not a short-term, one size fits all, top-down approach. Communities chosen for Justice Reinvestment must be supported to play a central role in the design, implementation and monitoring of local Justice Reinvestment plans.*

Cheryl Axelby, CEO Aboriginal Legal Rights Movement South Australia.

Health and wellbeing takes centre place in chapter six, **Focus in disabilities**. Failure to provide appropriate healthcare during incarceration is not only a human rights issue but can lead to lessened success rates of rehabilitation. Over-representation of Aboriginal and Torres Strait Islander people within court systems and prison is concerning enough, but more so for people with hearing loss, cognitive impairments, foetal alcohol spectrum disorder and other disabilities.

" *If one in five people with disability are diverted from detention and into a supported disability program, then the overall Aboriginal and Torres Strait Islander prison population could be reduced by 10 per cent.*

Scott Avery, Policy and Research Director at the First Peoples Disability Network.

Chapter seven, titled **Trauma-informed solutions**, highlights the impact of family violence and intergenerational trauma, as well as trauma associated with dealing with justice systems.

" *The criminal justice system is not necessarily considered the most appropriate means for dealing with family violence. Indigenous experiences of family violence and the justice system suggest that people are interested in programs that focus on preventing the transfer of violence, not just prosecuting or punishing people for being violent.*

Dr Anna Olsen, Visiting Fellow at the National Centre for Epidemiology and Population Health (NCEPH) at the Australian National University, and Dr Ray Lovett, Research Fellow at the Australian Institute of Aboriginal and Torres Strait Islander Studies and at the NCEPH.

In chapter eight, **Caring for youth**, there are strong calls for action to prevent more young people presenting before the criminal justice system.

> *It is abhorrent that there are approximately 450 Indigenous children in detention across Australia every night. Even more abhorrent is that we do very little to combat this when indeed we could. Be outraged at that!*

Darren Parker, Ngunawal man, PhD Candidate at the Melbourne Law School.

Young people are again a key focus in chapter nine, **Health leadership**, as are community-controlled approaches, evidence-based practices and government accountability. And there is a strong call for culturally safe approaches, taking in to account intersectionality.

> *When it comes to Indigenous LGBTQI people, very little is known about our interactions with policing and justice systems. We know even less about how policing and justice systems are responding to our particular needs.*

Dameyon Bonson, founder of Black Rainbow Living Well.

Chapter ten, **Addressing racism**, shines a light on themes that need to be discussed openly and honestly: institutional racism, power and privilege, human rights abuses, historical contributors to current inequities, and concerns over discriminatory practices in policing and law.

> *There won't be a single bullet that cures all areas of disadvantage faced by Aboriginal and Torres Strait Islander people, but real constitutional reform would have important symbolic significance to ensure that our foundational document removes the racist elements that still pervade our Aboriginal and Torres Strait Islander people and their communities.*

Eddie Cubillo, Executive Officer of the National Aboriginal & Torres Strait Islander Legal Service (NATSILS)

Chapter eleven sees a continuation of these themes, through the shocking human rights abuses that were exposed at **Don Dale** juvenile detention centre in Northern Territory. Graphic images of young detainees being treated roughly at the hands of staff caught the public's attention. The government response was to call for a Royal Commission into the Protection and Detention of Children in the Northern Territory.

> *We need to continue to express our disgust when we learn of abuse against children and young people and to speak up for those who do not have a voice. We also need to remember that a purely punitive, tough-on-crime response to youth offending can lead to unacceptable and shocking mistreatment of children, as well as being ineffective in making our community safer.*

Liana Buchanan, Victoria's Principal Commissioner for Children and Young People, and Andrew Jackomos, Commissioner for Aboriginal Children and Young People.

Whilst incidents at Don Dale gained broad public attention and a swift response from government, there were countless equally disturbing incidents during 2015 and 2016 that did not. With only a small number of recommendations from the 1987-1991 Royal Commission into Aboriginal Deaths in Custody having been actioned, it is easy to feel despondent.

This book encourages readers to acknowledge those feelings of being overwhelmed, but is also a call to not give up. It asks everyone, from politicians and policy makers to people working within health, social services and justice sectors, and the broader community, to listen.

Listen deeply to Aboriginal and Torres Strait Islander people, families and community-controlled organisations.

Hear the truth mirrored within the evidence-based research and the personal stories.

Develop a deeper understanding of the complex drivers of Aboriginal and Torres Strait Islander peoples' over-representation in the criminal justice system.

And respond to the call for collaborative, culturally safe, strength-based approaches for #JustJustice.

Karen Wyld is a freelance writer and consultant based in South Australia, with a background in Aboriginal health, research, community development and health workforce training.

• Read more about the back-story to the #JustJustice campaign on page 241.

Contextual timeline

23 April 2013: Long-standing campaign by Aboriginal and Torres Strait Islander groups for the Federal Government's Closing the Gap commitments to include justice target is backed by then Coalition Indigenous Affairs spokesman Nigel Scullion and later by Labor.

20 June 2013: Senate inquiry into Justice Reinvestment finds that in addressing the social determinants of crime – unemployment, homelessness, health and education issues – justice reinvestment has the potential to improve the life outcomes of individuals and build strong, safe and cohesive communities.

November 2014: Federal Government backs away from pre-election bipartisan support for a formal Closing the Gap justice target.

8-9 April 2015: The need for effective solutions to the "public health catastrophe" of the over-incarceration of Aboriginal and Torres Strait Islander people highlighted at the Prison Health: From the Inside Out conference held this week in Western Australia by the Geraldton Geraldton Regional Aboriginal Medical Service (GRAMS).

29 April 2015: Leading Aboriginal and Torres Strait Islander, community and human rights organisations launch the Change the Record campaign to end the over-representation of Aboriginal and Torres Strait Islander people in the justice system within a generation.

1 May 2015: Major and ongoing protests launched across the nation, spearheaded by the #SOSBlakAustralia movement on Facebook and Twitter, in protest at Western Australian Government's threat to close hundreds of remote Aboriginal communities.

June 2015: Inquiry into the harmful use of alcohol in Aboriginal and Torres Strait Islander communities: Alcohol, hurting people and harming communities. The inquiry noted that alcohol contributes to contact with the justice system, and found there is a strong link between FAS and FASD and contact with the criminal justice system. The inquiry was positive about justice reinvestment as one solution to issues relating to alcohol and contact with the justice system.

6 July 2015: Aboriginal Legal Service (NSW/ACT) secures six month funding reprieve for the acclaimed Custody Notification Service (CNS) following urgent campaign for funding from Federal and State Governments that attracts 50,000 petitioners.

September 2015: In a keynote speech to the Secretariat of National Aboriginal and Islander Child Care national conference in Perth, Marninwarntikura Fitzroy Women's Resource Centre leader June Oscar calls on new Prime Minister Malcolm Turnbull to abandon Tony Abbott's Indigenous Advancement Strategy (IAS), which she said had brought many child welfare and family centres to the brink of closure.

23 November 2015: Coronial inquest finally begins into death in custody of Yamatji woman Ms Dhu, following nationwide campaign by her family, backed by the Deaths in Custody Watch Committee, for answers about the circumstances of her death at Western Australia's South Hedland Police Station. It hears that WA police told hospital staff they thought Ms Dhu was "faking" when she was in the process of dying from septicaemia and pneumonia.

30 November 2016: The Change the Record Coalition launches the landmark 'Blueprint for Change', to meet two overarching aims: to close the gap in rates of imprisonment by 2040 and cut the disproportionate rates of violence to at least close the gap by 2040 with priority strategies for women and children.

3 December 2015: Law Council of Australia issues communique calling on Council of Australian Governments (COAG) to place 'reducing Indigenous imprisonment' as a key item on its 'Closing the Gap' agenda and establish specific targets.

7 December 2015: Cowra Shire Council declares unanimous support to pursue a Justice Reinvestment pilot, after a three year research project in the town by National Centre for Indigenous Studies at the Australian National University.

10 February 2016: Indigenous Affairs Minister rejects continuing calls from Indigenous and mainstream health and justice groups for a Closing the Gap justice target, saying it "makes no sense" as the "criminal justice system is a state and territory responsibility and the Commonwealth has no business interfering with the judiciary."

17 March 2016: Senate Inquiry into the Commonwealth Indigenous Advancement Strategy tendering processes finds they were deeply flawed and recommends dropping its "blanket competitive process" and awarding longer contracts to Indigenous organisations.

31 March 2016: Change the Record welcomes the report of the Victorian Royal Commission into Family Violence and its detailed recommendations around reducing violence against Aboriginal and Torres Strait Islander women, child protection, women in prison and investment in services, including legal support.

13 April 2016: Senator Pat Dodson, a commissioner at the Royal Commission into Aboriginal Deaths in Custody, marks the upcoming 25th anniversary of its final report with a National Press Club address, saying by and large the problems it was set up to examine have become worse. Amnesty International Australia reports that only a handful of the Royal Commission's hundreds of recommendations have been implemented by federal and state governments.

15 April 2016: 25th anniversary of handing down of the final report of the Royal Commission into Aboriginal Deaths in Custody, which found that 99 Indigenous deaths in custody in the 1980s were due to the combination of police and prisons failing their duty of care, and the high numbers of Indigenous people being arrested and incarcerated.

5-6 May 2016: The inaugural Aboriginal and Torres Strait Islander Suicide Prevention Conference held in Alice Springs.

9 June 2016: Redfern Statement issued for the 2016 federal election by an historic collaboration of 16 Aboriginal and Torres Strait Islander peak organisations, supported by many more health groups and NGOs, calling for Government action to "meaningfully address Aboriginal and Torres Strait Islander disadvantage", including over-incarceration.

2 July 2016: Three new Indigenous MPs elected to Federal Parliament – Labor Senators Patrick Dodson and Malarndirri McCarthy, and the first Indigenous woman elected to the House of Representatives, former New South Wales Minister Linda Burney.

14 July 2016: Aboriginal leaders and communities respond with some relief but continuing concern to Western Australian Government's 'Resilient Families; Strong Communities' roadmap which backs away from earlier threats to close hundreds of remote communities but leaves ongoing concerns about the future of many.

26 July 2016: Prime Minister Malcolm Turnbull announces Royal Commission into the abuse of young people in the Northern Territory corrections system following shocking footage broadcast on the ABC's *Four Corners* program.

1 August 2016: Indigenous and mainstream justice and rights leader welcome the appointment of Aboriginal and Torres Strait Islander Social Justice Commissioner Mick Gooda and former Queensland Supreme Court Justice Margaret White to lead the Royal Commission into abuse in juvenile justice in the Northern Territory.

Their appointments follow the resignation of former Northern Territory Chief Justice Brian Martin and widespread criticism from NT Indigenous groups about a lack of consultation over his appointment and concerns of potential conflict of interest.

7 August 2016: #IndigenousDads trends nationally with heartfelt tributes to Aboriginal and Torres Strait Islander men and their families to counter the racist stereotyping of a Bill Leak cartoon published in The Australian.

27 August 2016: Northern Territory Coalition Government headed by Aboriginal Chief Minister Adam Giles swept out of office.

6 September 2016: First public sitting of the Royal Commission into the Protection and Detention of Children in the Northern Territory held in Darwin.

21 October 2016: Indigenous Affairs Minister Nigel Scullion offers to fund a national roll out of the Custody Notification Service (CNS) – similar to the scheme that currently operates in New South Wales. He still says there is no role for the Commonwealth in declaring Closing the Gap justice targets, but says he will push the states to introduce targets.

New Western Australian Senator Pat Dodson, a commissioner of the Royal Commission into Aboriginal Deaths in Custody, describes evidence given by the Minister and others in a Senate Estimates hearing on Don Dale as "an appalling demonstration of ignorance about the criminal justice system and its interface with Aboriginal peoples".

26 October 2016: Release of the landmark Taskforce 1000 investigation into Victoria's child protection system by the Commissioner for Aboriginal Children and Young People Andrew Jackomos.

27 October 2016: Indigenous leaders, including Senator Pat Dodson, cautiously welcome Federal Government's request for the Australian Law Reform Commission to investigate the over-representation of Aboriginal and Torres Strait Islander people in the justice system which Attorney General George Brandis describes as a "national tragedy".

27 October 2016: High Court agrees to hear legal challenge brought by the North Australian Aboriginal Justice Agency (NAAJA) on behalf of Anthony Prior to the Northern Territory's harsh police protective custody powers.

10 November 2016: The Aboriginal and Torres Strait Islander Suicide Prevention Evaluation Project (ATSISPEP) releases its final report, *Solutions that work: what the evidence and our people tell us*. It provides a blueprint to improve suicide-prevention services and programmes for Aboriginal and Torres Strait Islander people based on the principle of prioritising community-led, culturally-appropriate services.

7 December 2016: The Australian Human Rights Commission launches the Social Justice and Native Title Report 2016, calling for a greater focus on alternatives to custody including investment in individuals, families and communities, and supporting Justice Reinvestment.

1. Cultural solutions

"Cultural identity and connectedness is vital to the best interests of Aboriginal children

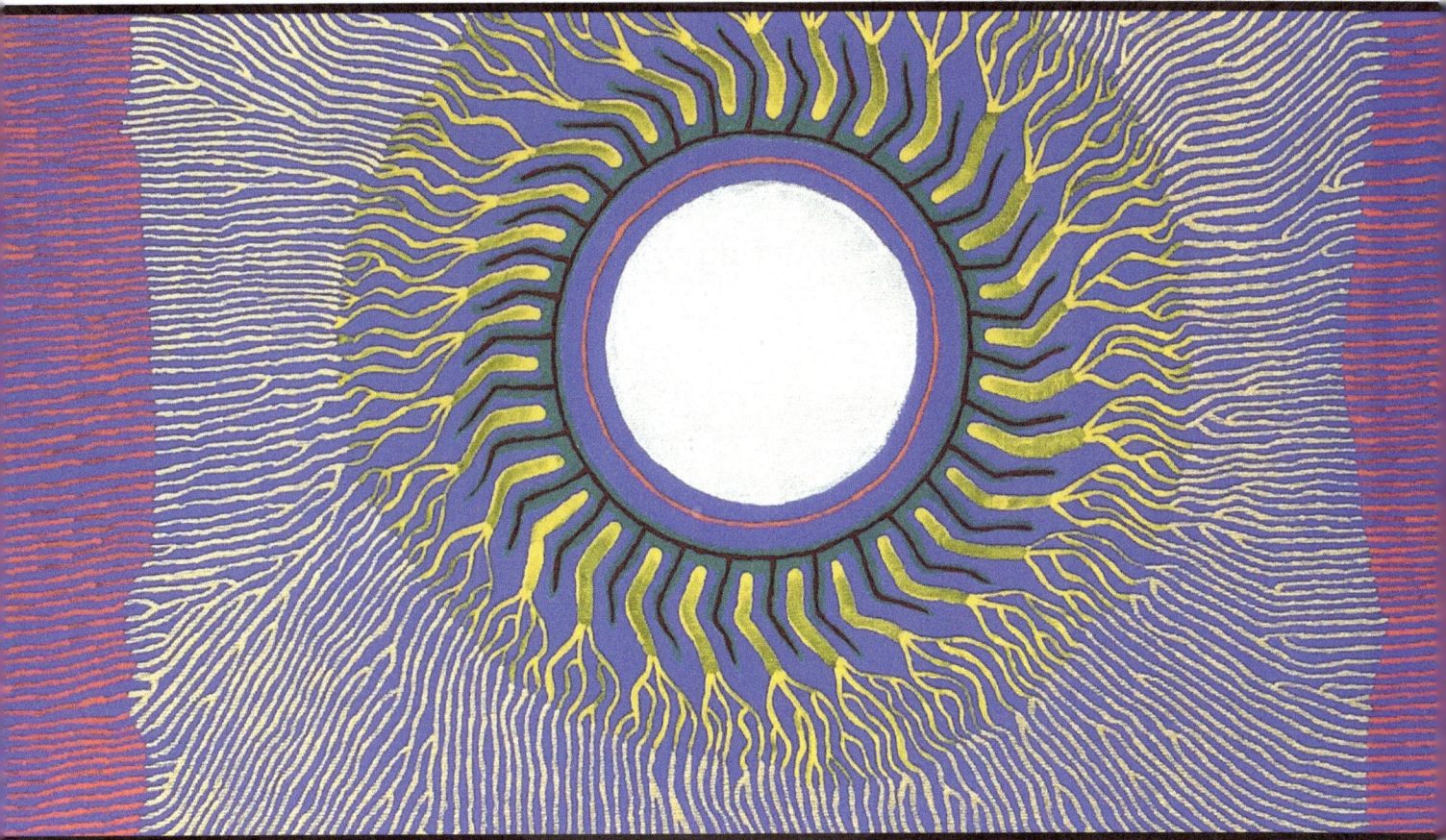

Andrew Jackomos: Culture is not a 'perk' for an Aboriginal child – it is a #JustJustice lifeline

Author:	Andrew Jackomos	Published:	September 01, 2015

Andrew Jackomos was appointed Australia's first Commissioner for Aboriginal Children and Young People in Victoria in 2013.

He came to the post with a **long family history** of activism on Aboriginal and Torres Strait Islander rights and a deep understanding of #JustJustice issues, as the former Director of the **Koori Justice Unit**, which coordinates the Victorian Aboriginal Justice Agreement – a formal partnership agreement between the Victorian Government and senior members of Victoria's Indigenous population set up in the wake of the Royal Commission into Aboriginal Deaths in Custody.

Under the **Taskforce 1000** project, he reviewed nearly **1,000 individual cases** of Aboriginal children in out-of-home care to examine the **systemic failings** that have produced steep increases in the number of children removed not just from parents, but from culture and community.

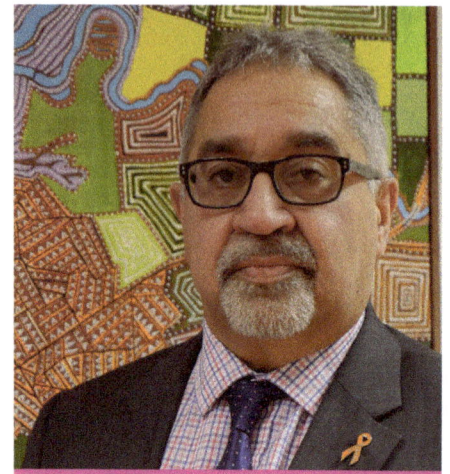

Andrew Jackomos

He outlines progress and priorities in the post below, which is an edited and updated version of his 2014 International Human Rights Day Oration and was first published in the Indigenous Law Bulletin, Volume 8 Issue 17, (Mar/Apr 2015).

See also his recent **speech** to the Victorian **Aboriginal Children's Summit**, which outlines some of the "systematic exclusion of our children from family, community and culture across the state".

Andrew Jackomos writes:

As the Commissioner for Aboriginal Children and Young People I have the great honour and privilege to be in a position to strongly advocate for all Koori children and young people; and to bring their lived experiences and their voices to the forefront. I have a role to particularly advocate for our most vulnerable babies, children and youth.

The right of Koori children to their culture, along with the other core human rights of children—to life, to family, to protection—was one of the immediate priorities I set when I commenced as Commissioner in August 2013. Cultural rights directly impact on a child's ability to meaningfully enjoy every other human right and freedom, let alone their health. Like all human rights, they are universal, indivisible and interdependent.

For Aboriginal and Torres Strait Islander peoples, Indigenous peoples, First Nations peoples, for Koories, this human right is crucial to our wellbeing, it is crucial to our sense of pride, to our sense of belonging. Culture is the most resilient factor protecting our children. Culture links us to our past so we can navigate our future.

Koori Culture

Our people, be they living on the Mornington Peninsula, or on the banks of the Murray River, will have a deep, rich, spiritual and emotional continuing connection to this land from time immemorial, which they will pass on to younger generations. It is who we are as people and who we are as a family and a community.

I am a Yorta Yorta man from the Murray River and the lands in north central Victoria and adjacent lands in New South Wales. I am also proud of my blood ties to the fighting Gunditjmara of the south west and the Taunarung peoples across the black spur, also of the greater Kulin.

Koori culture in Victoria, culture in my community, runs deep and strong and I see overwhelming evidence of this wherever I go. Our culture did not cease to exist when the Macassans first started to trade with our brothers and sisters up in the Top End. Both cultures adapted and changed with the times for the mutual benefit of both. Nor did the culture of Boon Wurrung end when the English invaded our shores and sailed through the heads. The Boon Wurrung culture adapted and changed with the times, as it had done for thousands of years, and as it has continued to do so ever since.

But I will tell you what happened after our exchanges with these newcomers. Our dynamic and flexible culture, for the most part, remained vibrant, alive and strong. It wasn't until Eddie (Koiki) Mabo, the great Torres Strait Islander warrior from the Meriam people of Murray Island, successfully challenged the Queensland government and the immoral myth of Terra Nullius in the High Court, that you might now know that this land here always was and always will be Boon Wurrung.

Unfortunately, it is not all good news. In my role I see the symptoms of past and failed government policies. I see the results of intergenerational trauma, grief and loss. I see this in many of our children who are over-represented in the child protection and youth justice systems, often creating the foundations for their future admission to the prison system.

Every day I hear sad and traumatic stories from one end of the state to the other. The evidence suggests that the communities that are faring the worst are those without strong and well-resourced community infrastructure. In these under-resourced communities, there is a lack of strong advocacy that would otherwise help prevent family violence and protect the rights of children and promote their culture.

What do I mean when I talk about culture in this context? The expression has infinite scope and will mean different things to different people. The enjoyment of "culture" holds a special significance for Aboriginal and Torres Strait Islander peoples, as it does for all First Nation peoples and communities.

Culture is not something that just stops in time, nor an ideal that can be bottled and measured against the past. In the words of the United Nations Committee on Economic, Social and Cultural Rights, culture 'is a living process, historical, dynamic and evolving, with a past, a present and a future.' Aboriginal and Torres Strait Islander peoples from time immemorial have been growing, evolving, adapting for over 40 000 years.

For us, culture is about our family networks, our Elders, our ancestors. It's about our relationships, our languages, our dance, our ceremonies, our heritage. Culture is about our spiritual connection to our lands, our waters. It is in the way we pass on stories and knowledge to our babies, our children; it is how our children embrace our knowledge to create their future. Culture is how we greet each other and look for connection. It is about all the parts that bind us together. It is the similarities in our songlines.

In communities where culture is strong, the force of identity and the knowledge of each other, the knowledge of our ancestors is a shield against racist remarks and negative stereotypes. Knowing family, community and connecting to culture, to land, to waters—these are the things that build up our young. As I travel the state and the nation I see and feel a great cultural revitalisation growing all around me and it fills me with hope. In my travels I am witnessing greater celebration of our diverse, vibrant and distinct cultures.

Impact of loss of culture

What happens when we destroy people's links with their culture and deprive them of their sense of identity, strip them of their dignity, of their sense of belonging? The results are catastrophic. We all know about the Royal Commission into Aboriginal Deaths in Custody. But you may not know that Indigenous incarceration rates across the country are higher now than then.

In 1991 the Royal Commission into Aboriginal Deaths in Custody handed down its final report. In undertaking its work across every jurisdiction, the Commission met with Aboriginal and Torres Strait Islander people who told them about the injustices they experienced in the justice system. Despite the glaring warnings and recommendations of the Royal Commission made over 20 years ago, more than 50 per cent of children and young people in youth detention in Australia are Aboriginal. For children under 18 years of age the rate is over 60 per cent!

The rate of detention of Aboriginal children and young people in Victoria is the lowest in the country, yet Koori children are still *13 times* more likely to be in custody that their non-Aboriginal brothers and sisters. This is simply unacceptable—not just to me, but it should be totally unacceptable to all Victorians.

The Commission for Children and Young People's independent visitors have frequently reported that the majority of children aged 10 to 14 at the Parkville Youth Justice Centre are Koori. Many of these children are in custodial facilities un-sentenced, awaiting their court hearing, because there are not sufficient diversionary options available to magistrates. We know of children aged under 14 years who are held incarcerated separately from their peers for days on end. We know that so many Koori children in detention have come from out-of-home care and remain child protection clients. They are in the vortex

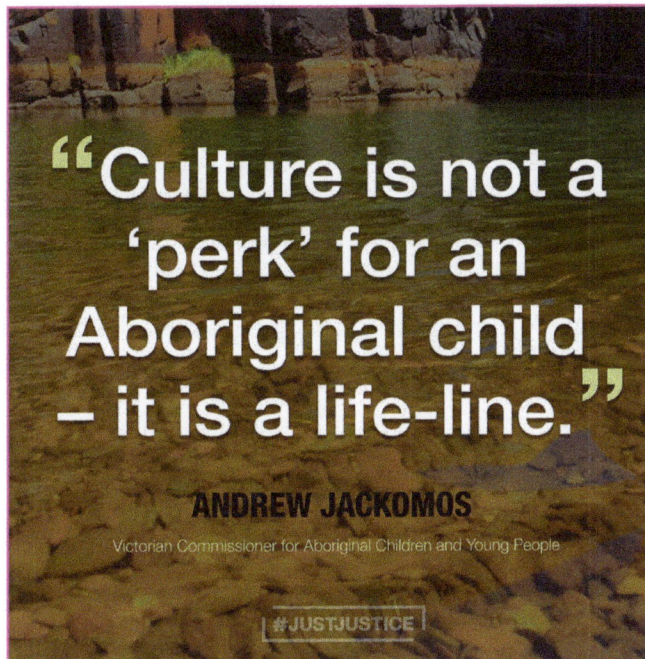

> " **Culture is not a 'perk' for an Aboriginal child – it is a life-line.** "

ANDREW JACKOMOS

Victorian Commissioner for Aboriginal Children and Young People

#JUSTJUSTICE

where the government has assumed the role as their parent but is at the same time their "jailer". Would this parent, being the government, advocate for their child with the same relentless passion as other parents to have the best legal representation, effective diversionary options, and the best possible outcome for them?

We know that children who become isolated from cultural and community networks when placed in out-of-home care are more vulnerable to being abused and less able to seek help. It is devastating to witness that some of our children being removed from a violent or turbulent home life for their 'protection' are placed in care that isolates them from relationships with their family, community and culture—the very things that would have otherwise grounded and shaped them. They can become disengaged and face further hardship and suffering.

The number of Aboriginal children in Victoria in out-of-home care today is greater than it has ever been. Of the approximately 6,500 children in the Victorian out-of-home care system, over 1,200 are Koori and growing. This is a staggering ratio when the Koori population in Victoria is only around 1 per cent.

Taskforce 1000

To provide better support to Koori children and their families and to reduce the level of their separation we must understand *why* Koori children are still being removed from home at such high rates.

Reports on Koori children are substantiated at a rate of 67.4 per 1000 compared to 7.2 per 1000 for non-Aboriginal children. We need to unpack how the system operates and how people in the services sector view Koori children; as well as confront the drivers that result in our babies, children and young people entering and languishing in care for many years. Most reports to child protection are for babies and preschoolers aged 1-4 years of age.

Taskforce 1000 was formed to critically review the case plans of 1000 Koori children and young people in out-of-home care. I have so far listened to the experiences of well over 500 children and young people from Sunraysia, Latrobe Valley, central and outer Gippsland, inner Barwon, Central Highlands, and across Melbourne.

Male-perpetrated family violence is the major reason these children have been removed from home. In most cases violence is coupled with alcohol and drug misuse. Other common themes in the cases we have reviewed are: intergenerational trauma driven by past government policies of child removal; prior parental involvement with child protection and the justice system; sexual abuse; mental health; incarceration; poor housing and transience. Learnings from the past are not changing the trajectory for our children. Generational cycles of poverty, disadvantage, disconnection and discrimination are not being broken.

Koori children and young people are progressing from the out-of-home care system to the youth justice system at alarming rates, further disconnecting them from their cultural ties and identity. The age of criminal responsibility in Victoria, as it is nationally, is just 10 years of age. We are all failing these children and establishing patterns of involvement with the criminal justice system before they are old enough to be a truant from school or drive a car.

A right to culture in legislation

It is the sad truth that not all our children have access to their culture, and many do not have access to cultural relationships. Many are being denied their basic human right to culture. Victoria, along with the ACT, is one of only two states or territories in Australia to have enacted human rights legislation.

The *Charter of Human Rights and Responsibilities* is important because it elevates many of Australia's international commitments to observe human rights principles to legal obligations at home. In Victoria law-makers must now consider human rights when enacting new laws; and public authorities must act and make decisions in a way that is compatible with human rights. This is an incredibly positive step. It is the right step.

The Charter also took an important step in recognising the unique rights of Koories in Victoria and in specifically recognising the importance of culture. Section 19 is modelled on the right to culture embodied in the *International Covenant on Civil and Political Rights* to which Australia became a party in 1980. As the United Nations Human Rights Committee has explained, this provision is directed towards 'the survival and continued development of the unique cultural identity of minorities, thus enriching society as a whole.' The Committee interpreted this right as extending to the cultural rights of Indigenous peoples.

Despite its initial resistance, Australia gave a formal statement of support for the United Nations Declaration on the Rights of Indigenous Peoples in April 2009. Whilst it is terrific that the right to culture is embedded in such documents, the challenge is what actually happens in the daily experience of Aboriginal people. How accessible are these rights and do they make a difference?

In Victoria, the human rights embodied in the Charter do not give rise to individual causes of action and the courts cannot strike down offending legislation – parliamentary sovereignty is maintained. In other words, the rights of minorities, our Aboriginal children, remain subject to the democratic process of majority decision-making.

The obligations relating to culture that are mandated in our child protection legislation—the *Children Youth and Families Act 2005* (Vic) – are not being implemented consistently or effectively, and there is no accountability when they are not implemented. Legislative entitlements give our children the right to demand that they be fulfilled.

Victoria's child protection regime is underpinned by a principle that prioritises the best interests of the child. You might think this is obvious and should go without saying, but we need to ensure a culturally-informed understanding of what a child's best interests are or the principle is completely meaningless.

The legislative provisions seek to foster and maintain cultural and kinship connections when Koori children are removed from home. One such provision is the Aboriginal Child Placement Principle as contained in the *Victorian Children Youth and Families Act*. We know, through Taskforce 1000, that the application of the principle has significant scope for improvement. The Commission is currently conducting an inquiry in relation to this.

Unfortunately government – the system – is failing in practice to acknowledge that cultural identity and connectedness is vital to the best interests of Aboriginal children. There is a legislative mandate to implement cultural support plans for all Aboriginal children under Victorian guardianship orders. As at June 2013, cultural plans were being implemented in less than 10 per cent of cases and many of these are lacking in substance and meaning.

There is a lot to be done between now and March 2016, when the obligation to implement cultural support plans will extend to all Koori children in out-of-home care. It is vital to be aware that a cultural support plan is not about just taking a child to a NAIDOC march, or sticking up an Aboriginal flag. Cultural meaning comes from connections, relationships and socialisation with other Koori children and role models who will inspire and support the child as their life unfolds.

Culture is not a 'perk' for an Aboriginal child – it is a life-line.

Andrew Jackomos is the Victorian Commissioner for Aboriginal Children and Young People. He has over 30 years' experience in Aboriginal affairs policy and administration.

This is an edited and updated version of the speech he delivered as the International Human Rights Day Oration in Victoria on 4 December 2014. It was first published in the Indigenous Law Bulletin, Volume 8 Issue 17, (Mar/Apr 2015).

Also since this speech was delivered, the Productivity Commission's latest national Report on Government Services showed that Aboriginal babies and children in Victoria removed and living away from immediate family homes rose by 42 per cent in just 12 months to 30 June 2014.

Be the best you can: solutions and hope for Indigenous men, families and communities

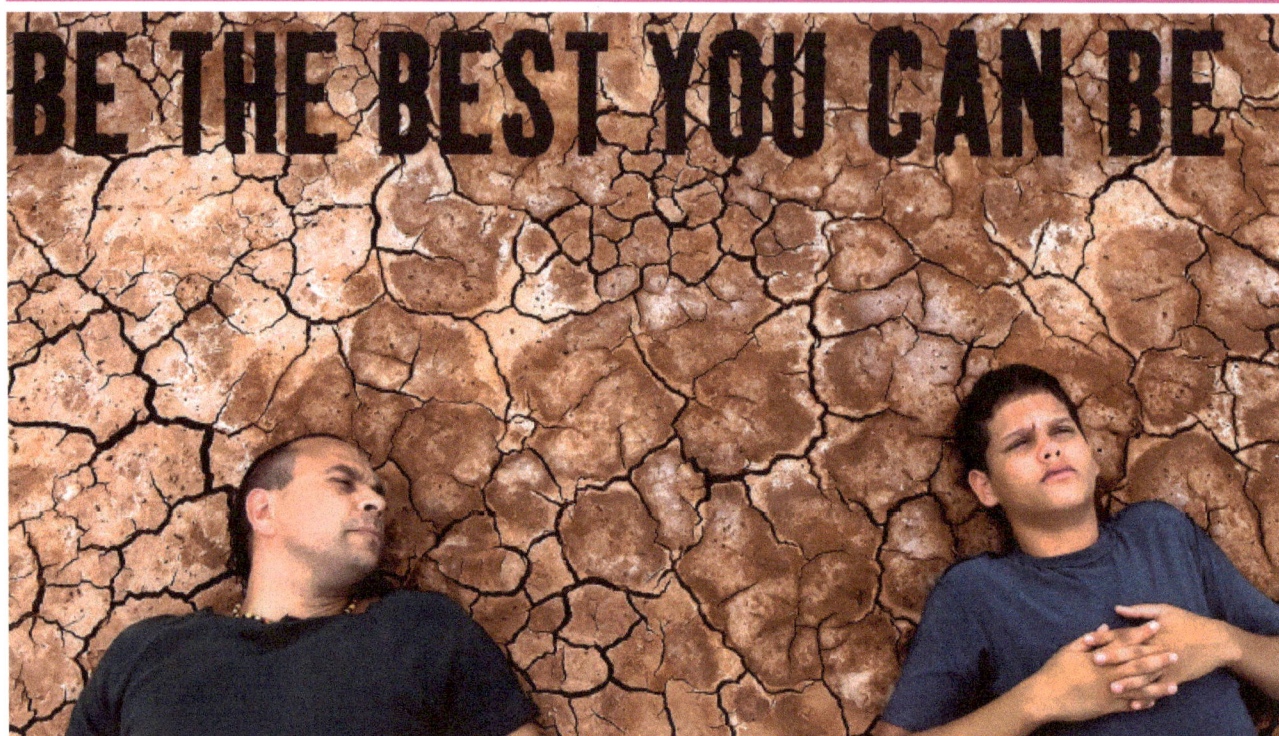

Author:	Megan Williams, Jack Bulman, Brendan Fletcher, Antony Stockdale and Christina Grant	Published:	November 04, 2016

An innovative men's health program is drawing on the outstanding Australian feature film Mad Bastards to address racism, trans-generational trauma, and loss of culture, identity and land that lie behind issues of over-incarceration, violence and alcohol abuse in Aboriginal and Torres Strait Islander communities.

The article below profiles the program and its impact across a range of groups and locations, from men's camps, in a correctional facility and among varied groups in remote, rural, regional and urban settings.

It is published as part of Croakey's #JustJustice series on the over-incarceration of Aboriginal and Torres Strait Islander people.

Our thanks to Bush Turkey Films for permission to use stills from the film.

Megan Williams, Jack Bulman, Brendan Fletcher, Antony Stockdale and Christina Grant write:

While Aboriginal and Torres Strait Islander men have among the worst health and social status of any population in Australia, including being over-represented in prisons and earlier age at death, they also have many solutions to the issues they face.

Further, Aboriginal and Torres Strait Islander men have solutions to benefit whole communities; without strong men, there is little chance for strong families or communities to develop and be sustained.

Many health organisations struggle to engage Aboriginal and Torres Strait Islander men in their activities. On the other hand, many Aboriginal and Torres Strait Islander men's programs are often overwhelmed by requests for support from men and their families, yet have limited resources and infrastructure to meet these.

There are many ways to strengthen Aboriginal and Torres Strait Islander men's groups and their leadership. This article describes a group-based program designed and delivered by Aboriginal men and their collaborators, drawing on the Australian feature film Mad Bastards as poignant stimulus.

"You need to sort out what you came here for. So don't go wandering off."

Mad Bastards: a story at the heart of Aboriginal men's health

The *Mad Bastards* film was developed during a 10-year collaboration between Brendan Fletcher from Bush Turkey films and Broome musicians Alan and Stephen Pigram, with Aboriginal men from the Kimberley and Nyoongar communities of Western Australia. It focuses on Aboriginal men and the challenges they face.

Mad Bastards is a story at the heart of Aboriginal men's health – a man battling his many difficulties in order to repair his relationship with his family. Cape York Health Council Public Health Medical Advisor Dr Mark Wenitong says:

" *The movie 'Mad Bastards' speaks to all of the key issues facing Aboriginal men and their relationships, as sons, uncles and partners … as well as the usual social issues of incarceration, violence and alcohol abuse. Most importantly, it brings a message of hope, an inspiration that they can break cycles and be the men they want to be.*

Since its release, Bush Turkey Films has received requests from all over Australia to show the film and engage with the men and stories behind the movie. In response, Bush Turkey films sought a process to respond to these requests in an integrated, strategic way, and called together a Working Group of diverse practitioners and researchers involved in Aboriginal and Torres Strait Islander men's healthcare.

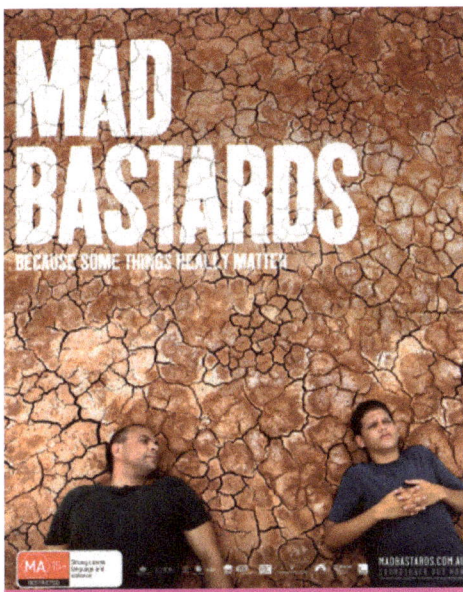

Official movie poster

Development of the Be the Best You Can Be program

Together the Mad Bastards Working Group decided to focus on several key themes of the film, and develop resources to explore these in group contexts. The themes were Deciding to Change, Relationships, Identity, Transformation, Taking Responsibility, and Staying Strong. For each theme, cards with *Mad Bastards* quotes were designed, along with still images and video clips from the film. A review of literature and theories relating to the themes was also generated, which contributed to identifying prompt questions to use in group discussion. A facilitator's guide was developed to introduce and support the group process, including for follow-up care.

The resulting program, entitled '*Be the Best You Can Be*' was piloted in an urban and regional site with around 100 men. Adaptations were then made, with leadership by **Mibbinbah Men's Spaces** health promotion charity, who now hold educational rights to the program.

One of the best features about the Mibbinbah Mad Bastards program is its flexibility – in terms of which themes groups choose to explore, or which resources they use. Also, group participants can choose whether they explore issues related to the characters in the film, or for themselves personally – depending on group safety and trust within the group context.

The program is suitable for a range of groups and locations. The program has been undertaken on men's camps in a correctional facility, used with young people and mixed groups of men and women – always with the support of local leaders. The program has been undertaken in remote, rural, regional and urban settings. It has been delivered in a weekend, or across several weeks, in a range of venues and with various group sizes. Programs have been paid for by organisations commissioning Mibbinbah for a local program, as well through Mibbinbah's various funding agreements. The program suits a range of health issues, such as for wellbeing and healing, self-care and chronic condition management, and cultural awareness training for general audiences.

" *In all the chaos and mess, someone's gotta be strong for everyone.*

The future

Mibbinbah holds close the vision of healthy Aboriginal and Torres Strait Islander men available for their families and communities. There are many well-established and fledgling Aboriginal and Torres Strait Islander men's groups across Australia to invest in. Mibbinbah aims to support and inspire these groups, to show the film, and train local facilitators to explore the themes in their communities. As lead character and strong Aboriginal man Texas says to men beginning to form a group together: '*This is about making you feel a little bit important, so you don't feel like no one cares about you*'.

Mibbinbah is focused on supporting Aboriginal and Torres Strait Islander males to take their rightful place in society, whatever that may be. By identifying and addressing common life factors affecting Aboriginal males such as racism, trans-generational trauma, loss of culture, identity and land, Mibbinbah seeks to take steps to support males with their journey.

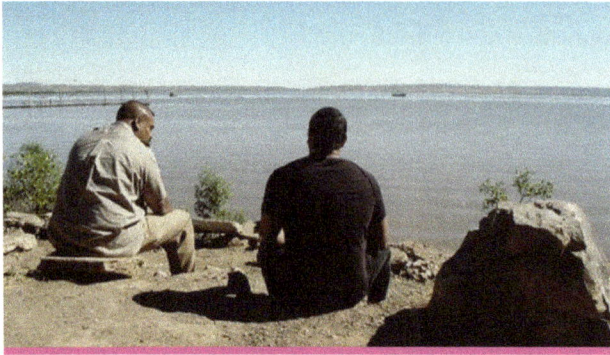

"You need to sort out what you came here for. So don't go wandering off."

Mibbinbah achieves this support through creating safe spaces and networks of support, education and training, empowerment strategies, research, transfer of knowledge, capacity development and celebration.

Dr Megan Williams is a member of the #JustJustice team, a Senior Research Fellow at the Aboriginal Health and Wellbeing Research team at Western Sydney University, and descendant of the Wiradjuri people through her father's family. She was a member of the Mad Bastards Working Group.

Jack Bulman is a Muthi Muthi man from South Western New South Wales, a co-founder of Mibbinbah, a member of the Mad Bastards Working Group and leads the Mibbinbah Mad Bastards: Be the best you can be program

Brendan Fletcher, from Bush Turkey Films, was writer and director of Mad Bastards which was nominated for the Grand Jury Prize at the 2011 Sundance Film Festival, won the Independent Spirit Award at the 2011 IF Awards; won Best Film at the Deadly Awards and garnered Film Critics and Director's Guild nominations for Best Director. Brendan was a member of the Mad Bastards Working Group and on behalf of the group won a 2012 National Child Abuse Prevention Network Play Your Part Award for enabling the film to be used in the Be the Best You Can be program.

Antony Stockdale and Christina Grant, also members of the Mad Bastards Working Group, are creative production consultants from the digital communications Pangea Collective.

Calling out from country for law reform for #JustJustice (and wonderful rock art photos)

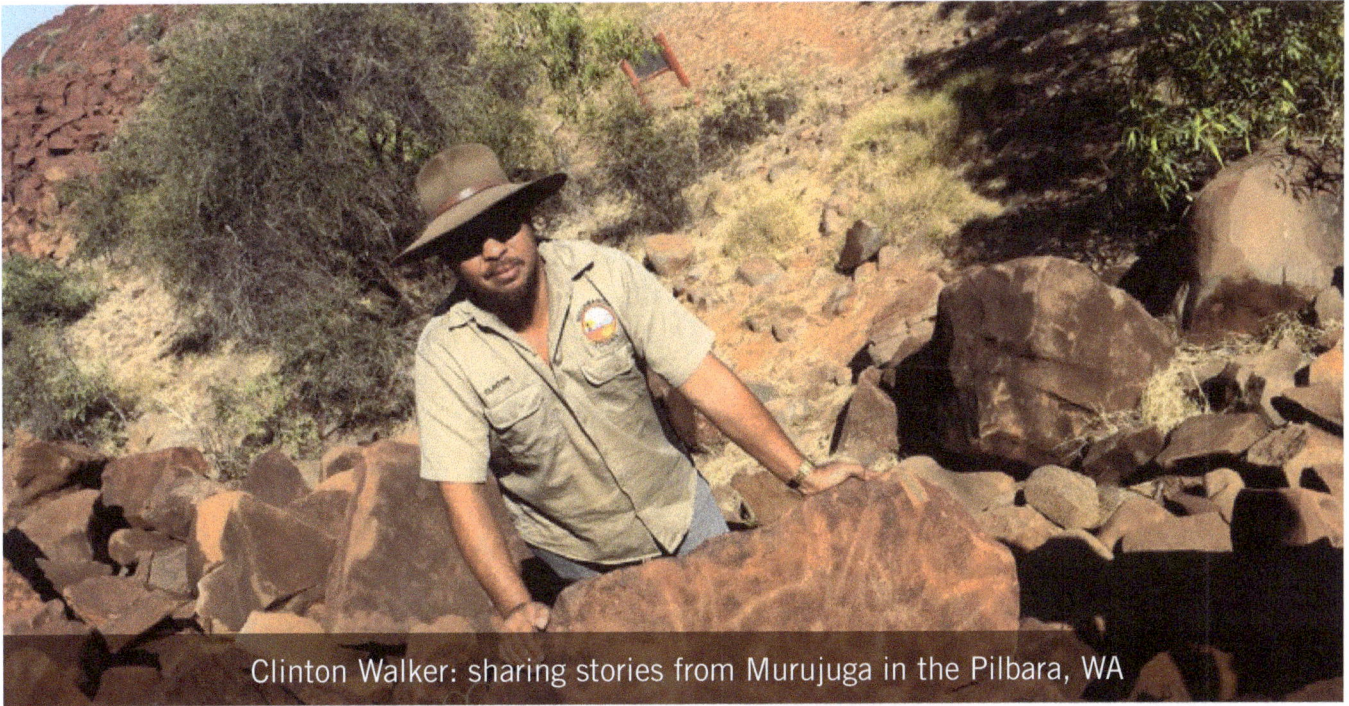
Clinton Walker: sharing stories from Murujuga in the Pilbara, WA

Author:	Melissa Sweet and Clinton Walker	Published:	July 06, 2016

As these photographs suggest, Murujuga or the Burrup Peninsula in the Pilbara region of Western Australia is simply stunning.

Murujuga is thought to have the world's highest concentration of engraved rock art or petroglyphs, and is a profoundly important place for the local Aboriginal people.

With #NAIDOC2016 celebrating "Songlines, The Living Narrative of our Nation", it is timely to bring you this interview below with Clinton Walker, a Ngarluma and Yindjibarndi man.

It was broadcast from Murujuga, where many songlines begin, according to Clinton.

In the clip below, he talks about the importance of fostering connection to culture and country as part of efforts to reduce the over-incarceration of Aboriginal and Torres Strait Islander people.

Watch the interview, which was streamed live via the Periscope app last year as part of Croakey's #JustJustice series.

Clinton, a cultural tour guide, says the justice system should be reformed as too many Aboriginal people are being imprisoned for petty crimes and unpaid fines.

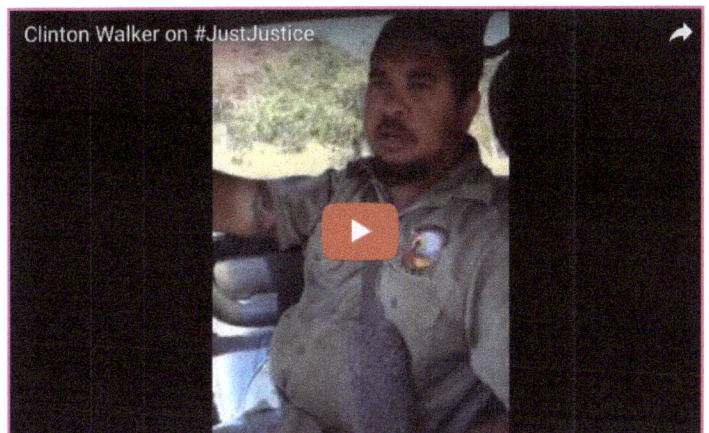
Clinton Walker on #JustJustice

He would like to see prisoners being put to work on country, helping with weeding and maintenance. Policymakers need to visit communities to learn first-hand about the need for law reform, he says.

Working on country would also enable spiritual healing.

Clinton also speaks of the importance of strong leaders and Elders to help young people growing up to be respectful and to avoid destructive cycles.

He recommends a DVD, which many Croakey readers might appreciate, Exile and the Kingdom, which was made with people from the Roebourne area.

The people of Roebourne are "taking our community back", he says, and have the solutions to the issues facing them.

Clinton Walker is a Ngarluma and Yindjibarndi man. Follow Clinton on Twitter @NgarlumaMan. And at Facebook Ngurrangga Tours – Aboriginal Cultural Tourism.

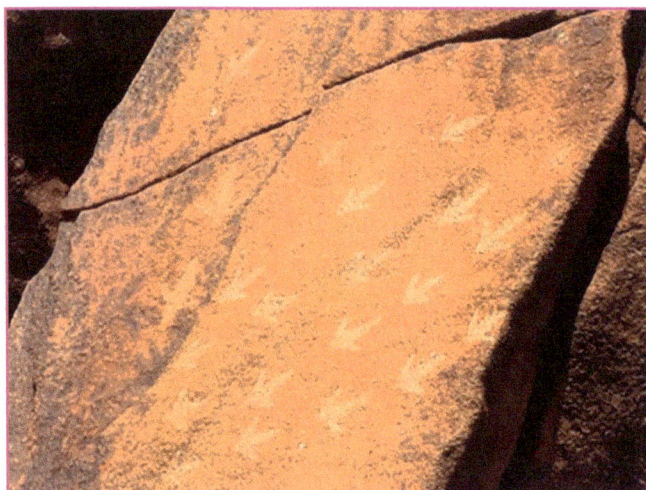

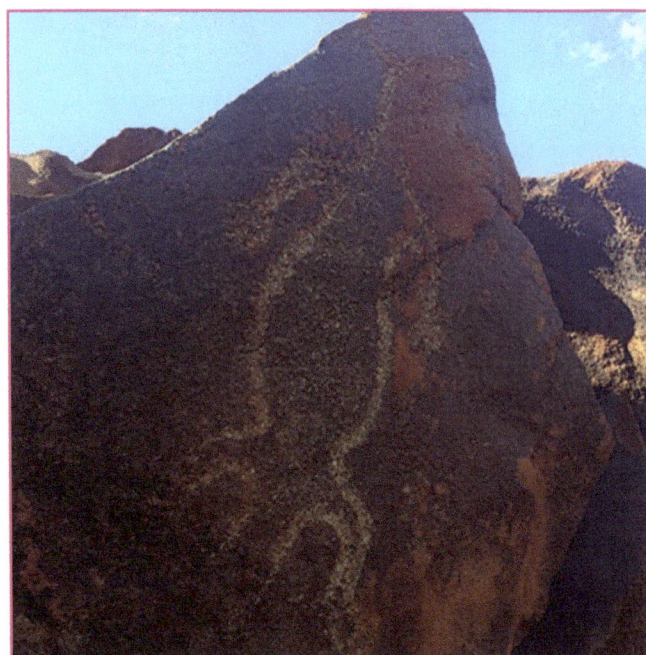

Sharing stories about the importance of safe spaces, when healing from family violence

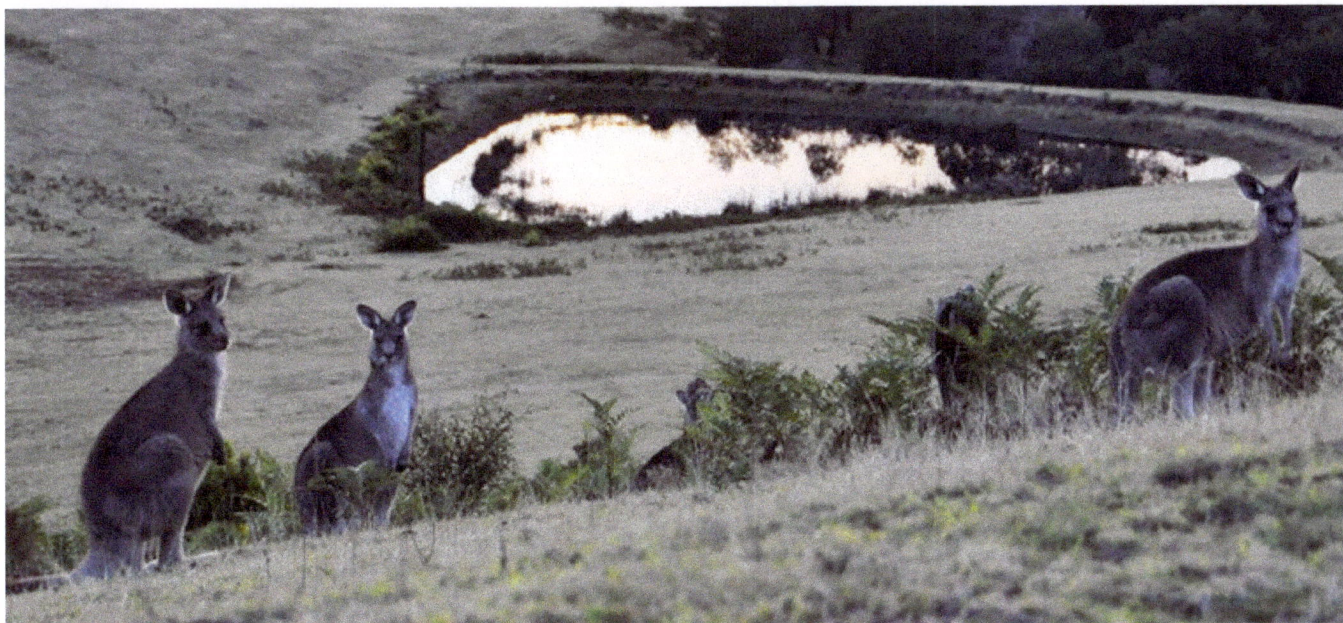

| Author: | Clinton, a Gamilaroi psychologist | Published: | January 28, 2016 |

As part of the #JustJustice series, Darren Parker, a Ngunawal man and PhD candidate at Melbourne Law School, shared a very personal account, *One man's story of surviving the trauma of family violence*. (See page 44).

The author of the article below, Clinton, a Gamilaroi psychologist, has also had to deal with the impacts of family violence upon his life. Much like Darren, he has channelled his experiences into his work. In Clinton's case, this is helping other men.

Below, Clinton reflects on Darren's story, the issues he has faced personally, and discusses the impact that family violence has on men, drawn from his experience as a psychologist. He talks about how men can turn to "negative coping mechanisms" to deal with their pain, and how culture can improve Aboriginal and Torres Strait Islander men's wellbeing.

Clinton writes:

Like Darren, I too have experienced the full brunt of domestic and family violence and completely understand the scars it leaves. I have also had the dark beast of depression chase me throughout my life, and was at the brink of suicide on several occasions in my younger years. I have had to work through my own scars over the years.

I engaged in almost 20 years of negative coping after negative coping strategy and am definitely someone, like Darren, who managed to be high functioning throughout these years. I managed to successfully complete my entire university degree and honours year in a messed-up state of negative coping. It allowed me to escape, or so I thought at the time.

I acknowledge that it is only through sheer luck that I did not end up as another Aboriginal male incarcerated or suicide statistic, and thank those who have helped me on my healing journey thus far and those who will help me into the future.

My name is Clinton and I am a Gamilaroi man and a psychologist by trade.

Most of my current work happens in the area of men's wellbeing including: drug and alcohol rehabilitation, and loss and grief work. I am a current PhD candidate and have been investigating Aboriginal and Torres Strait Islander culturally bound mechanisms for protecting wellbeing.

I completely acknowledge the pain caused by some men through the perpetration of family violence; however, I do not believe that men are inherently violent or that those who may perpetuate violence are necessarily "evil men".

I do, however, believe we have a lot of men who are very damaged and disconnected, lost and scared of them themselves and the world around them. Men who grew up witnessing negative coping mechanisms have been left with imprints of "how we survive", which become the driving force behind "bad behaviours".

I believe many of our men have not had the opportunity to engage with the positive and protective factors of our true Lore and culture, and that a loss of Lore and culture is the greatest issue we face as Aboriginal peoples. This loss contributes to the high rates of incarceration of Aboriginal and Torres Strait Islander people.

While media and government policy may cause hysterical stereotypical images of Aboriginal society in the minds of unknowing Australians, our culture and our Lore is positive and, if utilised, can keep us strong, safe and secure as Aboriginal peoples. It can build and maintain strong positive men, women and families. It can keep us out of jail.

We often hear of the physical scarring caused by domestic violence and family violence, yet rarely is the equally damaging impact on our emotional, psychological and spiritual self acknowledged. For many who have experienced domestic violence or family violence, they will have had multiple attempts at "fighting" the threats of the past.

This is often through drug or alcohol abuse, through gambling or withdrawing from society. Or unfortunately through perpetuating the exact same violence onto their loved ones.

On holistic healing

We don't often take the time to find our "safe place": that space in which we feel connected, stable, supported, and where we are able to fight our problems.

If you watch a kangaroo when it is threatened by wild dogs or dingoes, you will notice, more often than not, it will head for water if it is available. Water is the kangaroo's "safe place"; here it is balanced, empowered and strong, and can size up and tackle the threats (the dogs) that chase it.

We need to find our "water" – that place where we can be strong and empowered to tackle our "dogs". Just like dingoes, social determinants and negative life events hunt in packs. You will not find someone struggling to cope who has only been impacted negatively by a single social determinant or has only experienced a single negative life event in recent times.

I now spend much of my days guiding other men who have had similar life experiences to me and my family, on their journeys, helping them learn how to be positive, fathers, husbands, workers and men

Again not dissimilar to Darren, despite my ability to carry on with the day-to-day grind at a high level, I was struggling beyond explanation inside. I mostly chose drugs and alcohol, but the drug and alcohol use generally led to other negative behaviours.

To heal, I needed to heal as a whole being. From an Aboriginal perspective, this is largely yarned of as having to heal my social and emotional wellbeing. I needed to accept my scars, all of them, and to learn from them. I needed to accept I couldn't erase the past or the wrongs, both those created by me and those by others towards me, my family and my mob.

I needed to take responsibility for the pain I'd caused others, I needed to take control of my thoughts and actions and to empty myself of negativity, to allow space for positivity. I needed to learn from the lived experiences and knowledge of others in a positive way, and I needed to learn and return to cultural epistemologies and ontologies, or ways of knowing and being. I had to learn to truly respect myself with all my scars to be able to truly love and respect others.

Most of all, I needed to stop trying to escape through a bottle or baggie and to find my "safe places".

I now spend much of my days guiding other men who have had similar life experiences to me and my family, on their journeys, helping them learn how to be positive, fathers, husbands, workers and men.

Positive principles

I do this by allowing them an opportunity to learn positive principles of being. Principles such as respect, responsibility, empathy, acceptance, gratitude and most importantly, truth. I've been fortunate to learn these from an Aboriginal perspective, yet do not see these as Aboriginal specific but rather underlying concepts practised by all spiritual belief systems across many cultures.

As people we strive to experience acceptance in all aspects of our lives, we want to be loved and nurtured, we want to have friendships, we want to be positively recognised for our work and most of all we want to feel safe in our identity.

However, often what we witness and experience is rejection, including neglect, disregard, disrespect and constant identity conflict or confusion. This was something I initially learnt from Uncle Tommy Powell, a founder of a successful Aboriginal wellbeing program called Red Dust Healing.

Our striving for acceptance, which brings the rush of the so called "happy brain chemicals", leads us to chase acceptance in the most unlikely of places, and yet our desire to be free from rejection is often what leads us to reject others. Often young men who have experienced frequent rejection or domestic violence and who feel disconnected will search for acceptance elsewhere.

They may already be using negative coping strategies such as drug and alcohol use, petty crime, the disrespect of others, fighting. While these young people perceive a sense of satisfaction (through the release of serotonin and other "happy" hormones) that comes with feeling accepted, they don't realise the rejection they are causing toward themselves (largely through a lack of self-respect) and for others such as family, teachers, employers.

They don't find the opportunities to learn truthful respect or absorb how to fulfil responsibilities and obligations in a purposeful, respectful and meaningful way. This conflict drives the young person to want to "escape" again and again, furthering the negative coping. Things can then quickly spiral out of control for many.

The young person grows and the cycle becomes more entrenched. The negative life events increase in frequency and compound. Drinking a little turns into drinking a lot, marijuana use leads to harder drug use, petty crime morphs to serious crime and abuse becomes more violent.

How do I know this?

Because I lived it and witness it every day in the lives of almost all those I now work with.

Where opportunities and resources are scarce, where oppression is a continued lived experience and where loss is frequent, negative life events and negative coping will go hand-in-hand.

It is no surprise then that we see such high rates of offender behaviour, such as family violence, and therefore incarceration rates amongst groups of society in which we know there has been and continues to be such concerns.

For instance, Aboriginal and Torres Strait Islander peoples make up only 3 percent of our national population, yet our incarceration rates sit at nearly 10 times this rate. And a report from an Amnesty International investigation found that our children are 24 times more likely to be incarcerated than other Australian children.

Incarceration leads to further disconnect – leads to further need to cope – leads to further negative coping – leads to further offender behaviour – leads to further incarceration, and the cycle continues.

An Australian Institute of Health and Welfare report indicated as many a quarter of Aboriginal and Torres Strait Islander women will report having experienced domestic or family violence in the past 12 months.

A large proportion of these will report having experienced such violence from someone who was intoxicated or under the influence of drugs. Women reported that 30 percent of these attacks came from a current or ex-spouse (commonly categorised under domestic violence) while as much as 40 percent of these came from relatives (commonly categorised under family violence).

This is not at all to say men do not experience violence, it absolutely must be acknowledged that men experience high rates of both physical and psychological domestic and/or family violence also.

It is, however, much more difficult to obtain accurate data on men's experiences with family violence and domestic violence. With each of these offences, comes further incarceration and again further disconnection. The cycle continues as the problems continue.

So what is the answer?

Well to me that's a complex question, and one that I personally believe most in positions of power do not truly want to explore, because it challenges the very societal structures that keep them in such positions of influence.

- Why is one man worth 10-fold of another?

- Why is the day-to-day effort of a minimal wage shift worker worth less than that of a politician or GP?

- Why is opportunity plentiful for some and not others?

- Why as a nation can we not recognise our own naivety and dis-truth?

- What really is a "fair go for all"?

We need to be truthful as people and as societies. We need to break the cycle of disconnect. We need to increase opportunities and resources for all people within society.

There's a desperate need to assist people to learn to positively cope in times of distress and disconnect to enable them to replace negative coping strategies.

We need to assist people to find their "safe places", where they can stand and fight their problems and heal. We need to re-educate ourselves and our children on positive living, and not allow ourselves to be continuously caught up in the negative, self-centred whirlwind that is Western capitalism and all its consumerist values.

As Aboriginal peoples we need to get back to Lore and Culture and to heal our spirits.

I congratulate you Darren on your honesty, thank you for your strength in sharing your yarn, and wish you all the best in your journey.

- For more information on Aboriginal family violence and working with those who have experienced such please refer to – **Working Together: Aboriginal mental health principles and practice 2nd Ed**.

- Read Darren's story on page 44.

- For descriptions of Aboriginal healing models see Part six of this text (chapters 24-31). Links to free downloads of all these chapters can be found **here**.

Clinton is a Gamilaroi man and registered psychologist with a keen interest in holistic wellness. He is undertaking a PhD with Griffith University, researching factors of holistic wellbeing for members of the Aboriginal and Torres Strait Islander health workforce. Clinton founded Marumali Consultations in 2010 and continues to run this business along with Stacey Vervoort.

Marumali Consultations specialises in: providing holistic counselling services for Aboriginal workers; in specific men's and women's wellbeing; cultural competence auditing and training; cross cultural psychological and business management services; and wellness focused mentoring and professional supervision.

Putting culture and community at the heart of #JustJustice for Aboriginal and Torres Strait Islander youth

Author:	Marie McInerney	Published:	March 11, 2016

Journalist Marie McInerney visits a Koori cultural program for young offenders in a youth justice facility at Parkville in inner suburban Melbourne.

Marie McInerney writes:

On this grey, chilly Melbourne morning, it looks for a while like the spark won't catch, but soon the familiar smell of burning eucalypt wafts across the grounds.

"Put the smoke through your hair, under your feet," urges Clayton, an Aboriginal liaison worker, as he explains the significance of the different gum leaves he is burning to the group of youth justice clients and other staff members. They are sitting around a makeshift campfire on the edge of the high security facility .

First he lays on the leaves from a sheoak, to represent slow growth and the strength of Elders. Then the yellow wattle, significant to the local area. He talks about how, at home, his mob burns the leaves of the cherry ballart, whose roots attach themselves to those of other plants, "representing kids holding onto mothers".

This Aboriginal smoking ceremony is short and sweet, but it's deep with meaning and purpose here at the Parkville Youth Justice Precinct, in inner suburban Melbourne.

The smoking gum leaves seem worlds away from the high-tech retina scans that visitors undergo on the way into the facility and from the six-metre fence that winds its way across the precinct, dividing those who are here on remand and those who are serving sentences.

It's a ceremony that's far away too from daily reality for the many young Aboriginal and Torres Strait Islander offenders who have lost contact with, or confidence in their culture through difficult, often traumatic, childhood experiences.

"Knowing who and what you are is the first step forward," says Gunditjmara Elder Uncle Jim Berg as the two-hour Koori Cultural Program held here every Monday, gets underway on this day.

Much has already been written in Victoria about the transformation that has taken place at Parkville since a damning Ombudsman's report was published in 2010.

A big part of the change has been the establishment of Parkville College, an official Victorian Government school based within the facility. Parkville College holds classes seven days a week for every young person held at Parkville and boasts some outstanding results.

There are sceptics, and the facility is currently being challenged to the hilt by "unintended consequences" of tough on crime policies that have changed the mix of the facility, but the College – championed by then Victorian Coalition Community Services Minister Mary Wooldridge – has put education at the heart of rehabilitation for young offenders.

The Koori Cultural Program has now added cultural education to the Parkville College curriculum. It became part of the College's offering last year, at the urging of local community members and in recognition that young Aboriginal and Torres Strait Islander people make up 15-20 per cent of the Parkville Youth Precinct population.

The Archie Roach connection

Shane Evans is the Manager of Student Engagement at Parkville College's Education Justice Initiative (EJI), based at the Melbourne Children's Court, who works with young people who have disengaged from education.

Different threads of his family, life and work came together at the 2014 NAIDOC celebrations at Parkville, when the College announced the start of the Koori Cultural Program.

The NAIDOC concert featured his uncle Archie Roach, who has since become the patron at Parkville College and a big supporter of the Koori program.

At the event the legendary Aboriginal singer songwriter revealed a painful personal connection to Parkville.

"We had a bit of a stroll around the grounds and my uncle Archie was frozen by the trauma," Evans recalls. "I hadn't known that he was processed there (for foster care) when he was taken off Framingham mission, separated from his mother," he said.

"That's a story in itself, that goes to the very heart of what we do," he said.

Parkville is familiar ground in a different sense for Uncle Jim Berg who worked for more than 40 years in Victoria's legal system, including as founding CEO for the Victorian Aboriginal

Legal Service (VALS). He's been an official prison visitor and sat on the Parole Board for 13 years.

He laughs that he was "coaxed" out of retirement by Shane and Archie, and by Parkville College Executive Principal Brendan Murray, whose father-in-law is former Federal Court Judge Ron Merkel, another important figure in the founding of VALS.

These connections have ensured the Koori Cultural Program has had big firepower from the start. Guest speakers have included judges, magistrates, public servants, footballers, musicians and researchers in languages and geneology. Over the past year the program has settled into themes: the Stolen Generation, identity, culture. Each session starts with a yarning circle, but the curriculum aims of the day's program are also inked on the whiteboard to provide structure.

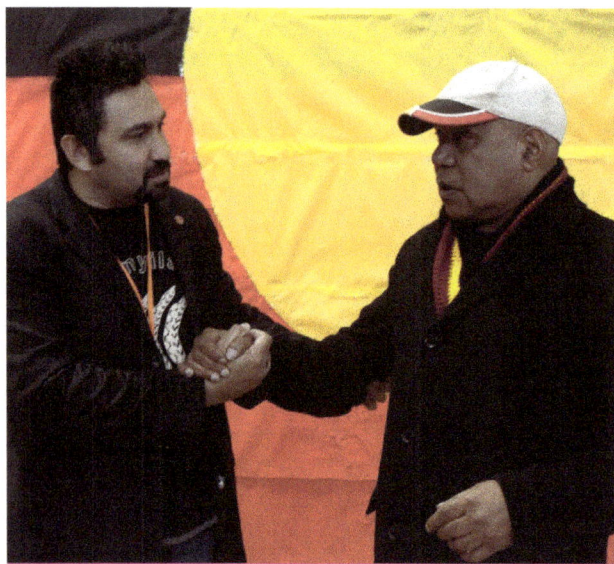

Shane Evans and his uncle, Archie Roach

Except, he adds, that it's not been the reality till now for many of the kids in Parkville. Other staff talk also about the damage to identity and sense of belonging of many of the kids who have grown up in out-of-home-care, away from community, culture and country.

One of their guest speakers, Andrew Jackomos, the Victorian Commissioner for Aboriginal Children and Young People, has been sounding the alarm for years about the highly vulnerable 'second stolen generation' of young Aboriginal kids who are removed from kin at increasingly high rates.

He called for urgent action as the number of Aboriginal children in out-of-home care soared by 42 per cent in Victoria. It makes for a terrible pathway to prison: according to Victoria's Youth Parole Board, 62 per cent of its clients are or have been under Child Protection.

Still, Uncle Jim reckons he can trace the family tree for 99 per cent of the kids who come into the program. It gives them a bit of confidence, some pride to know that they belong somewhere, he says. "Some may not talk up a lot but they listen and learn."

Harsh impact of rising remand numbers

Victor Hugo's famous quote – "He who opens a school door, closes a prison" – provides inspiration on the wall at Parkville.

But these words do not reflect the reality of growing numbers of remand prisoners in the wake of the former Coalition State Government's changes to the Bail Act and justice diversion options that have sent many more young people to Parkville ahead of their day in court.

Victoria's former Commissioner for Children and Young People Bernie Geary last year said the numbers languishing on remand were "absolutely scandalous"; of the 83 young people at Parkville the week before he spoke out, only 19 had been sentenced; 10 of those on remand, or 15 per cent, were aged between 10 and 14 years old.

Jesuit Social Services recently released a report – An escalating problem: Responding to the increased remand of children in Victoria – showing a 57 per cent rise in the number of children in remand in Victoria over 12 months (from 112 to 176), including a significant increase in the number of Aboriginal and Torres Strait Island children (from 12 to 32). The number of those aged between 10-14 years rose from 1 to 12.

The numbers have been significantly driven, it says, by breaches of bail conditions that apply equally to children as well as adults (despite many warnings of the potential implications) such as residing at a particular address, being subject to a curfew or geographical exclusion zone, not driving a motor vehicle, and not contacting specified persons or classes of persons.

There's been major relief this year with the passage last month (February) by the Victorian Labor Government of bail amendments, which are expected to significantly reduce the number of children ending up in detention on remand. But they will take time to come into effect, "so it will be a while before we see the effect in Parkville," says Smart Justice for Young People convenor Tiffany Overall.

The rising remand numbers were breaching the recommendation from the Royal Commission in Aboriginal Deaths in Custody that prison should be a "last resort". From the Parkville College perspective, they have also disrupted education and rehabilitation.

"Trauma saturated"

Simon Lenten, Director of Strategy & Services at Parkville College, says the College operates with a careful understanding of how to work in a context that is "trauma saturated", informed by attachment theory and the work of John Bowlby, along with a humanistic physiological approach championed by Carl Rogers.

The College has also tapped into the work of US psychiatrist Dr Bruce Perry from the Child Trauma Academy, which has close links in Melbourne with the Berry Street Childhood Institute. Perry's work is focused on what happens to a child's mind when he or she is traumatised, and what is needed for healing. He spoke last year in Melbourne to community sector workers about how hard it is, neurologically, for traumatised kids to think and learn when they live in 'fight or flight' mode.

Parkville staff and visitors say that being on remand only exacerbates that, and they ask how can the College meaningfully engage young offenders in education and create a therapeutic environment of learning, when so many are cycling in and out on average for just three weeks.

"If it's their first time in, they're pretty much poo-ing their pants (about just being here) – it's a very daunting place, a maximum security facility," Evans said. "The sentenced kids are more settled, they're not awaiting their fate. The brain can't concentrate when it's in panic mode."

Lenten says the rising remand numbers "fundamentally changed the way the place runs".

He says: "The issue with remand is the terrible waste of resources and the terrible impact it has, to have a huge group there for a very short time: the remand group really only has the opportunity to experience disruption, without the opportunities to add value, rehabilitate or educate because most remand children aren't there very long. It has changed the nature of the place because it creates the dominant theme as that of a churn of students entering and re-entering the College...and that impacts disproportionately on Aboriginal children."

"Everyone is learning"

At the end of today's session, the Koori Cultural Program group gets together for a party pie lunch. At the end of each term there's a barbecue. For some kids it's the first steak they've ever had.

Today it's cold outside, so everyone squashes in together in the kitchen and yarning room: five Parkville students – two girls and three boys, Shane and Uncle Jim, three Aboriginal Liaison Officers and two non-Indigenous Secure Services staff (employed by the Victorian Department of Health and Human Services which manages security at Parkville and Malmsbury). It's one of the few occasions at Parkville where the boys and girls, and remand and sentenced students mix.

I'm welcome to speak to the young people but asked not to try to find out why they're in there. Shane Evans says he's never queried that: "I want to have a clear mind, not judge."

It's a bit awkward, interrupting what is clearly a welcome break from prison routine, but I ask one of the girls what she likes about the Koori Cultural Program. "There's lots of jokes and laughter, and good food," she says.

One of the non-Aboriginal Secure Services staff members is also on board with the program. "I can see how important it is for them to come (each week), they get really upset if we're short-staffed (and they can't). Whether they're coming for the culture or interaction with other Aboriginal people, I hope it works for them."

In fact, the cultural learning is also aimed at him – staff as well as students.

"It's important to have non-Aboriginal teachers and others working alongside Uncle Jim and me," Evans says after the group has left. "Everyone is learning, not only the students. I'm learning from Uncle Jim: I learn wisdom, how to be humble, professionalism, integrity. I learn the old stories, the old ways that my mum talks about. For me it fills in pieces of the jigsaw puzzle."

For rehabilitation, he says, education is key. "We have to make that a priority, a protective factor, alongside and interconnected with healthy culture, families and relationships."

Evans talks about his own early years, of growing up in a public housing estate in inner city Melbourne, one of six kids; his Dad was Welsh Irish mix, his mum Gunditjmara, born and bred on Framingham. He admits to having got into "heaps of trouble" with police. "I was no angel, got into some petty stuff, on the perimeters of gangs, drove cars illegally. I make no bones about that."

He also copped abuse, discrimination and assault "for the colour of my skin", including being allegedly bashed by police on Smith Street in Fitzroy for wearing an Aboriginal T-shirt in 1988, the Bicentennial year. "I got assaulted, handcuffed, bashed in the back of a divvy van," he said. "It really traumatised me".

So, given the pathways in the justice system, how has he ended up on the other side of the fence at Parkville?

"Call it lucky", he says. He credits a number of interventions along the way: a couple of very good PE teachers "who cared for us kids from the Commission flats when no-one else did"; youth clubs that "kept us engaged in sport"; and a strong family, "grounded, embedded in culture".

The importance of those "protective factors" are underlined when his Parkville colleague Clayton talks about what some of the kids experience on their way into prison, and which is likely

> *It has changed the nature of the place because it creates the dominant theme as that of a churn of students entering and re-entering the College... and that impacts disproportionately on Aboriginal children*

to lead to a cycle of offending. There's also the question of what support is around for detained children and young people on their release.

"For some, this is a better home than they've ever had," Clayton says. "When you've come through residential care, even the best one in the world is not necessarily going to be 'home' for you. With one guy, we had to talk him into going to court to apply for bail because it was better for him here than on the outside."

Accountable to Elders and community

Simon Lenten makes the point that the Koori Cultural Program was set up in consultation with and at the urging of Aboriginal Elders and the local Aboriginal community, and that the College knows it must be accountable.

The program has now been expanded to the Malmsbury Youth Justice Precinct, set up under Victoria's unique dual track system to allow adult courts to sentence young offenders aged 18-20 to serve custodial sentences in youth detention instead of adult prison.

Lenten says it's early days yet for the program but the "hope and desire" is to see Koori education embedded formally in Parkville programs, to become a formal Victorian Certificate of Applied Learning (VCAL) vocational subject, and to drive content in other subject areas.

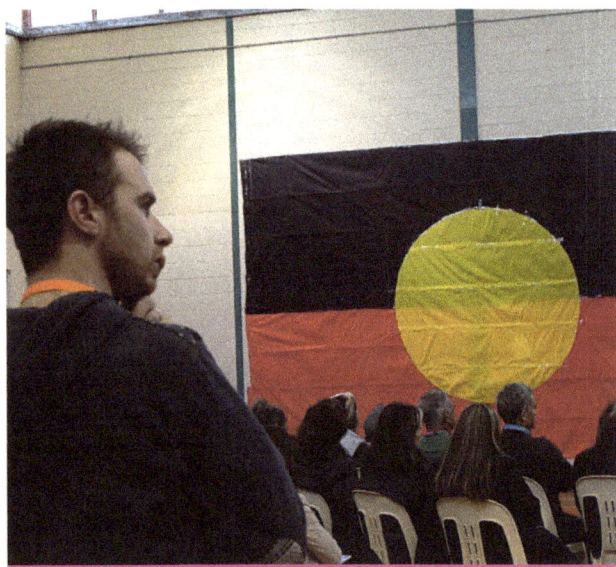

NAIDOC event at Parkville. Photograph credits: Parkville College photography teacher Lesley Turnball

"We want that to be formal, thoughtful and properly resourced, connected to communities and Elders, and guided by people who understand that space well," he said. "I think it's really good (so far) but I think we can get better and better at it."

"Aboriginal students are such a big group in our school community that we needed to respect and honour that in a way. The Elders and community members had indicated it

was important to do, as had lots of literature and research of course."

In her recent report on the State's prisons, Victoria's Ombudsman Deborah Glass focused on the need for and efficacy of cultural programs for Aboriginal and Torres Strait Islander prisoners, saying they were currently run "haphazardly" in the prison system.

There's been no formal evaluation yet of the Koori Cultural Program at Parkville, though that will come, Lenten said. For the moment, the College assesses its value in the willingness of young Aboriginal people to participate.

But it fits firmly inside the school's rights platform that sees the role of education – particularly in a youth justice context – as much more than just learning content or curriculum.

"Numeracy and literacy are important and will always be measured and valued by us as a school but we also have a much bigger responsibility and purpose in developing young people who have been denied access to education previously," Lenten said.

"And that's the truth of our students if you like, along with almost universal experience of trauma, abuse and neglect in their backgrounds, along with a lot of other complex issues in terms of family dynamics and other issues around mental health, disability presentations, drug and alcohol issues…. So when that's applied to particular groups of cultural over-representation, led by Indigenous Australians and compounded by the fact that it's their country too, that asks of us to understand and think carefully about how we offer that to our students. For Aboriginal children, it also means understanding of identity and where they come from as a really valuable part of building a relationship which is a great vehicle for all learning."

Uncle Jim and Shane Evans have documented all that they've done from the beginning. They want, Evans says, to develop a best practice cultural program that can be shared with any school in the state, whether there are Aboriginal kids there or not, "that accurately tells the story of this country" and that builds pride and identity early.

"You need goodwill and people that really value that white Australia has a black history. I think our school is heading in the right direction, it's profound what we've achieved in a year but we're only scratching the surface. Koori cultural programs should be in every school in the state, in the country."

"Listen to Us": This report deserves a wide readership #JustJustice

| Author: | Summer May Finlay | Published: | August 13, 2015 |

Summer May Finlay writes:

Western Australia is often in the headlines for policies that are harmful for Aboriginal and Torres Strait Islander people, including for hurtful comments by the Western Australian Chief Justice.

But the State also recently produced a fantastic report: *"Listen to Us: Using the views of WA Aboriginal and Torres Strait Islander children and young people to improve policy and service delivery"*.

Published by the Commissioner for Children and Young People, WA, the report outlines ways of improving young Aboriginal peoples' wellbeing. It is based upon consultations with 1,217 children and young people across the state.

This report is powerful because it shows the difference that it makes when people listen to us, and respect our views and knowledge.

While the Chief Justice's stereotyping comments were reported by mainstream media, it is disappointing that that the "Listen to Us" report didn't attract so much attention.

The report takes a holistic approach; if its recommendations are widely implemented by governments and other service providers, perhaps this would help to create some #JustJustice, and to reduce the over-incarceration of Aboriginal and Torres Strait Islander people.

Hopefully, the Chief Justice will take note. And listen – especially to the young people telling us about the harmful impacts of stereotyping and racism.

Below are some of the important messages from the report.

Key approaches: *"local, cooperative and, ultimately, community-led and controlled"*

Drawing from identified good practice, relevant research and evidence, the work of the office of the Commissioner for Children and Young People, the guiding principles under the legislation and listening to the voices of the children and young people, there needs to be a collective commitment to the following four approaches.

1. Improving outcomes for Aboriginal children and young people, and their families, must be seen as core business for all agencies as there is an imperative to achieve truly integrated planning, funding and delivery of programs and services. This requires genuine partnerships between all levels of government, the community and private sectors.

2. Programs and services need to be flexible, understand and respect the diversity of Aboriginal children and young people and their communities, their language, their culture and their histories, and be able to respond to their unique circumstances, needs, strengths and capacities. This requires approaches that are local, cooperative and, ultimately, community-led and controlled.

3. Programs and services must recognise the importance of, and build on the strengths of, Aboriginal family and kinship.

4. Services and programs to support the safety and wellbeing of children and young people must be evidence-based and outcomes focused. This does not mean compromising the capacity to be innovative and try new approaches, but rather a commitment from service funders and providers to measure, evaluate and define meaningful and sustainable outcomes, to relinquish what does not work, and focus on what does.

Key strategies: *"an ongoing commitment to listening and responding"*

In responding directly to the views expressed by Aboriginal children and young people in this consultation, more focused investment is required in the following eight strategies.

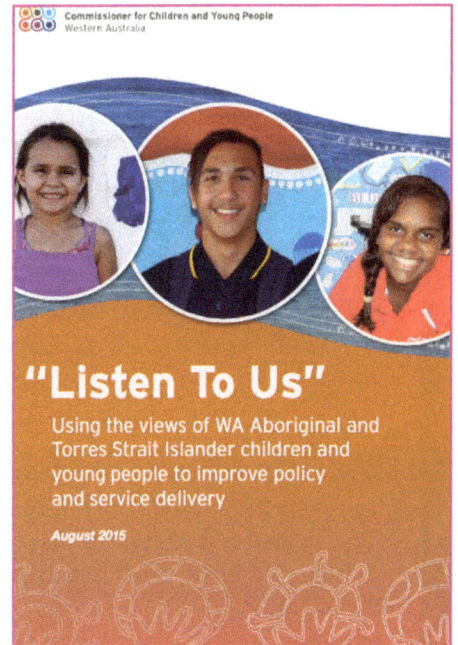

1. Supporting the role and capacity of parents by investing in culturally appropriate early childhood services – including pre-natal support, universal and targeted parenting programs, child health and allied health services jointly delivered and co-located on or near school sites – must be a priority.

2. Recognising that culture is important to individual and community resilience, Aboriginal children and young people must be supported to learn and practice their culture, and communities supported to restore, strengthen and celebrate their culture.

3. There needs to be greater efforts to address racism and support reconciliation with a focus on building cross-cultural understanding and connection with all Western Australians, with schools being an important setting for this work.

4. Multiple strategies are needed across agencies to support engagement and participation in education, which include strong partnerships between schools, families and communities, and work to better identify and remove the barriers to school engagement.

5. Better access to mentoring, role modelling and support programs is required to provide long-term support and advice regarding education and pathways to post-school education, training and employment options.

6. Aboriginal culture, knowledge and identity need to be integrated more widely into educational programs and philosophies.

7. Neighbourhoods and physical spaces need to be designed with and for children and young people to support their development, encourage community cohesion and positive interaction.

8. All children and young people need to have access to a diverse range of age-appropriate, low-cost recreation, sport and cultural activities to support their active engagement and social participation. It is important to recognise these programs can and do provide an effective vehicle to access other supports that impact positively on the wellbeing of children and young people. Fundamentally, programs and services need to be underpinned by an ongoing commitment to listening and responding to the views of Aboriginal children and young people, and it is the role of all organisations that work with Aboriginal children and young people to ensure these meaningful conversations continue.

Summer May Finlay is a Yorta Yorta woman, a public health practitioner and a PhD candidate.

Reviewing a brilliant series from Vice – "Over Represented"

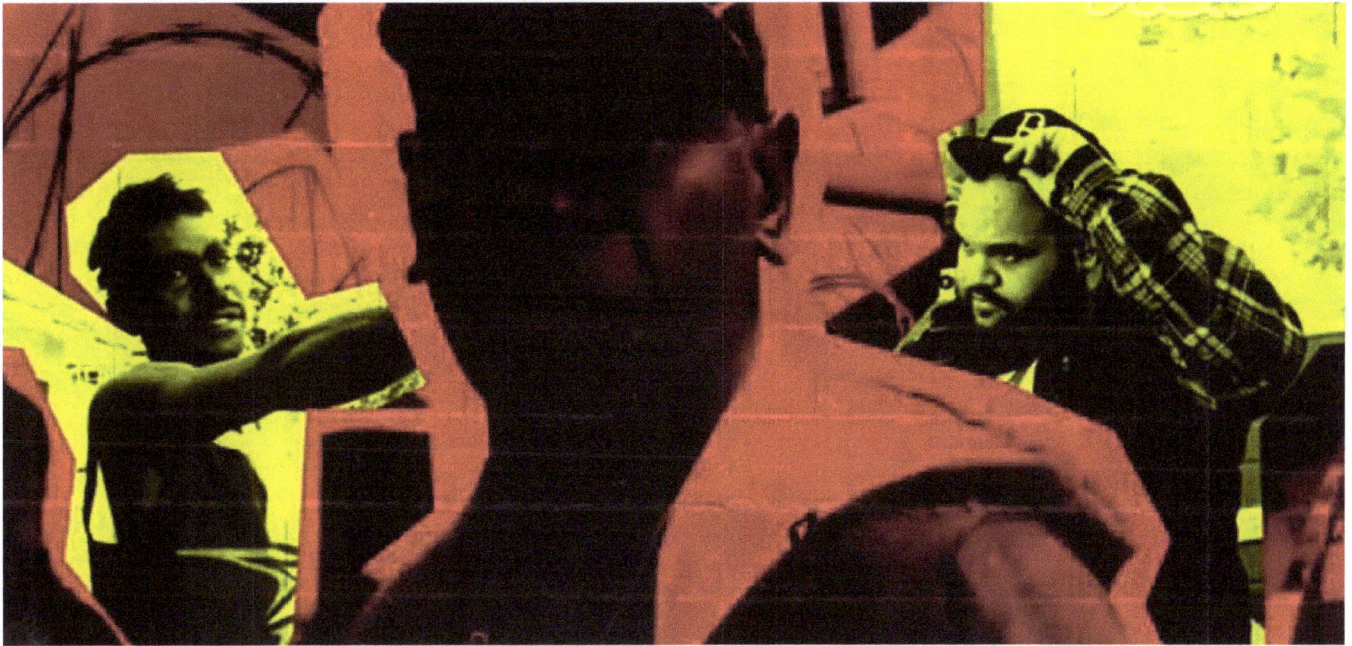

| Author: | Julian Cleary | Published: | November 09, 2015 |

Julian Cleary writes:

Amnesty recently partnered with Vice Magazine to screen their powerful three-part series that looks at Aboriginal and Torres Strait Islander experiences of the justice system in Australia – **Over Represented**.

The series presents three snapshots from around the country of Aboriginal people visiting, being caught up in, and working in the justice system. Throughout the series, Vice lets these people do the talking – no voice-overs or corny analysis.

The series kicks off by following Yorta Yorta rapper **Briggs as he visits kids in juvie in south-west Sydney**.

As one of the staff at the Reiby Youth Detention Centre points out, 60-70 per cent of the kids (aged 10 to 17) at the centre are Aboriginal. Aboriginal kids make up about 5 per cent of the total population in this age bracket – the over-representation is staggering.

The most compelling thing about the series opener for me is it shows that the boys at Reiby are just kids. Too often that gets lost in the abstract talk about the stats and 'juvenile justice.'

Briggs puts it well when he says that "there's a lot of potential behind this razor wire." That potential is far too often overlooked to the detriment of these kids and the rest of us too.

Briggs has an amazing rapport with these young fellas. It seems like it comes from a place of mutual respect, and from his understanding of where they are coming from and what they might have been through.

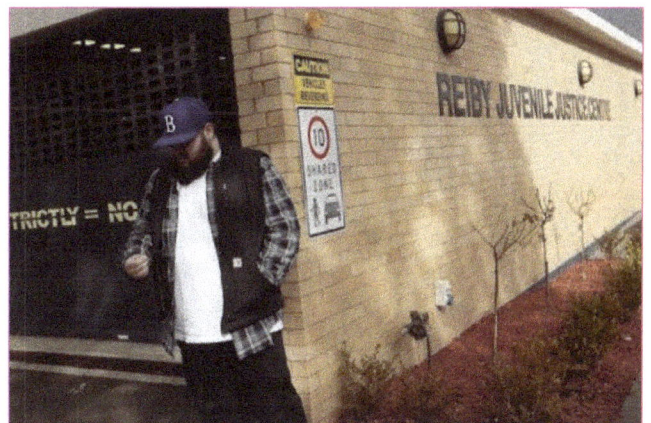

You can sense how much Briggs cares about these kids and wants them to recognise that potential and succeed – as Briggs himself is succeeding.

As a long-time local hip hop fan, I first saw Briggs on stage as hype man for Melbourne hip hop icon 'Reason' maybe 10 years ago. He had plenty of stage presence even back then.

But I didn't have any inkling of how much of an impact he would have on the hip hop scene, on young guys like those at Reiby, or on me for that matter.

Since then, Briggs has grown in stature and confidence to the point where he is now a role model and emerging leader.

Like many people, I was blown away by Briggs' homage to Archie Roach released this past NAIDOC week: The Children Came Back. It is an awesome celebration of some remarkable Aboriginal leaders and legends: from Sir Douglas Nicholls (and Lady Gladys Nicholls in the film clip) to William Cooper, Cathy Freeman and Adam Goodes.

I was lucky to also catch the Melbourne launch of Briggs' music label: Bad Apples. The label roster is made up of eloquent and outspoken young Aboriginal rappers whose talents Briggs is helping to cultivate and whose voices he intends to amplify (Nookie, Philly and Birdz). Also under Bad Apples is his own collaboration, the A.B Originals, with Ngarrindjeri rapper and producer Trials, best known for his work with Adelaide hip hop group the Funkoars.

The atmosphere at that show was different to most other Australian hip hop shows I've been to. It felt like a celebration of black excellence.

'Briggs Live at Juvie' seems like an extension of these other developments. He is evidently aware of the courage and strength of those Aboriginal leaders that have come before him and is carrying on that legacy in his own unique and charismatic way.

As Victorian Aboriginal Children's Commissioner Andrew Jackomos, another Yorta Yorta man, recently wrote on this blog: culture is far more than a perk for young Koori kids; it is a lifeline. He wrote that "cultural rights directly impact on a child's ability to meaningfully enjoy every other human right and freedom, let alone their health."

There needs to be more opportunities for role models like Briggs and countless other passionate, committed Aboriginal and Torres Strait Islander people all over Australia to work with kids whose reality they understand far better than the outsiders often drafted in to do this kind of work.

It is crucial that this happens in youth detention centres, but it has to happen much earlier too, to turn around what is now a youth detention epidemic among Aboriginal and Torres Strait Islander kids in Australia.

Next stop, Darwin

From Reiby in Sydney, Vice take us up to Darwin to ride along with the Larrakia Night Patrol.

This second part to the series is confronting. It deals with the carnage wrought by alcohol among marginalised and maligned Aboriginal people living in the long grass on the fringes of Darwin.

Tauto Sansbury gives some context in the film, explaining that invasion, dispossession and forced child-removal has resulted in widespread intergenerational trauma that needs to be better acknowledged and addressed.

What shines through in this documentary, though, is the commitment, care and compassion that Larrakia staff bring to their work for their people.

Larrakia Nations, among many other things, play a vital role by providing care, support and assistance to the 'long grassers' in Darwin (where the Indigenous homeless population are colloquially referred to by this name).

This documentary highlights the need to respond to alcohol and drug abuse through better investment in therapeutic community-led approaches, rather than the failed law and order response that is currently dominant in the Northern Territory.

I couldn't help but think of the tragic story of Kumanjayi Langdon when I watched this documentary. Mr Langdon was a Warlpiri Elder who recently died in a police cell in Darwin where he had been locked up for public drinking under the NT's new paperless arrest laws.

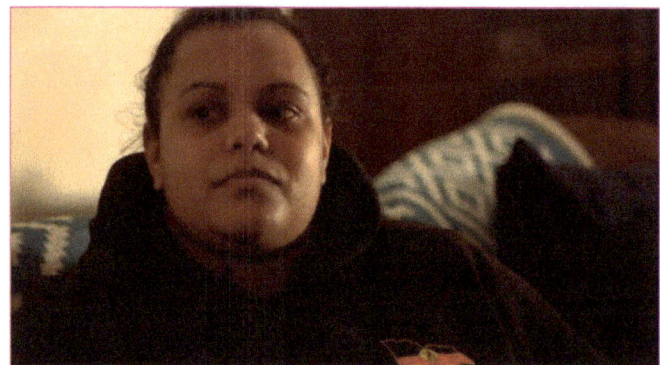

This film describes the cycle that starts with a fine. Yet under the new laws a person can be arrested and detained in a police cell immediately for what used to result in only such a fine.

Kumanjayi Langdon had been drinking, but was described by police at the inquest into his death as being at all times polite and cooperative with police; there was no justifiable reason for his arrest and detention.

The Coroner put it as follows:

" Kumanjayi Langdon, a sick middle-aged Aboriginal man, was treated like a criminal and incarcerated like a criminal; he died in a police cell which was built to house criminals. He died in his sleep with strangers in this cold and concrete cell. He died of natural causes and was always likely to die suddenly due to chronic and serious heart disease, but he was entitled to die in peace, in the comfort of family and friends. In my view, he was entitled to die as a free man.

The Coroner found that these paperless arrest laws were putting such a massive burden on police and nurses at the watchouse that they couldn't properly care for the flood of Aboriginal people now being targeted and locked up for offences that would never carry a prison sentence.

The coroner urged the government to scrap these laws before they led to more deaths – a call that has so far been ignored. The North Australian Aboriginal Justice Agency have led the charge to see these laws repealed and are currently awaiting the decision of the High Court.

Former Police Union President Vince Kelly said that "we can't arrest ourselves out of this mess." He is right. Yet Larrakia Night Patrol suffered funding cuts under this NT Government, at the same time as they increased police powers to arrest people for extremely minor offences.

The same NT Government has transferred kids to a former adult detention centre and treated them horrifically. These retrograde steps fail everyone, including those people who demand tough responses to crime.

These kids in detention far too often become more hardened and marginalised; the community at large becomes less safe and more Aboriginal people face death in custody, while the underlying problems go unresolved.

Saving lives

The third and final documentary, Barred Calls, follows the incredibly patient and caring Elva from the Victorian Aboriginal Legal Service as she is notified of, and phones to check after the welfare of every Aboriginal person taken into police custody in Victoria and Tasmania.

This life-saving service provides a stark contrast to the "lock em up" approach that is putting Aboriginal lives at risk in the Northern Territory.

Elva's tireless work is one example of how the Victorian Aboriginal Legal Services, and Aboriginal and Torres Strait Islander Legal Services generally, go far beyond the usual transactional legal relationship.

Being controlled by and run for Aboriginal people, they look at the bigger picture and do vital work in the face of constant funding shortages.

Despite having been a recommendation of the Royal Commission into Aboriginal Deaths in Custody, custody notification services like this are only in place in New South Wales, the Australian Capital Territory, Victoria and Tasmania. And only the Aboriginal Legal Service (NSW/ACT) receive federal funding to deliver it.

Many Aboriginal deaths in custody, like those of Kwementyaye Briscoe, Ms Dhu and Kumanjayi Langdon might have been avoided if such a system were in place in the Northern Territory and Western Australia. A program like this should be funded by the federal government in place in all states and territories.

The Vice Over Represented series provides some brilliant insights into some of the issues and solutions in the justice system.

They are well worth checking out. So too is Vice's recent edition devoted to the issue of incarceration that touches on a range of related issues.

Julian Cleary is a researcher/campaigner with Amnesty International's Indigenous Rights team. In this role, he has done extensive research into Aboriginal and Torres Strait Islander youth justice issues across Australia. Julian also worked for several years in advocacy and research roles with the Central Land Council in Alice Springs. In his downtime, Julian makes hip hop music under the pseudonym Jules Berne and as part of Renovators Dream. In April 2015 he released debut solo EP Escapades.

Sharing solutions

Author:	Lynda Ryder and Michelle Adams	Published:	November 22, 2016

Lynda Ryder and Michelle Adams, two Yindjibarndi women from Karratha with many years of experience in cultural community development, share their suggestions for a fairer justice system in the interview below.

Among their suggestions are:

- Local cultural competence training for police and others involved in the justice system, including judges and magistrates.

- Western law and justice system should learn from Aboriginal knowledges and cultural practices.

- Courts should employ Aboriginal advocates to assist offenders and families.

- Culturally appropriate alternatives must be found to locking up people when this is not needed for community safety. Too many people are locked up for repeat driving offences, that could be better dealt with in other ways.

- Policing should work with the community to keep the community safe, rather than take a punitive focus.

- Policing and justice systems need to be work with the families of offenders. Families should be supported to assist family members through rehabilitation and to rebuild their lives post prison release.

- An end to the problematising of Aboriginal people by colonial structures and systems.

- Address racism within the criminal justice system.

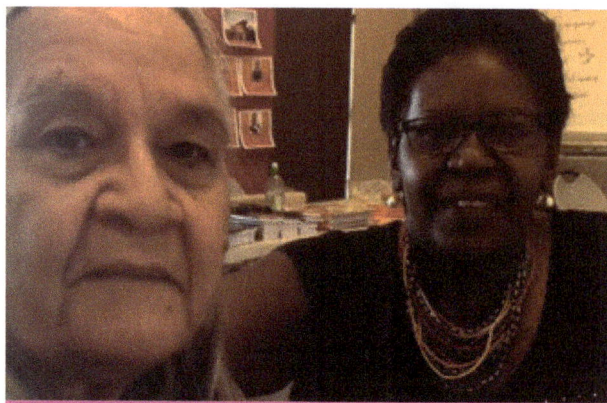

Lynda Ryder (left) and Michelle Adams

Lynda Ryder concluded the interview by saying:

"I hope that anything we've said can be taken in the way that it was given and it's shared. And it helps somewhere along the way to get people to think differently, about a lot of things, not just the justice system. There's justice in education, there's justice in housing, there's justice right across the board. Are we being just to everyone? I would say, probably not.

Watch the interview here:
https://www.youtube.com/watch?v=enrL-7b3RR4

Lynda Ryder and Michelle Adams are Yindjibarndi women from Karratha.

2. Stories from the heart

" Cultural integrity and respect is the cup I now sup from

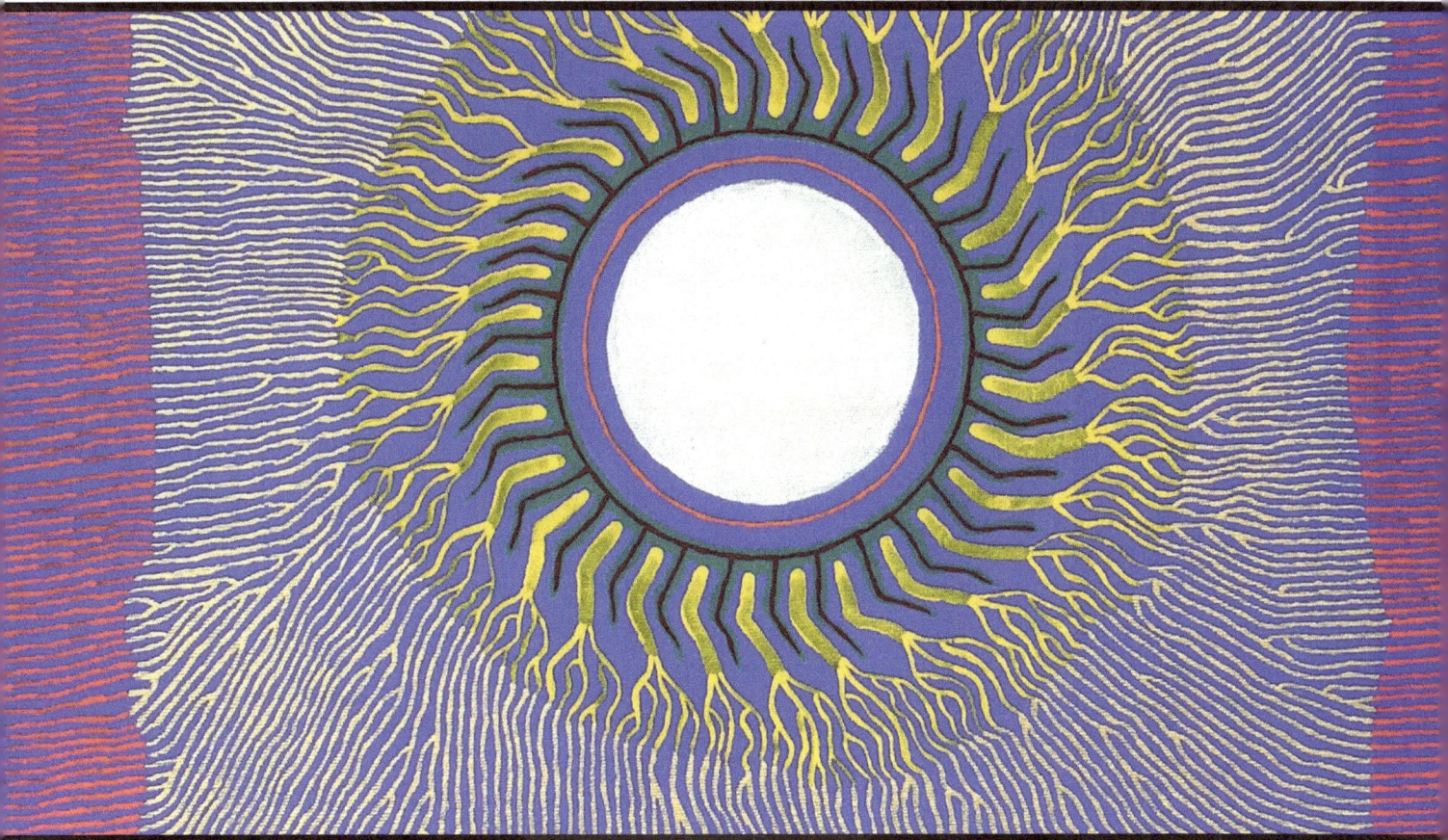

Sandy: a dear friend, condemned by harmful systems

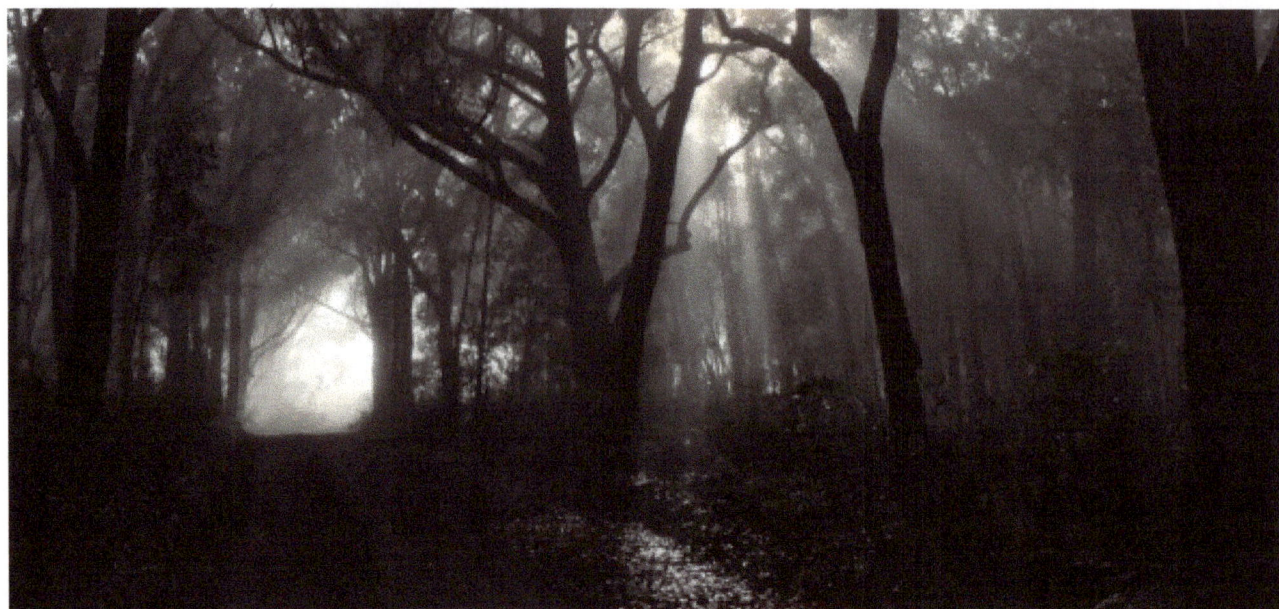

| Author: | Megan Williams | Published: | April 27, 2016 |

Dr Megan Williams tells the story of her friend Sandy, an Aboriginal man who has been in and out of prison many times, and explores how punitive, disconnected systems contribute to recidivism.

Williams is a Senior Research Fellow at the Aboriginal Health and Wellbeing Research team at Western Sydney University. Through her father's family, she is a descendent of the Wiradjuri people of the NSW Riverine.

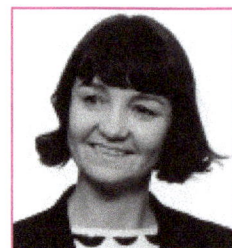

She has worked for 20 years in community health, evaluation and research, and completed a PhD investigating the role of social support to prevent re-incarceration among urban Aboriginal people.

Megan Williams writes:

I've known my dear friend Sandy for several years. He's been like an angel in my life – kind, supportive and trustworthy.

But his life has been punctuated with prison sentences and justice system nightmares, showing how remarkably easily he has been caught in the cycle of re-incarceration and poverty, over and over again.

Last year showed the most promise for Sandy. After being in and out of prison for two decades, desperation led him to again try long-term residential drug and alcohol rehabilitation.

He hated his case worker and other residents, but he persevered because he couldn't see any other option for escaping the violence he'd experienced in prison, the risks he'd experienced with drugs, or the deep sense of failure that he carried around.

Little by little, Sandy's resistance to being helped shifted, ironically only because of the actual experience of being helped. There was no one magic solution. Several different types of support worked together for him – Sandy connected with older Aboriginal men, who talked with him openly about forgiveness, self-acceptance, and his value to other people. Psychology and counselling helped him better understand the anger and grief at his family situation, and the way their trauma conditioned his own beliefs and actions.

Sandy was supported to enrol in a TAFE course, earned his driver's licence and rented his own low-cost housing as part of a prison after-care program. He kept connected to an Aboriginal men's group, 12-Step programs and a relapse prevention program. With some new and old friends he went to social events, spent time in nature and keeping active, and enjoyed being a much-loved uncle.

By all accounts Sandy finally started living a 'normal', 'reintegrated' life.

Life changes in a moment

One unexpected knock at the door changed all that in an instant. He was issued with yet another summons to appear in court, for charges which preceded his last period in prison, and which had breached his good behaviour bond. He, his caseworker and legal representation all believed these matters had been dealt with by his last prison sentence.

In court, the presiding magistrate said he had no choice but to re-sentence Sandy. He handed over his wallet and phone, was handcuffed and immediately removed to the underground watch-house.

Inflexible policies meant he lost his place in both the aftercare program and TAFE, and he was separated from all the community support he relied on to cope with addiction, anxiety and depression.

Sandy wasn't eligible for any programs or drug and alcohol-related support in prison because of his short sentence. During his sentence he worked and received a few visitors, although was moved between three different correctional centres. He spent many hours indoors, became unfit and underweight and very depressed amidst hostilities of other prisoners.

Post-prison accommodation was arranged by a custodial officer with Sandy's family, among whom he had experienced childhood abuse and neglect. When the day of release came, friends arranged to pick Sandy up. He was released several hours earlier than expected and rather than waiting on the footpath, walked several kilometres to catch a bus to the Parole Office, carrying a garbage bag of a tracksuit and a few letters he'd received.

Sandy met his parole conditions well, despite being stressed by how impractical they were, because of public transport gaps and poor treatment by one staff member in particular.

Sandy stayed drug and alcohol free for a few months, but didn't make the same progress that he had before. Within months he went back to prison, yet again for drug possession charges.

No reference was made by Sandy's lawyers or presiding magistrates to the Royal Commission into Aboriginal Deaths in Custody, which recommended prison as a last resort, particularly if rehabilitation was available and the person was willing to attend.

Sandy was just another person to process according to the letter of the law. He wasn't treated as someone suffering from chronic and risky health conditions, and he wasn't seen as someone who had progressed well when a range of supports were put in place.

Systemic gaps

Sandy seemed to slip through gaps in systems which are touted as being integrated. In his case, the justice system didn't match with health, which didn't match with accommodation, which didn't match with education, which didn't match with income support.

All these government departments were all dealing with Sandy, but in disconnected ways, which saw him move from satisfying to inappropriate housing, from having a stable income to living in poverty, from being enrolled in study to not enrolled, and from being physically and emotionally healthy to being unhealthy and very vulnerable.

Stories like my dear friend Sandy's highlight that the real issues he faced were administrative. They weren't really anything to do with him as a person, or his actions apart from drug use, which was about addiction and his way of coping.

He didn't want his life to go this way, he didn't want to be back in prison, he wasn't in there with his family and he didn't prefer it to life on the outside.

But, without a sustained opportunity to be well supported in the community, Sandy struggled in daily life, destabilised by so many periods of incarceration.

Sandy's crimes were against himself, but so obviously exacerbated by falling through the cracks of systems designed to help him. There is no need for a 'tough on crime' approach here.

A moment that could have made a positive change for Sandy would have been one particular magistrate having the power and knowledge to order a suspended sentence, with appropriate reporting conditions, rather than another prison sentence.

I can only imagine that if Sandy hadn't returned to prison, he would have finished his study and gained his qualifications. He would have kept building on all the various types of supports he so gratefully accessed. He was a blessing to be around.

I can't imagine how many more times Sandy can handle the court and prison cycle before he gives up, one way or another.

> *I can only imagine that if Sandy hadn't returned to prison, he would have finished his study and gained his qualifications*

Dr Megan Williams is a Senior Research Fellow at the Aboriginal Health and Wellbeing Research team at Western Sydney University. Through her father's family she is a descendent of the Wiradjuri people of the NSW riverine.

Invest in communities, not prisons

| Author: | Michaela Crowe | Published: | October 20, 2015 |

Michaela Crowe is a 26-year-old Yinggarda woman from Carnarvon in Western Australia, where the state government recently invested more than $52 million in a new police and justice centre. Meanwhile the Gwoonwardu Mia Cultural Centre, over the road, has closed.

Rather than spending on prisons, Crowe would like to see greater investment in community development, and activities and programs for young people. She knows from personal experience of seeing relatives and community members locked up, often for minor infringements, that the impacts upon families and communities are devastating.

Listen to her tell this story here.

Michaela Crowe writes:

When my car was broken into recently, I didn't ring the police. I went and found the young children who were responsible – they are younger than 12 – and gave them a talking to.

I didn't want to ring the police because there are too many young people being locked up already. They would have ended up behind bars, sent away to a detention centre, because they already had a record.

Locking them up wouldn't have solved anything. It would have only caused more problems, and it takes away their childhood. They are only kids.

It's causing so much sorrow for old people, seeing the young ones locked up. It's bringing the elder people to their graves, knowing their children and grannies [grandchildren] are in and out of prison.

It causes terrible problems within families too; if someone can't get to a family member's funeral because they are in prison, this can cause rifts within families.

I'm not saying that jail is not a good thing for bad people, but too many are going to jail over silly little things, like not paying fines, or stealing a bottle of alcohol or a feed.

What the young people around here need are more activities and programs to keep them out of trouble. They need to be put in touch with culture, not drugs and alcohol.

It would help stop people drinking so much if we could have a youth centre with activities, and more family events, sports carnivals and cultural activities that are affordable for people.

I know of young men who have been in and out of jail because of neglect from family; they just need help to get their lives together. There's no support for the young men who need the help. There's a lot of mistrust of the police.

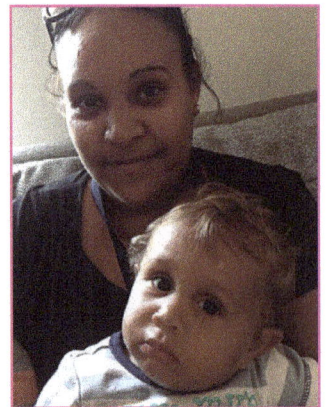

I've heard stories of people being bashed and threatened. To get a fairer system, we need more Aboriginal police and social workers, and just more Aboriginal people in the system generally.

There's also a lot of racism in the police and justice system. There should be a specific number you can call to make complaints that will take the matter seriously.

My late grandfather, Mr Crowe, used to go to court to fight for the young people. He'd ask the magistrate not to lock them up, that he'd take them out bush and teach them some culture. We need to see that happening again.

I have got two young children. I grew up with violence and alcohol. I don't want that for them. I'd like to see a change in this town. If my son is naughty, I tell him where the uncles have been and what it does to them. Jail takes away their pride and happiness. It causes so much grieving to the family.

For my family, we keep them strong by going bush and connecting them with culture. We go fishing all the time. If we get a lot of fish, we go out to the community and share it out with the old people.

We even get wood so they can sit around a fire because that's giving them peace, they can have a grill, cook their meat, keep warm, tell a yarn and have a cup of tea out of the house.

We're teaching the little ones how to make a fire, the bush way. We teach them how to survive, how to dig a soak near a river, how to cook in the ground, how to make dampers. They love the kangaroo tails.

The best thing is to get them in the outdoors, and teach them your way.

If I could talk to the PM, I'd say, "Lend a hand. Be more supportive and think not only of politics, but think of the Aboriginal people."

A visit to the Old Derby Gaol provides critical historical insights for #JustJustice

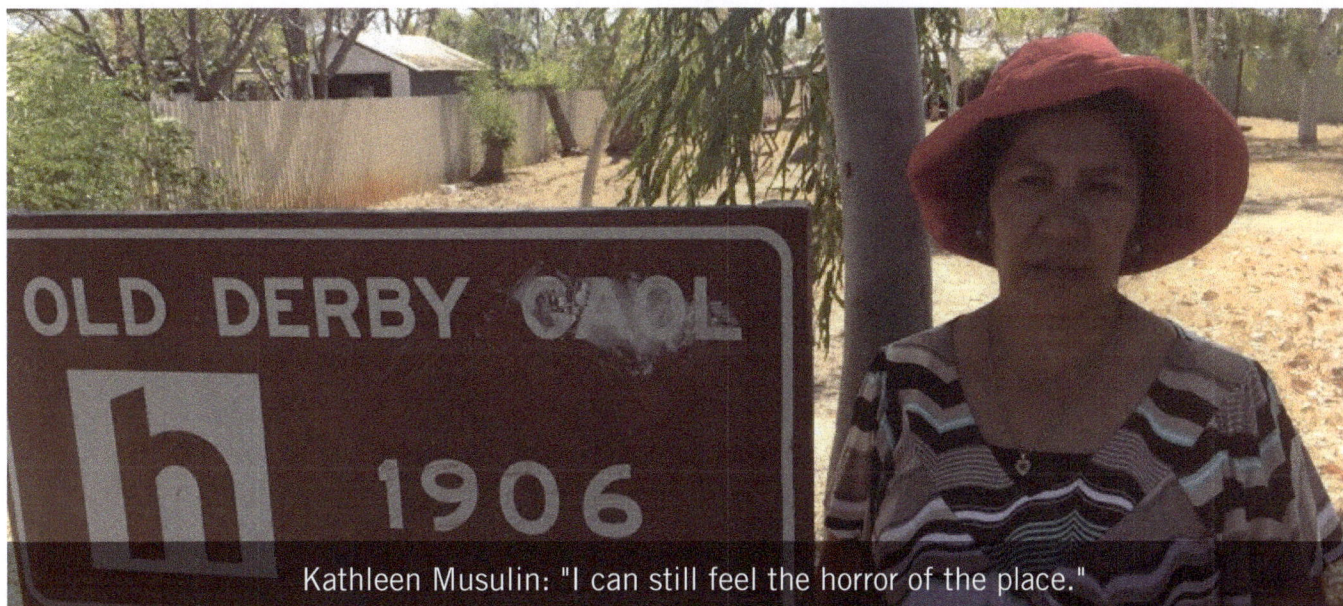

OLD DERBY GAOL
h 1906

Kathleen Musulin: "I can still feel the horror of the place."

Author:	Kathleen Musulin	Published:	November 01, 2016

***Caution to Aboriginal and Torres Strait Islander readers: This post contains images and details of people who have passed away, and of traumatic history ***

A visit to the Old Derby Gaol in Western Australia gives harsh insights into how the criminalisation and incarceration of Aboriginal people have been such a central strategy of colonisation, from its earliest days.

Kathleen Musulin, a Malgana and Yawuru woman, describes her deeply distressing visit to the gaol, a National Trust registered site, in the article below for Croakey's #JustJustice project.

The gaol, which operated from 1906 to 1975, was designed for 30 people but at times held more than 100 Aboriginal people, chained and crowded in the most appalling conditions, in open-air cells, each about the size of a suburban garage.

Below her article are extracts from the Roth Royal Commission of 1904, revealing the harsh treatment of Aboriginal prisoners and the links between incarceration and dispossession.

Kathleen Musulin writes:

It is more than a year since I visited the Old Derby Gaol site for the first time, but I can still feel the horror of the place, and how overcome I was by sadness and grief.

There is a very powerful historical display that tells visitors something of the history of this gaol and, most importantly, includes some of the stories and memories of Aboriginal people.

Men, women and children were held here, on their way to other gaols and institutions. The cells were meant to provide only temporary accommodation, but sometimes people were chained here for months at a time.

These cells don't even have proper walls. Iron bars provided the only "protection" from the elements.

The most common reason for incarceration in those days was for "cattle killing" – as people fought for survival as pastoral expansion stole their country and degraded their food and water.

Many people ended up in this place, on their way to other gaols, because they were hunting for the survival of their families and communities on the land that was being stolen from them.

On the display is a list of the names of more than 100 Aboriginal people who were sentenced to two or three years with hard labour in 1907-1908 for being "in possession of stolen beef".

In 1907, there were up to 61 people detained here at any one time; the display says the cell was designed for 30 people but to my mind not even one person should ever have been held in such conditions.

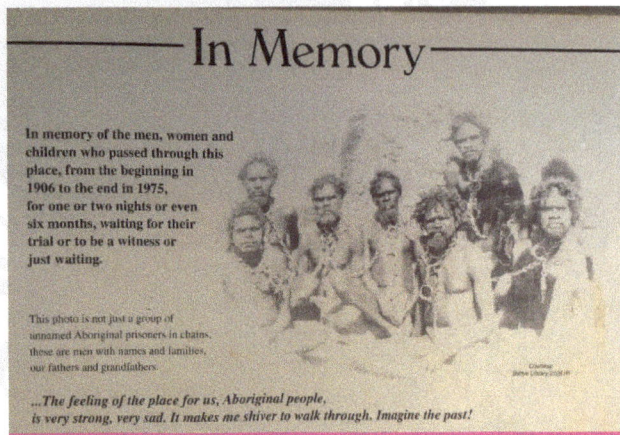

In memory of the men, women and children who passed through this place, from the beginning in 1906 to the end in 1975, for one or two nights or even six months, waiting for their trial or to be a witness or just waiting.

This photo is not just a group of unnamed Aboriginal prisoners in chains, these are men with names and families, our fathers and grandfathers.

...The feeling of the place for us, Aboriginal people, is very strong, very sad. It makes me shiver to walk through. Imagine the past!

Sign at the Old Derby Gaol

I stood and looked at the photo of several men, the chains looped around their necks, tying them together, and read these words:

"In memory of the men, women and children, who passed through this place, from the beginning in 1906 to the end in 1975, for one or two nights or even six months, waiting for their trial or to be a witness or just waiting.

This photo is not just a group of unnamed Aboriginal prisoners in chains, these are men with names and families, our fathers and grandfathers."

It was impossible not to choke up reading some of the stories on the plaque, in the words of Aboriginal people:

"...The feeling of the place for us, Aboriginal people, is very strong, very sad. It makes me shiver to walk through. Imagine the past!!

...To think of the figures lying in here, sitting down, so frustrating. Why were we treated like this? Not only to be taken away from their home and put in the cell but not knowing that they were going to be shipped off and taken further away from their families...

People's spirits are roaming still after dying away from their country.

...Cold times, the wind would blow the rain inside and they'd be huddled together in a corner just to keep themselves warm. That's how we lost a lot of people through prisons like this..."

"...Go back in the beginning when people didn't know why they were having chains around them in the first place. They didn't understand. They were probably wondering what's happening? Why are they doing these things?"

As I read more from the display, I lost my power to speak. I couldn't find the words to describe how upsetting it was. This is what the display said:

"Prisoners were held by neck chains, which were secured by handcuffs to the ring bolts in the floor. They slept on the concrete and in winter sometimes had only a single blanket to protect them from the chill of the floor and the wind.

Clothing and blankets were never cleaned and the cells lacked any form of sanitation. This caused a serious health threat. An influenza epidemic that claimed the life of one prisoner in 1908 prompted an inquiry into living conditions. No improvements were made.

In 1926 the overnight sanitary facilities comprised a covered pan for 'nightsoil' and guttering that lead to outside urinal buckets. In 1950 a storm blew the roof off the Gaol, which finally prompted structural and sanitary improvements for the prisoners."

In 1959, there were 26 male inmates and three women; in 1966, there were 109 men and women held here.

These are the memories of someone who spent a night in the gaol in the late 1960s:

"There was a drum in the corner for the toilet area blocked off by a blanket. You just tried to jump over to get to the toilet and there were bodies there. No mattress. I remember the smell and stuff you know. I remember bodies were everywhere on the floor."

I was horrified when I read the gaol did not close until 1975. In that year, I was in grade five at school.

> I was horrified when I read the gaol did not close until 1975. In that year, I was in grade five at school

It just shows how close this horrific history is to our present. It just shows that if you want to understand the reasons for the over-incarceration of Aboriginal people today, you don't need to look too far back into the past to see where this problem began.

Visiting this place has left a lasting impression on me. It really brings home the message that gaol should be the very last resort.

Too many of our young people are being locked up for driving offences or for not paying fines, and for other things that should not result in a gaol sentence. Just like those old people should not have been locked up, for the "crime" of trying to feed their families at such a traumatic time.

There has to be another way. We have to stop this history being repeated, and repeated. We have to work with people and communities, rather than building more and more prisons.

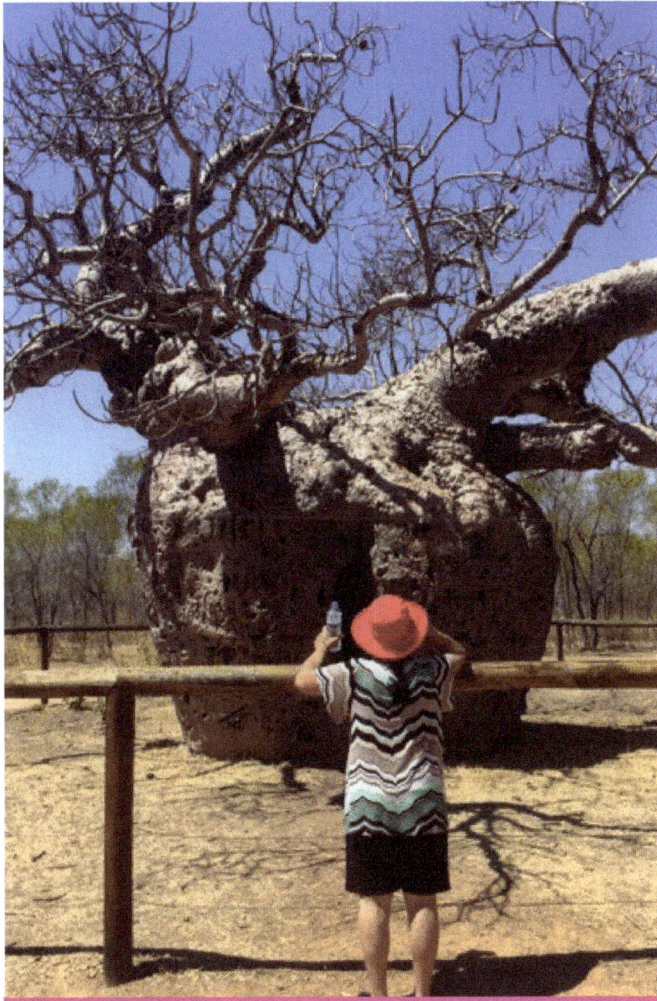

Kathleen Musulin is photographed above at the Derby boab prison tree, where Aboriginal prisoners were held in chains on their way to other gaols. According to a display at the site, prisoners were often marched 24 to 48 kilometres a day, in chains, on their way to gaols

Extracts from the Roth Royal Commission findings

In August 1904, Dr Walter Edmund Roth was appointed Royal Commissioner to inquire into the condition of the "natives" in WA, and his report gives chilling insights into the experiences of Aboriginal people at the hands of police and the "justice" system.

Roth visited gaols at Carnarvon, Broome, Wyndham and Roebourne. There were about 300 Aboriginal people in WA gaols at the time. He was told they were neck-chained from the day they arrived until they left (except in times of sickness), sometimes for more than two or three years. The prisoners also worked in neck chains on the roads at Broome, Carnarvon, Roebourne, and Wyndham. The neck chains ranged in weight from 2 to almost 6 lbs.

His report, "*Royal Commission on the Condition of the Natives*", dated 29 December 1904, records that he heard evidence of:

- Children as young as 10 being black-birded to work in the pearling industry and being indentured to work on the boats for years, without education or payment.

- Police bringing in groups of 20-30 people at a time, walking long distances, in neck chains. The prisoners were chained, as well as the women brought in as unwilling witnesses. There are reports of police raping these women while they were chained. The chains were not taken off when people were crossing creeks and rivers and there were reports of several people having drowned this way. The Commissioner of Police gave evidence that he had never heard of neck chains being used on Europeans. Commissioner Roth recommended the abolition of neck chains but this recommendation was over-ridden.

- The system incentivised police to maximise their arrests, as they received per capita ration payments for prisoners. Roth recommended the end of these "blood money" payments to police, and this system was changed.

- One gaolor told the Commission that of 20 Aboriginal people in his charge, not one really knew why he was there. Another, with 72 prisoners in his charge, thought one-third understood. Another gaolor said the prisoners thought they were brought for road building, not cattle killing. Dr Dodwell Browne, the Resident Magistrate and District Medical Officer at Wyndham, gave evidence that many of those charged with cattle killing did not understand what they were being charged with and did not get justice.

Kathleen Musulin is a Malgana and Yawuru woman living in Carnarvon, Western Australia.

Photos and Roth Royal Commission extracts by Melissa Sweet.

One man's story of surviving the trauma of family violence

| Author: | Darren Parker | Published: | July 17, 2015 |

Caution to readers: this article contains graphic detail of family violence

This is the first in a two-part series by Darren Parker, a Ngunawal man and Phd candidate at Melbourne Law School, as part of the crowdfunded #JustJustice project.

In sharing some experiences of racism and violence within his family as a young boy, Darren Parker highlights the importance of the social and cultural determinants of health in any discussion about the over-incarceration of Aboriginal and Torres Strait Islander people.

His story also highlights how traumatic early childhood experiences can set young people upon a pathway that increases their chances of coming into contact with the criminal justice system, as well as the strength that can be found through family and cultural connections.

In the second instalment, he will explore whether decolonising Australian law will assist Aboriginal and Torres Strait Islander people in attaining justice.

Darren Parker writes:

As children we all want the love, nurture and respect of both of our parents, but sadly not all of us are provided with such. This is part of my story of domestic violence as I experienced it growing up. (There is more to tell but, not here, not yet.)

I firmly believe there is strength in publicly sharing experiences like these both, individually and collectively. However, critically, what everyone must keep in mind whilst reading or hearing these experiences is that they are deeply personal – as well as political in many regards – and that the author has to be totally respected. Meaning, allow the person whose experience you are listening to or reading about, to speak, without inquisitive questioning along the lines "and what else….".

This is just one story. It forms a part of the seas of tragedy that are the lived experiences of family violence. Moreover, this story is part of a greater narrative of the direct and indirect effects of the horrors of violence in my family. Miserably, it appears, according to numerous official reports that these seas are rising.

However, this story leads onto a much longer story of resilience, a story that is continuing to this day for my family – with my Mum and me. Yet, it felt the resilience was perhaps a long time coming for me.

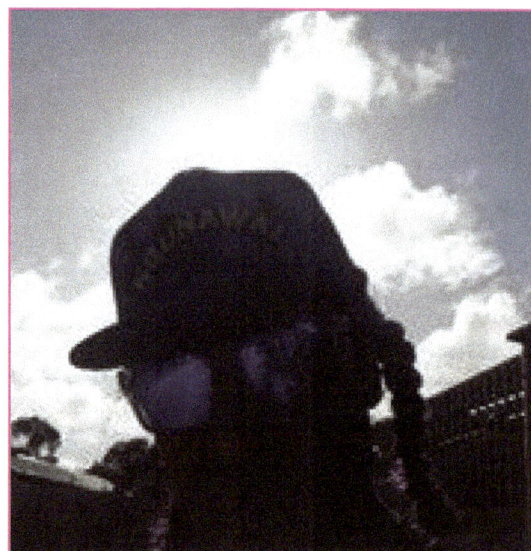

My Mother on the other hand was, is and will always be the rock of resilience, of whom I am in complete awe. Though, I am sure if you asked her, she would downplay that point.

All that being said, each one of us in my family have dealt with the aftermath of those experiences, both individually and collectively over the course of our lives – and we continue to do so.

Before we proceed, some clarifiers. The following is told from my perspective and memory of events – obviously there are other perspectives and memories, but they are not transcribed here. These memories are inscribed into my mind as if they happened yesterday. The only person from whom I sought approval in writing this was my mother. I have no idea whether my father is still alive or not – and frankly, I do not care. And a trigger warning: if the realities of domestic violence are viscerally or psychologically difficult for you to stomach, I advise you stop reading this now, or at least read it with your own 'safety-net'.

Earliest memories of childhood are the stuff of Disney; the warm embrace of a parent, their loving direction, being cajoled to sleep….not so, for me. One of my earliest memories is more like a horror movie – being trapped beneath a bed with a monster desperately reaching out to grab hold of me. That monster was my father. A monster fuelled by alcohol, as well as a deep-seated anger – an anger that had overt racial connotations. It was his anger that I remember most, long after the bruises and breaks had healed.

My father was a white male (Irish/Australian), who married my amazing and resilient mother (Ngunawal) after wooing her at the local dance, as the story goes. An Indigenous/non-Indigenous union is not uncommon in many communities throughout Australia. Yet, what in many ways may seem counter-intuitive is that my father was a racist of Australian proportions and as such, particularly racist about Aboriginals – or "boongs", as he would call us – and I acknowledge the psychological violence in this.

But for now, here, I will simply concern myself with discussing the bodily violence, while recognising, of course, the intrinsic link between psychological and bodily violence.

Back to that earlier memory of my childhood and the preceding events. In short, I spilt my father's coffee – that was it. That was all it took on this occasion. Sometimes it was even less.

It was a Saturday morning, the night after another drunken rampage by him that had terrorised my Mother, my sisters and myself. On that particular morning, my sisters were readying themselves for dance classes, whilst I had no such commitments as a four-year-old, and played and joked with Mum on the bed in her room.

At this point, I should inform you, that he had expressly forbidden me from precisely this type of behaviour. That I was doing this whilst he was preoccupied with his hangover in the bathroom had inherent risks. Even then, I realised that my (natural) behaviour was perilous and potentially injurious. Only much later did I realise how this 'reality' was a conditioning point for the 'normalising' of domestic violence (DV) for its victims. That is, the "walking on eggshells" routine became so ingrained that to break that norm was to risk an actual break.

The reason for my "risky" behaviour was simple. As mentioned, the night before had been filled with another of his drunken rampages, and I wanted to console my Mother and make her laugh and to help her forget. So, I was laughing and joking with her (showing off as four-year-olds tend to do) and jumping around the bed. I over-balanced and began to fall, though catching myself with the wad of blankets, I managed to stay somewhat upright and on the bed.

However, in my scramble I had inadvertently knocked over my father's coffee. It made a mess, sure, but nothing that couldn't be fixed. A couple of blankets would need a wash and the bedside table a wipe-down. And a new coffee would need to be made. Like I said, nothing irreparable.

In all of this, however, there is a moment that I remember vividly (one that which has caused me a great recurring dread). It was the moment when my Mother's eyes and my own locked, with a look of terror on both of our faces. We both knew. As such, we acted fast.

In a coordinated scramble that was both clinically precise and frenetic, my Mother and I moved with absolute purpose. We both knew. I began grabbing up the blankets with Mum's help, whilst she also took the cup to the kitchen to then return with a dishtowel to wipe up the excess. We dumped the blankets in the laundry (under the pretext of 'weekend washing' – if asked) and cleaned the residue of the coffee from the side table. My sisters were unwarily recruited into this 'weekend washing' alibi by my Mother, by directing them both to take their blankets off their beds and deposit them in the laundry.

My sisters had no idea what was going on – and it was better that way – but us kids were all acutely attuned to motherly housekeeping instructions, regardless. After helping clean up the coffee and removing signs of any spillage (and on being satisfied there weren't any) both Mum and I began making the bed anew – new sheets, pillowcases, covers and blankets. The bed looked good and everything was squared-away.

The old man was still in the bathroom and oblivious to what was going on. We had gone undetected. Sweet.

Mum sat on the edge of the freshly made bed and was doing her hair. Stupidly, I thought I would repeat my earlier antics with her – bad move on my part, that's for sure. I had just made it onto the bed and, standing behind my mother, was about to…."Boy!!" and the simultaneous shove.

I don't recall even seeing him. I remember just hearing him shout and the feel of his hand pushing across my lower back. I went flying. Instantly, I was off the bed and smashing into the window frame and the wall. I didn't cry, I couldn't. I knew (even at four) better than that. But, I did feel the blood. I had caught the corner of the window frame just behind my left ear above the hairline. It wasn't a large gash but the blood poured freely. Instantaneously, I put my hand up to stem the blood and rushed to scramble under the bed. I centred myself beneath the bed and scrunched my t-shirt to my head as a makeshift bandage.

To say that I was scared would be an understatement of serious proportions. I was terrified. Not for being caught doing something expressly forbidden. Not of bleeding and leaving blood spatter across the wall or on my clothes. No, I was terrified of what I knew was to come.

He attempted to grab me before I disappeared under the bed, but feeble in his effort my foot slipped his grip. And that was what terrified me. That I dared to disobey, that I dared to 'react' to his monstrosity. Ironically, it was having a reaction to

> *To say that I was scared would be an understatement of serious proportions. I was terrified*

his outrage, which instigated his most vile retribution. That was something I had witnessed and experienced numerous before, even at my tender age.

I huddled under the bed, looking at the specks of blood – my blood – flecked upon the white paint of the wall above the skirting board and holding my scrunched t-shirt up to cover my cut. I could hear my poor panicked Mother trying to reason with him, to absolutely no avail. Mum's pleas to leave me alone were ignored and met with more threats against her and my sisters (I only found out much later that they had huddled in one of my sister's rooms – for the relative comfort of being terrorised together).

My Mother tried in vain to stop his one-way express to 'Terrorville', but this merely escalated his anger. I curled there beneath the bed, shivering with the foreboding of not 'knowing' what I should do. That's when it happened.

As I lay curled in the foetal-position staring at the blood flecks, it suddenly became a whole lot brighter "under" the bed. When people talk about moments in time that seem to occur at "slow-speed", this is a moment that I recall, among others. And yet, it took me by total surprise. In his venomous rage, he grabbed the side of the bed and ferociously lifted. It completely over-turned the bed onto its side, blocking my mother from what was now our side of the room – just him and me.

I recall him taking a single step and reaching down to grab me, lifting me up by my already scrunched up shirt and spitting, directly into my face, the words "you stupid little f*ck! I was just trying to see if you were alright." There is more that happened here but, I am not yet comfortable with committing that to the page – not yet anyway.

That is just one story of how he showed his 'love' to me over the course of the next six to eleven years. My Mum divorced him when I was ten but I had court-ordered 'visits' until I was fifteen, and then decided I had finally had enough. The experience I have written here is but one of my experiences of family violence. Wretchedly, there are many others.

One absolute constant throughout these years growing up was my Mother. It was her inner strength that she passed onto me that helped then, for the most part, and is certainly assisting me now. Mum was the one who, whilst working two jobs and raising three kids, kept me in line as best she could. I am forever in a debt to her for this. Mum always stressed the importance and vitality of our culture, as well as the necessity of an education. Both of these I have grasped on to tightly, even during the lowest ebbs of my life, and pursue with even more vigour now. It was at her direction that I completed maths 'quizzes' every school

night and 'book-reports' most weeks, which has instilled in me a deep love of reading and learning.

Moving away from this particular experience, I'd like to just briefly speak of the effects of growing up within a violent household. I am not speaking for either of my sisters or my Mum – those stories and experiences are theirs, not mine.

The repercussions of growing up under such conditions are as varied as some of them are deep-seated. I have an automatic unspoken distrust of people, particularly men – and that has to be repeatedly proven to be unfounded before I relinquish that distrust. I don't feel completely at ease in social gatherings – this is in spite of always being labelled a "rambunctious" person. You know the old trope of the loudest person is often the one craving the most silence. Yet, being labelled rambunctious is completely incongruous with how I feel inside – quiet and solitary. There are other effects too, but I merely proffer those ones for the time being.

However, I will now speak to two very intense and very deep effects I laboured with for years – alcoholism and suicidal tendencies. Thankfully, I have put one of them "back in its box" or "pissed it out of my life", as I enjoy saying, that being alcohol. Whilst I no longer drink grog, I have not turned into anything resembling a puritan in this regard. I do not deride anyone who does drink, as it is none of my business.

One of the great positives of ceasing drinking, and there are a few, is that my mental health has noticeably improved

In terms of my own personal autonomy, I have finally made what I feel is the best life-course for myself. But I am forever vigilant, knowing that another bottle is just around the corner if I want it to be and that patently, I am an alcoholic. I am learning my triggers and what sets them off, realising that I must be constantly aware of them. Being a non-practising alcoholic requires a never-ending awareness of self and is easily one of the hardest challenges I have ever encountered, particularly as alcohol is so ubiquitous in this society.

One of the great positives of ceasing drinking, and there are a few, is that my mental health has noticeably improved. Now, I'm not talking about others noticing and/or commenting, I'm speaking about how I have noticed within myself the psychological upside of pissing off the grog. Whilst I have no illusions of being 'cured', I have not entertained such self-destructive thoughts for some time. However, ridding myself of that foul inner-voice that has, in the past, screamed my 'unworthiness' at me is always an on-going process.

I would love to tell you that I have a number of years of sobriety and with it a well-developed positive mental health outlook under my belt. But I do not. It has only been a matter of months since I began this journey. However, the differences are already quite noticeable, to me.

When I was immersed in the bottle and/or feeling like death, you would have to have known me exceptionally well to see it, and even then it was not always possible. I was what might be called a "high-functioning" alcoholic.

I did not acknowledge the self-destructiveness that arose out of those childhood experiences of psychological bombardment and physical assault. That lack of self-worth was 'blackened out' by alcohol, and binges of drinking the pain away, and waking to a new day in a "shame-spiral". At points throughout my life, it seemed that this was "my lot", that I would continue on such a path until my eventual and perhaps premature death.

Thankfully, I have chosen a different path, one that is not fraught with: drunken messes; blackouts; police cells; courts; fines; mania; depression; suicidal plans; hospital visits; and the like. While there was not a single event that broke this pattern, it was just after the last time I went home on one of my regular visits to see Mum for a catch up and something – something – just didn't feel right. Something in her voice that I couldn't quite pick…. Anyway, after spending a few days at home, catching up, making food and eating, hanging out, I had to return to my place.

It was on the drive back that I committed myself to the course I have recently set upon. I made that choice in silence and did not voice it for at least a month. By then I was already experiencing the positive effects of my choice. Then on one of our regular phone calls I finally told Mum, and instantly I could hear and feel the change in her – and that confirmed it for me. That Mum then spoke, in an abstract way, about our cultural resilience merely reinforced that confirmation.

Knowing that I am truly starting to fulfil my cultural obligations and the cultural respect for my Mother and my ancestors – those who have sacrificed so much for me to be where I am today – is a touchstone with a force incomparable to any bottle. Cultural integrity and respect is the cup I now sup from.

Now I feel ready, willing and able to move forward in the most positive of ways I can. That is, to move with the respect for others and myself that for many years was despicably masked by the horrors of family violence.

Darren Parker is a Ngunawal man and Phd candidate at Melbourne Law School. Follow him on Twitter @Darren_Parker

Caring for people in prison

Author:	Phyllis Simmons	Published:	November 20, 2016

Phyllis Simmons, who for many years was an Aboriginal visitor at the Roebourne Regional Prison in Western Australia, gives some insights into the system issues that contribute to over-incarceration, and offers practical advice for preventing people winding up in prison.

Phyllis Simmons writes:

For 18 years, up until 2014, I visited Aboriginal prisoners at the Roebourne Regional Prison, providing support and practical help.

As an Aboriginal visitor at the prison, I did everything I possibly could to keep prisoners safe and well.

My role was making sure prisoners in custody, in lock ups and the prison didn't self-harm, take their lives or take someone else's life through the frustration of being incarcerated.

And a lot of other things it entailed, like family visits, making sure they had spends from family. Making sure they had medical treatment.

Q: What are some of the solutions to preventing over-incarceration?

Stop locking people up for petty driving fines! Help people get their drivers licences, so they are not driving around without a licence and get thrown back in prison.

Instead of sentencing them to jail for drug and alcohol related things, sentence them to an alcohol and drug rehab centre [where shown to be effective] – where they can get the proper treatment and get over their addictions. And they can get treatment, not only for their addictions, but general medical treatment as well.

Where they can go back and get their drivers licence, so they are not driving around without a licence and get thrown back into prison

Justices of the Peace also need to stop remanding people out of the towns from where they come. If they're sent to court in Karratha, they're told they're not allowed to go back to Roebourne until after the next court, which is two weeks away.

So they just wander around...they can't go back to their own homes where they're paying rent. It is setting people up to fail. Anything could happen to them if they end up sleeping in the creek. This happens all around the Pilbara. It is very disruptive for their families.

Why don't they let them stay in their own houses?

A lot of the people who come into prison for fines are brought in from Tom Price, Hedland, Newman, wherever

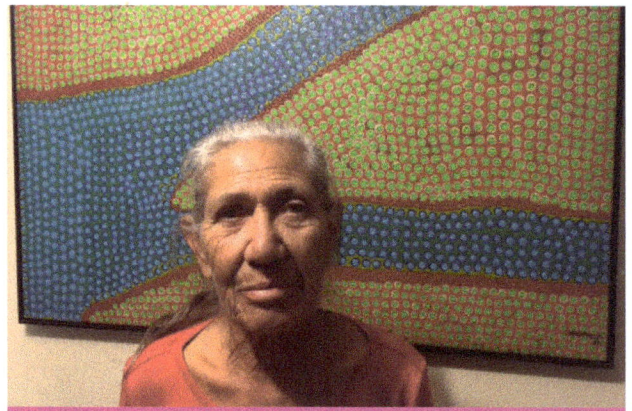

Phyllis Simmons: the vital importance of Aboriginal visitor schemes

they are picked up. Sometimes they are brought over on a Friday to be released on a Sunday. It just doesn't make sense. They have got no way of getting back to where they come from.

> *They really do need the Aboriginal visitors scheme in prisons. They have to have Aboriginal people based in these places. It's the same at Roebourne, it's critical to have the Aboriginal visitors there.*

I saw people that are sentenced to prison and on medication. The doctor that comes to the prison changes the medication; a lot of our people see a different tablet or a different package and they won't take it. Many times I have sat with different prisoners over the years to tell them the benefits of taking their medication – that that tablet was as good as the one they were taking before.

Mental health problems are common; I'd say 90 percent of them [the prisoners] were mentally struggling. The other thing we always said to the officers was, have the medical centre check them out because they could be people with FASD. It was really very frustrating because some of them would come up and ask us when they had to go to court. They'd get about 10 feet away from us, and come back and say, what date was that? That's heartbreaking.

> *They need to have the medical treatment from the doctors in the Aboriginal medical service and the health workers. They need to have the treatment from the people who know the people.*

It wasn't like a job, I loved working there, I loved every minute of it but, believe me, my days never started at nine and finished at three, because it's so hard to find family in Wickham and Roebourne, so I'd use my own time, sometimes I'd go looking for them early in the morning or after work or at night.

Some of the guys who didn't come from this area or had no family, we would actually put money out of our own pockets into their spends [accounts].

We'd say to the Super [Superintendent] – 'look, they haven't got enough money for tobacco or toiletries, can we please leave them some of our money?' He'd say, 'well it's your money', so we'd...just to help people out'.

Q: Big picture, what would be a fair justice system?

"How long is the Aboriginal legal service going, trying to get justice for us? How long have the people been lobbying for justice for us? There is no justice for us.

If people say, the law is there for everybody – no, it's not. They still have the black law, the white law and the kangaroo courts.

Phyllis Simmons was an Aboriginal visitor at the Roebourne Regional Prison for 18 years.

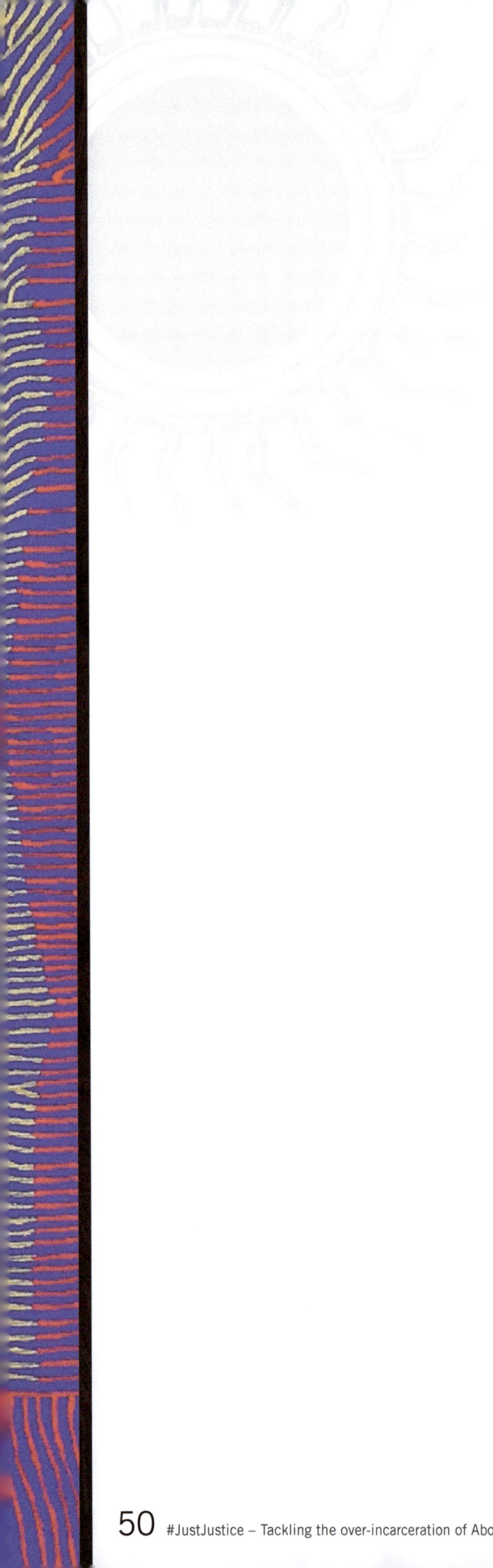

3. Landmarks in advocacy

" *Invest in communities, not prisons*

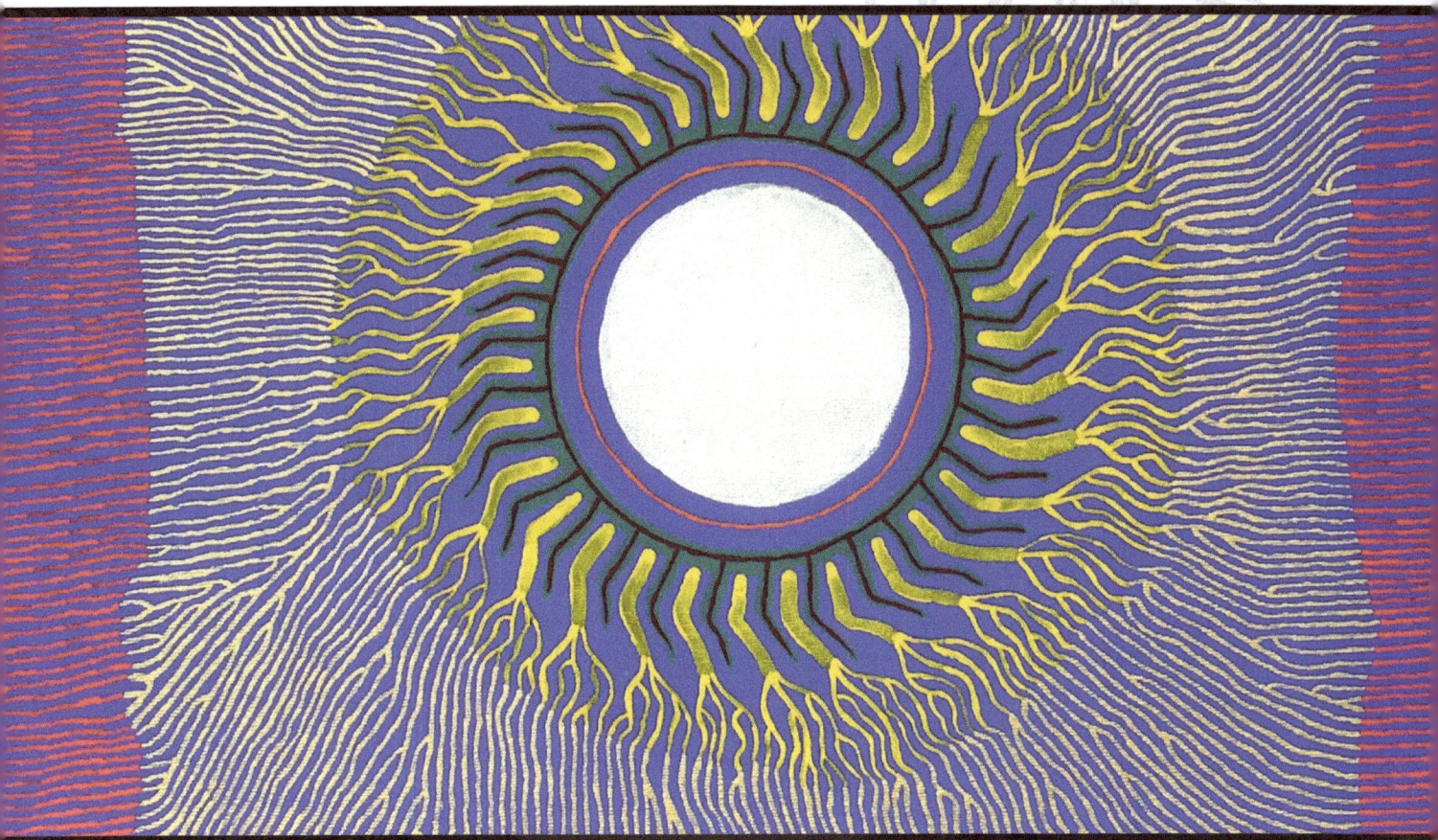

"We have barely seen a mention of Aboriginal and Torres Strait Islander policy or issues this election campaign. That changes today" – the Redfern Statement

Author:	Melissa Sweet	Published:	June 09, 2016

Aboriginal and Torres Strait Islander organisations have come together, with the backing of many health groups and NGOs, to issue a landmark election challenge calling for transformative action to address structural inequalities, and to improve the lives of Aboriginal and Torres Strait Islander people.

The Redfern Statement amounts to a scathing indictment of the Federal Government's efforts to date, describing the 2014 Federal Budget as "a disaster" for Aboriginal and Torres Strait Islander people, as well as noting the damage caused by policy upheaval and instability.

The Statement, calls for:

- Restoration of $534m cut from the Indigenous Affairs Portfolio by the 2014 Budget.

- Funding of the Implementation Plan for the National Aboriginal and Torres Strait Islander Health Plan (2013–2023).

- Aboriginal Community Controlled Services (ACCHS) to be the preferred providers for health services for Aboriginal and Torres Strait Islander people.

- Creation of guidelines for Primary Health Networks to ensure they engage with ACCHS and Indigenous health experts to ensure the best primary health care is delivered in a culturally safe manner. There should be mandated formal agreements between PHNs and ACCHS to ensure Aboriginal and Torres Strait Islander leadership.

- An end to the freeze on Medicare rebates, which has caused "profound pressure" on ACCHS and "adversely and disproportionately affected Aboriginal and Torres Strait Islander people and their ability to afford and access the required medical care".

- Reform of the Indigenous Advancement Strategy – "The next Federal Government must fix the IAS as an immediate priority and restore the funding that has been stripped from key services through the flawed tendering process."

- Funding of an Implementation Plan for the National Aboriginal and Torres Strait Islander Suicide Prevention Strategy.

- Development of a long-term National Aboriginal and Torres Strait Islander Social Determinants of Health Strategy. "The siloed approach to strategy and planning for the issues that Aboriginal and Torres Strait Islander people face is a barrier to improvement."

The Redfern Statement also calls for action to address the "national crisis" of the over-incarceration of Aboriginal and Torres Strait Islander people, including the adoption of justice targets as part of the Close the Gap framework, proper funding for Aboriginal and Torres Strait Islander Community Controlled front-line legal services, and implementation of the Change the Record Coalition's Blueprint for Change.

Read more in the media release below, and in the full Redfern Statement.

MEDIA RELEASE: Launch of the Redfern Statement 2016

National Aboriginal and Torres Strait Islander leadership organisations come together today to call on all parties to tackle inequality and disadvantage facing Australia's First People as a federal election priority.

"Today we launch the Redfern Statement 2016. This is the first time national Aboriginal and Torres Strait Islander leadership organisations have put this kind of united call to an incoming government," said Dr Jackie Huggins, co-chair of the National Congress of Australia's First Peoples.

Supported by mainstream non-government-organisations, the alliance is calling for an immediate restoration of the $534 million funding cut from the Indigenous Affairs Portfolio, to be invested into meaningful engagement, health, justice, preventing violence, early childhood and disability.

"We have barely seen a mention of Aboriginal and Torres Strait Islander policy or issues this election campaign. That changes today. Aboriginal and Torres Strait Islander groups have come together to demand urgent action. It is time that Aboriginal and Torres Strait Islander voices are heard and respected. It is time for action.

"The regular upheaval of major policy changes, significant budget cuts and changing governments in the short election cycles at all levels, are major impediments to improving life outcomes for Aboriginal and Torres Strait Islander peoples.

"This policy instability must stop and Aboriginal and Torres Strait Islander affairs must be brought in from the margins of national debate to the mainstream centre in order to end the unacceptable disadvantage experienced by First Peoples. This is the task at hand for the next Federal Government."

The alliance's plan for urgent government action calls for the following reforms:

To achieve meaningful engagement with government, industry and the non-government sector, it is critical that Aboriginal and Torres Strait Islander peoples are properly represented at the national level. National Congress of Australia's First Peoples (Congress) has fulfilled this role since 2010 and funding cuts to it should be reversed.

In the area of health, the alliance calls on all parties to recommit to Closing the Gap in order to achieve health equality in this generation. The alliance views funding the Implementation Plan for the National Aboriginal and Torres Strait Islander Health Plan (2013–2023), a policy developed through best-practice community consultation, as a priority. The alliance also recommends making Aboriginal Community Controlled Services (ACCHS) the preferred providers for health services, a measure which would promote self-determination essential to closing the gap in life outcomes for First Peoples.

The state of access to justice for Aboriginal and Torres Strait Islander people and their over-representation in the criminal justice system is a national crisis, as is violence against Indigenous women and children. To make headway in justice and violence prevention, the alliance calls on the next Federal Government to adopt justice targets as part of the Closing the

Gap framework, to overturn funding cuts to the Aboriginal and Torres Strait Islander Legal Services and to reinstate the National Family Violence Prevention Legal Services Program.

The alliance also champions the addition of disability access targets to the Closing the Gap framework to improve outcomes for the approximately 45 per cent of Aboriginal and Torres Strait Islander people identifying as having some form of disability.

Research demonstrates that early childhood services have the greatest impacts for vulnerable families, providing long-term wellbeing, productivity and cost benefits for society. However, the fact remains that Aboriginal and Torres Strait Islander children are half as likely to access early learning as non-Indigenous children. To rectify this inequality in early childhood education, the alliance urges the next Federal government to subsidise access to early childhood education and care for all Aboriginal and Torres Strait Islander children. The over-representation of Aboriginal and Torres Strait Islander children in out-of-home care, currently one in every three children, must be remedied. The alliance requests the development of a national strategy and target to reduce this over-representation.

"If the next Federal Government heeds the advice put forward in The Redfern Statement today, it will have an unprecedented nation-building opportunity and a chance to meaningfully address Aboriginal and Torres Strait Islander disadvantage. Improving the life outcomes of First Peoples is also fundamental to progressing the unfinished business of reconciliation," said Dr Huggins.

"We have laid out a clear roadmap today. We invite all those seeking election on July 2 to respond," said Dr Jackie Huggins.

The Redfern Statement (The Statement) has been developed by national Aboriginal and Torres Strait Islander peak and representative bodies including: National Congress of Australia's First Peoples, First Peoples Disability Network (FPDN), National Aboriginal and Torres Strait Islander Legal Services (NATSILS), National Aboriginal Community Controlled Health Organisations (NACCHO), National Family Violence Prevention Legal Services (FVPLS), Secretariat for National Aboriginal and Islander Child Care (SNAICC), The Healing Foundation, and National Health Leadership Forum (NHLF). The Statement also has the overarching support of The Change the Record Coalition, Close the Gap Steering Committee, and Family Matters campaigns. The Statement also has been endorsed by Reconciliation Australia and over 20 mainstream organisations, including the Australian Medical Association and Law Council.

Here you can see a list of dozens of organisations supporting the statement.

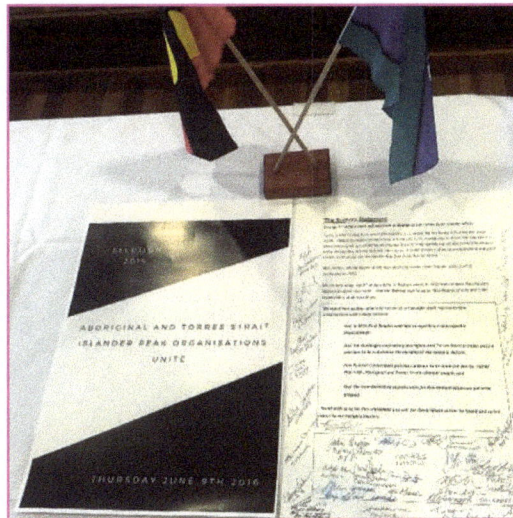

Governments now have a blueprint for action; it's time to Change the Record

| Author: | Melissa Sweet | Published: | November 30, 2015 |

Federal, State and Territory Governments have been handed **a detailed blueprint** for achieving justice targets, with the aim of closing the gap in the rates of imprisonment of Aboriginal and Torres Strait Islander people by 2040.

The Blueprint for Change, released today in Canberra by the **Change the Record campaign**, also outlines whole-of-government approaches for reducing the disproportionate rates of violence against Aboriginal and Torres Strait Islander people.

The recommendations for a whole-of-government approach through COAG aim to promote community safety and reduce the rates at which Aboriginal and Torres Strait Islander people come into contact with the criminal justice system.

They highlight the importance of health services, disability supports, drug treatment and affordable housing in helping to meet justice targets, and are underpinned by the following 12 principles:

1. Invest in communities, not prisons.

2. Local communities have the answers.

3. Recognise the driving factors of imprisonment and violence – including poverty and disadvantage, with early intervention aimed at stopping family violence and avoiding exposure to the child protection system, by supporting families and strengthening communities.

4. Focus on safety. The impacts of crime are felt most strongly by people in that community, particularly women and children. Successful early intervention and prevention strategies will not only cut offending and imprisonment rates, but importantly will increase safety by addressing the root causes of violence against women and children.

5. Services, not sentences. The criminal justice system is often an ineffective or inappropriate way to respond to people who have a disability or are experiencing poverty, mental illness, drug or alcohol addiction, homelessness or unemployment. A social policy and public health response to such issues is needed – not a criminal justice one.

6. Community-oriented policing. Many communities describe experiences of over or under policing, harassment or racism, which can sometimes exacerbate the situation for already marginalised and disadvantaged communities. Changes to the ways police interact with and enforce the law in communities experiencing poverty and disadvantage, as well as a greater level of cultural awareness, can play a vital role in building trust, promoting safety, reducing crime and building stronger communities.

7. Smarter sentencing. Harsher sentences and laws that strip judges of their ability to make the sentence fit the crime, such as mandatory sentencing, need to be changed. A wider range of sentencing alternatives encompassing non-custodial options enables judges to ensure that sentences are tailored, fair and appropriate.

8. Eliminate unnecessary imprisonment and consider more effective community options. Many people are imprisoned due to an inability to pay fines or are convicted for relatively minor offences. In many instances, sending a person to prison is unnecessary and can contribute to further involvement in the criminal justice system.

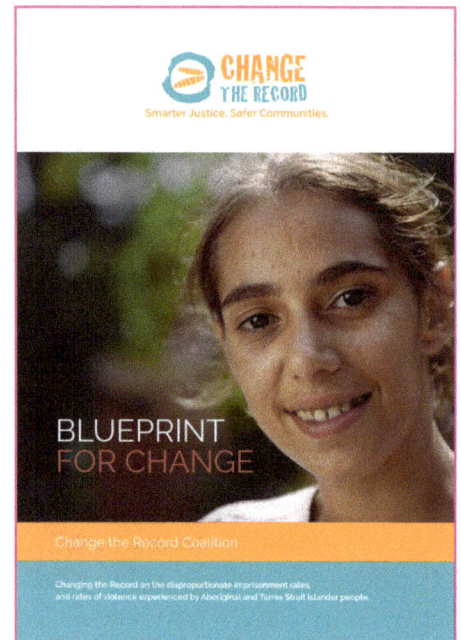

9. Adopt community justice approaches. Therapeutic and restorative processes, such as Koori and Murri courts, drugs courts and healing circles, are ways in which the criminal justice system can help to rebuild relationships and deliver positive outcomes for the entire community. Investing in early intervention and prevention activities, such as community legal education, is more cost effective and prevents offending occurring in the first place.

10. Young people don't belong in prison. Punitive 'tough on crime' approaches to youth offending and misbehaviour fail to recognise that young people are still developing and that far more appropriate opportunities for support and positive reinforcement exist than putting children behind bars. Exposure to youth detention also substantially increases the likelihood of involvement in crime as an adult.

11. Rehabilitation is in all our interests. Effective rehabilitation includes education and programs and support services to increase peoples' capacity to reintegrate into the community following release.

12. Reintegration not recidivism. Unfortunately, far too many people fall back into crime soon after being released from prison. This tells us that not enough support is being provided to people while in prison and during their transition back into the community. Better support needs to be provided to assist people to lead productive lives and fulfil their potential, which includes the provision of affordable housing, health care, and training and employment.

The Blueprint also calls for the establishment of an independent central agency with Aboriginal and Torres Strait Islander oversight, to co-ordinate a comprehensive, current and consistent national approach to related data collection and policy development.

Change the Record is a coalition of leading Aboriginal and Torres Strait Islander, human rights, legal and community organisations calling for urgent and coordinated national action to close the gap in imprisonment rates of Aboriginal and Torres Strait Islander people and cut disproportionate rates of violence experienced by Aboriginal and Torres Strait Islander people, particularly women and children. Take the Change the Record pledge here.

#JustJustice concerns: making global news and hitting the election trail

Author:	Melissa Sweet	Published:	June 05, 2016

A scathing indictment of Australia's failure to address the high incarceration rates of Aboriginal and Torres Strait Islander people has been published in an international journal, **BMJ Global Health**.

Researchers from the George Institute for Global Health at the University of Sydney have analysed the Australian Government's response to criticisms made as part of the UN-led Universal Periodic Review (UPR) process, which scrutinises countries' records on human rights.

Australia's UPR completed in November 2015 showed it had made little progress in addressing concerns about Aboriginal and Torres Strait Islander incarceration rates that had been raised in its inaugural UPR in 2011, according to an analysis by PhD candidates Janani Muhunthan and Anne-Marie Eades, and Professor Stephen Jan.

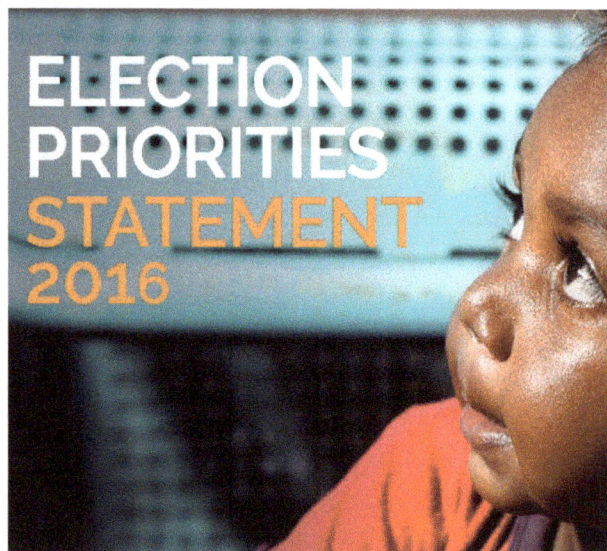

Image from Change the Record website

They describe Australia's "recalcitrance" and "underwhelming" efforts, compared with progress made by comparable countries such as NZ, the USA and Canada, which had introduced legislation or policy initiatives to facilitate effective, culturally sensitive crime prevention with Aboriginal and Torres Strait Islander communities at the forefront of decision-making.

As well as cutting funds to Aboriginal and Torres Strait Islander services, the Australian Government had dismantled preventive agencies, such as the Australian National Preventative Health Agency and the National Indigenous Drug and Alcohol Committee, the researchers noted.

Meanwhile, excessive policing and mandatory sentencing in a number of jurisdictions were worsening the problem.

The researchers also said it was concerning that the Australian Government's report to the UPR had not acknowledged increasing rates of Aboriginal and Torres Strait Islander incarceration and deaths in custody.

They called for the introduction of justice targets, investment into generating evidence for policy innovations, and sustainable funding for Aboriginal and Torres Strait Islander programs in order to reduce Indigenous incarceration rates.

They said it was "imperative" that potentially effective interventions such as the justice reinvestment model are trialled at scale, and that this would require cross-jurisdictional government support, leadership and coordination.

However, the researchers were pessimistic about whether the Australian Government would respond appropriately to the UPR processes:

The defiance evident in Australia's response to the first cycle of UPR in 2011, characterised by its lack of progress and failure to implement recommendations it has previously accepted, highlights the challenges ahead in promoting international collective action as a means of protecting the human rights and health of disadvantaged minorities such as Australia's First Peoples.

Change the Record election priorities

Meanwhile, the Change the Record Coalition has **released its election priorities**, calling on all parties to make it a national priority to address over-imprisonment and the disproportionate rates of violence experienced by Aboriginal and Torres Strait Islander women and children.

The Coalition's election priorities are:

1. A national evidence-based action plan

Governments should work through COAG to establish a national, holistic and whole-of-government plan to address imprisonment and violence rates, with a concrete implementation plan and justice targets. They should establish, or task, an independent agency with Aboriginal and Torres Strait Islander oversight to co-ordinate a comprehensive, current and consistent approach to data collection and policy development relating to Aboriginal and Torres Strait Islander imprisonment and violence rates.

2. Resourcing Aboriginal and Torres Strait Islander communities

Governments should support capacity building, and provide ongoing resourcing of Aboriginal and Torres Strait Islander communities, their organisations and representative bodies to ensure that policy solutions are underpinned by the principle of self-determination, respect for Aboriginal and Torres Strait Islander people's culture and identity, and recognition of the history of dispossession and trauma experienced by many communities.

They should ensure that laws, policies and strategies aimed at, and related to, reducing Aboriginal and Torres Strait imprisonment and violence rates are underpinned by a human-rights approach, and have in place a clear process to ensure they are designed in consultation and partnership with Aboriginal and Torres Strait Islander communities, their organisations and representative bodies.

Governments should also work in partnership with Aboriginal and Torres Strait Islander communities, their organisations and representative bodies to support the identification and development of place-based justice reinvestment trial sites.

3. Prioritise investment in early intervention and prevention strategies

Governments should invest in early intervention and prevention services commensurate with need, with priority for services that are Aboriginal and Torres Strait Islander community controlled.

This should include a focus on:

– Support for the development of holistic, integrated community-controlled early years' child and family services in all communities in need, and investment in culturally strong and intensive family support services.

– Increasing access to culturally-appropriate early intervention and support programs, with a focus on:

- Family violence
- Voluntary drug and alcohol issues;
- Mental health issues;

- Employment and training; and
- Support for people with a disability

Read more here.

Where do the parties stand?

The LNP Coalition: Withdrew their support for justice targets in August 2013, after previously committing to provide bipartisan support for Labor's proposed Closing the Gap targets on incarceration rates (read more here).

Labor: Does not mention justice issues in its Indigenous health election statement but Opposition leader Bill Shorten pledged last November to set justice targets with a focus on community safety, preventing crime and reducing incarceration, and to support research into justice reinvestment.

The Greens: Have pledged to adopt Change the Record campaign recommendations, including:

- Setting a national target to reduce incarceration of Aboriginal and Torres Strait Islander peoples.

- Developing a national, whole of government strategy to address incarceration rates.

- Undertaking an independent review of laws and policies which contribute to unequal incarceration rates, working to fix the problems in the system.

- Providing $40 million in grant funding for projects to help reduce the rate of incarceration.

- Providing $30 million to Aboriginal and Torres Strait Islander individuals, organisations and communities to help advance the national conversation on sovereignty and treaties.

New report reveals litany of failures by governments in response to Royal Commission into Aboriginal Deaths in Custody

| Author: | Melissa Sweet and Amnesty International Australia | Published: | April 14, 2016 |

On 15 April, 2016, it was 25 years since the report of the **Royal Commission Into Aboriginal Deaths In Custody** (RCIADIC) was presented to governments.

The Commission was convened in response to 99 deaths in prison, police custody or juvenile detention institutions, during the period 1 January 1980 to 31 May 1989.

To mark the anniversary, Amnesty International Australia has released a comprehensive, **871-page report** examining governments' progress (or lack thereof) in implementing the Commission's recommendations (some of which related to the health sector).

The report was commissioned by Katie Wood of Amnesty International Australia, and drafted by Clayton Utz on an entirely pro bono basis.

Professor Pat Dodson calls for accountability from legislators at National Press Club

Below is an edited extract from a section of the report detailing how governments have largely failed to comply with their commitments to report annually on implementation of the recommendations.

This failure is symptomatic of wider failures to systematically implement the recommendations; efforts have been patchy, to say the least, suggests the full report, which is **available here**.

Its findings add significant weight to calls for the Council of Australian Governments to adopt justice targets as part of the Closing the Gap agenda, to help improve accountability of governments and service providers in related areas.

(And here is **an Amnesty petition** calling for justice targets.)

The Change the Record campaign will also be highlighting the need for action at a series of events in Canberra tomorrow. Meanwhile, the National Press Club yesterday heard a powerful indictment of legislators from Professor Pat Dodson, who was one of the Royal Commissioners.

Professor Dodson said mandatory sentencing, imprisonment for fine defaults, "paperless" arrest laws, tough bail and parole conditions and punitive sentencing regimes had all contributed to high incarceration rates, along with funding cuts to frontline legal services and inadequate resourcing for much needed diversionary programs (read more **here** in the Fairfax report of his speech).

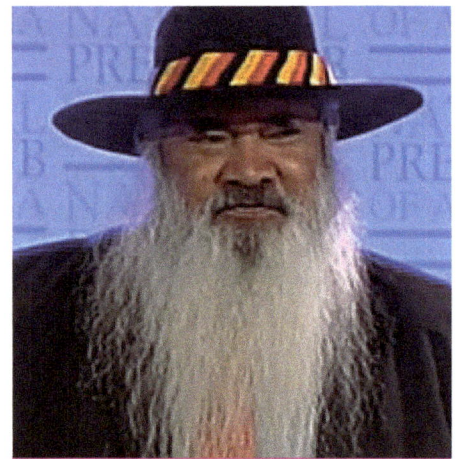

Documenting governments' failures in accountability

(Edited extract from a section of the Amnesty Review of the Implementation of RCIADIC)

In 1992, Federal and State Governments agreed to report annually on their progress in implementing the recommendations of the Royal Commission.

Not only have governments generally failed to provide these annual reports, they have also failed to implement most of the recommendations.

There was strong initial government support for the implementation of the Report and its Recommendations.

At a meeting of the Ministerial Council on Aboriginal and Torres Strait Islander Affairs in August 1992, the States (upon receiving funding from the Commonwealth) and Commonwealth agreed to report annually on the adoption and implementation of the Recommendations of the RCIADIC.

In response to concerns about the outcomes of the RCIADIC and the consistently high rates of Indigenous incarcerations and deaths in custody, a Ministerial Summit on Indigenous Deaths in Custody was held in July 1997 in which Commonwealth, State and Territory Ministers met with representatives of ATSIC, the Aboriginal and Torres Strait Islander Social Justice Commission and the National Aboriginal Justice Advisory Committee.

At this Summit, there was a renewed commitment to the full implementation of the RCIADIC Recommendations. In particular, all Australian governments (except for the NT Government) agreed to develop, in partnership with the Indigenous people, jurisdictional-based agreements (i.e. IJAs) with the aim of addressing these issues and improving the overall delivery of justice to Indigenous people.

The recommendation that ATSIC be given special responsibility and funding applied specifically to the Commonwealth Government. Although the body was formed in 1999, ATSIC was later disbanded in 2005.

Although a Royal Commission Response Monitoring Unit ('RCGRMU') was established in 1992 in direct response to Recommendation 1 following the downsizing and restructuring of ATSIC in July 1996, the functions of the RCGRMU were incorporated into ATSIC's Monitoring and Reporting Section ('MARS').

By October 1996, the ATSIC Social Justice Commissioner reported that

" Recommendation 1: "...had not been meaningfully implemented. Unfortunately, accountability for the implementation of recommendations of the Royal Commission is still unacceptably poor.

After ATSIC was disbanded in 2005, some of its duties were transferred to the Office of Indigenous Policy Coordination. However it is unclear whether there is any coordinated monitoring effort in regards to the implementation of the Recommendations.

For example, the Australian Institute of Criminology monitors and reports on trends in Australian deaths in prison, police custody and juvenile detention.

Since 2003, the AIC has published a number of reports concerning deaths in custody in Australia, with a major report published in 2013 covering all deaths that have occurred to 30 June 2011.

The AIC's reports, however, do not refer to the implementation of the RCIADIC Recommendations.

This report finds that that annual reporting on the implementation of the RCIADIC recommendations has been lacking or patchy in most jurisdictions, including NSW, WA, the ACT, and the NT.

Out of all jurisdictions, reporting by the Victorian Government has been the most comprehensive, despite not occurring on an annual basis as recommended.

In the period immediately following the RCADIC, all Australian States and Territories established their own respective Aboriginal Justice Advisory Committees ('AJACs'). In four of the five States with Aboriginal and Torres Strait Islander Agreements, an Indigenous peak advisory body was instrumental in its conception.

However, in subsequent years, many of the AJACs were either abolished or allowed to collapse by governments.

Overall, the implementation of the Commission's findings, across diverse sectors and agencies, from policing to health and criminal justice systems, has been patchy.

The report also covers the Commission's recommendations in the following areas:

* Deaths (recommendations 4-5)

* Post-death investigations (recommendations 6-40)

* Adequacy of information (recommendations 41-47).

* Aboriginal society today (recommendations 48-57)

* Relations with the non-Aboriginal community (recommendations 58-59)

* The criminal justice system: relations with police (recommendations 60-61).

* Young Aboriginal people and the juvenile justice and welfare systems (recommendation 62)

* The harmful use of alcohol and other drugs (recommendations 63-71)

* Schooling: responding to truancy rates (recommendation 72)

- Housing and infrastructure (recommendations 73-76)

- Self-determination and local government (recommendations 77-78)

- Diversion from police custody (recommendations 79-91)

- Imprisonment as a last resort (recommendations 92-121)

- Custodial health and safety (recommendations 122-167)

- The prison experience (recommendations 168-187)

- The path to self-determination (recommendations 188-204)

- Accommodating difference: relations between Aboriginal and non-Aboriginal people (recommendations 205-213)

- Improving the criminal justice system: Aboriginal people and the police (recommendations 214-233)

- Breaking the cycle: programs for Aboriginal youth (recommendations 234-245)

- Towards better health (recommendations 246-271).

- Coping with alcohol and other drugs: strategies for change (recommendations 272-288)

- Educating for the future (recommendations 289-299)

- Increasing economic opportunity (recommendations 300-320)

- Improving the living environment: housing and infrastructure (recommendations 321-327)

- Conforming with international obligations (recommendations 328-333)

- Addressing land needs (recommendations (334-338)

- The process of reconciliation (recommendation 339).

"330 deaths later: our justice system terrifies me"

| Author: | Kelly Briggs | Published: | November 23, 2016 |

In the 25 years since the Royal Commission Into Aboriginal Deaths in Custody (RCIADIC), more than 330 Indigenous people have died in custody. It's proof that our justice system doesn't care about me, my children and the hundreds of thousands of Aboriginal and Torres Strait Islander people, writes Kelly Briggs.

A man died alone in a cell from head injuries

At 7.30pm on a balmy night in 1980, police officers, unable to rouse a man on a sidewalk, dragged him unconscious into the back of a police van. The officers assumed he was too drunk to be woken.

They drove him to the station and dragged him into a holding cell. They then left him unchecked until 5am, when they found him dead.

The doctor called to assess the man concluded he had died during the night of a subdural haematoma, which is usually the result of a serious head injury. While this man was imprisoned and dying – his brain rapidly filling with blood and compressing tissue – police officers assumed he was too drunk to wake.

A woman's cries of agony were ignored

One hot January morning in 1984, police officers encountered an allegedly intoxicated woman at an intersection. They asked her questions and her replies were incoherent. She could not stand so they carried her into the car.

Records show this woman entered the watchhouse at 7.10am. At around 10am, a man in another cell banged on the door to tell staff that the woman was moaning and rolling around in pain, and that she needed medical attention. Nothing was done.

A short time later an officer noticed the imprisoned woman had defecated on her blanket and moved to the floor. The officer called out to her and she moaned. Still, nothing was deemed amiss.

At 2.25pm a friend of the woman came to bail her out but after failing to wake her, was told to come back later.

The officer went back to the woman's cell; he could not find a pulse. She was dead on a cold concrete floor, beside a blanket covered in her own faeces.

The cause of death was ruled as a haemorrhage from an ovarian cyst, consequent of advanced liver disease. The pain from a ruptured ovarian cyst is described as a sword rammed through your back, repeatedly.

A sick man is dismissed from hospital to die in a cell

At 5am on a Saturday morning in 1984, a man awoke and told his nephew his chest was feeling crook. He was picked up by family members and taken to hospital.

The doctor who attended the sick man prescribed aspirin and rest until he "looked" well. The nurse charged with overseeing the patient stated she saw him as a drunk with a hangover and wanted to be rid of him as soon as possible.

In evidence to the Commission, the nurse admitted that he was still complaining of pain when he was discharged, and was unable to give any satisfactory explanation for letting a very sick man leave. The nurse said she tried to reach family members to come and pick him up – however, only the police were contacted.

The patient was arrested for drunkenness and 27 hours later, he was dead. The coroner's report stated he had died from lobar pneumonia. It is easily diagnosed, either with a stethoscope or a chest X-ray.

This case was hindered by the fact the arresting officer claimed all documents relating to the case were stolen from his car. No charges of hindering an investigation or neglect were ever brought against the officer or hospital staff.

25 years later, we're still dying in custody

These are just three of the 99 Aboriginal deaths between 1 January 1980 and 31 May 1989, which became the subject of the Royal Commission into Aboriginal Deaths in Custody (RCIADIC). Its findings were handed down in 1991 and much to the surprise of many, no criminal charges were filed against any police officers. Not even one charge of criminal neglect.

But 25 years on, and armed with 339 recommendations from RCIADIC, are we any better at stopping preventable deaths in custody?

But 25 years on, and armed with 339 recommendations from RCIADIC, are we any better at stopping preventable deaths in custody?

To this day, most states have only adopted some of the recommendations, with no states or territories implementing them all.

Since RCIADIC, over 330 Aboriginal people have died in custody. Today Aboriginals are jailed at an even higher rate than when the RCIADIC commenced. These are damning statistics for our judiciary system, which has chosen to ignore its very own recommendations.

Only in the last six months, a young Aboriginal woman in Western Australia lost her life in custody, writhing in agony on a cold jailhouse floor. Another entirely preventable death – a parent's worst nightmare.

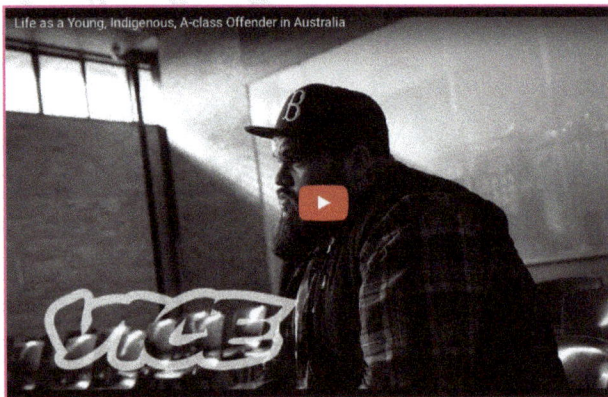

Life as a Young, Indigenous, A-class Offender in Australia

See the video here: https://youtu.be/UCJYlFHvlYU

"Numerous studies have shown that people believe black people do not feel pain in the same way as white people do. There is a very real empathy gap when Aboriginal people display signs of pain as opposed to white people.

In the past year the Northern Territory has introduced paperless arrest laws, which fly in the face of RCIADIC's recommendations.. There has already been at least one death in custody in the Northern Territory as a result of arrests for incredibly minor infractions.

My takeaways

When I look past my anger I feel deep sorrow – sorrow that this country for over 220 years has not valued Aboriginal lives. If it did, this article would not have to be written.

I would not lie in bed fearing for my family members that are imprisoned, that the next time I see them will be at their funerals. I wouldn't be terrified that my own children will one day make a mistake that puts them in a harmful judicial system.

This country must do better. Conversations are taking place but there must be a sense of urgency because as it stands, Aboriginal people are still dying entirely preventable deaths while incarcerated.

Kelly Briggs is an award-winning writer and social commentator. A Gomeroi woman living in Moree in rural NSW, Kelly brings a deep personal and political perspective to her work illuminating the determinants of the social and emotional wellbeing of Aboriginal and Torres Strait Islander people. Follow her on Twitter: @TheKooriWoman

Federal budget fails to deliver for Indigenous health (to put it politely)

Author:	VACCHO, Change the Record, Congress, Oxfam, IAHA, FVPLS	Published:	May 05, 2016

In the Federal Budget, the Prime Minister has failed to "walk the talk" of his Closing the Gap speech; instead, the Budget is widely seen as extremely disappointing for the health of Aboriginal and Torres Strait Islander peoples.

Below are statements from key organisations, including:

Victorian Aboriginal Community Controlled Health Organisation (VACCHO): Cuts bad news for health

Change the Record Coalition: Extreme disappointment at lack of action on justice concerns

National Congress of Australia's First Peoples: The pain continues for Aboriginal and Torres Strait Islander peoples

Oxfam Australia: Turnbull Government snubs Indigenous affairs

Indigenous Allied Health Australia (IAHA): Equity not a priority in Budget

Family Violence Prevention and Legal Service (FVPLS): Inaction on violence.

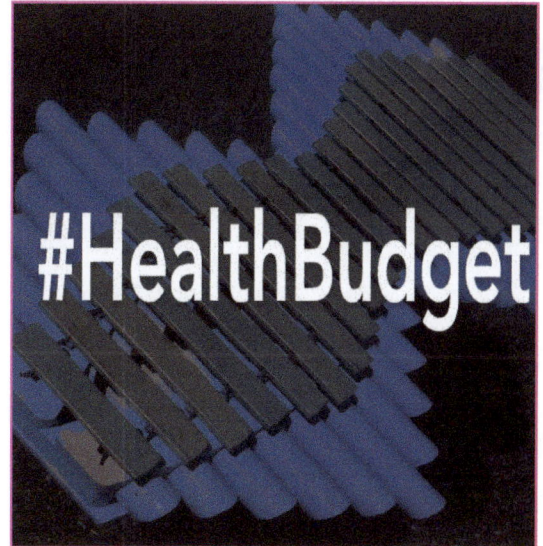

VACCHO statement: Smokes and mirror budget fails to heal previous health funding cuts

From VACCHO's perspective there are two related deficiencies in this year's Federal Budget.

- The lack of funding to implement the National Aboriginal and Torres Strait Islander Health Plan

- Failure to reverse all the hidden cuts to Aboriginal Primary Health funding caused by the freezing of Medicare rebates and the establishment of the Indigenous Advancement Strategy (IAS).

Jill Gallagher AO, VACCHO CEO says "We're not fooled, the end result of all this is that ongoing, unnecessary slashing of health funding has serious implications for Aboriginal peoples."

VACCHO as a partner of the National Close the Gap Campaign supports the ask of Government to provide details on resourcing for the Implementation Plan for the National Aboriginal and Torres Strait Islander Health Plan 2013-2023.

There is no allocation of funds in the Budget Portfolio Statement for the Implementation Plan and yet long term, sustainable funding for Aboriginal and Torres Strait Islander health is what is so desperately needed.

There is no sustainable support for Aboriginal Community Controlled Health Services still reeling from $534 million cuts to funding due to the IAS and continued funding deficits resulting from freezes to Medicare rebates introduced in 2014.

For our Member organisations who have a proven track record of improved health outcomes, this limits service provision to their most vulnerable community members. However, $21.3 million has been allocated to trial "medical homes" funding packages for people with chronic and complex conditions.

"The truth is, the vicious budgetary measures of 2014 still remain. You can't 'cut' your way to Closing the Gap" says Jill Gallagher AO.

There is no attempt in the current budget to repair damage caused by the IAS via funding cuts and the poorly targeted distribution of resources, despite severe criticism recently tabled by the Finance and Public Administration References Committee Inquiry.

VACCHO welcomes continued implementation on Palliative Care and National Blood Borne Virus strategies 2014-17 and the addition of new medications on the PBS including Hepatitis B and cancer drugs.

However, we want to see additional implementation measures and call on the Government to take action that:

- Allocates increased tobacco tax revenue to preventative health initiatives.

- Increases hospital investments which are reflective of the amounts cut in the 2014 budget with indexation.

- Expands the new dental scheme for adults and children beyond publicly funded dental services to increase access by vulnerable communities.

- Maintains accessibility of medications through the recommendations of the Medicare Review.

Prime Minister Turnbull has failed on his Close the Gap promise of "it is time for Governments to 'do things with Aboriginal people, not do things to them'."

"We know all too well that you can't have jobs and growth if you don't have fundamental investment in health and education," says Jill Gallagher AO.

Change the Record statement: Federal Budget fails to prioritise Aboriginal and Torres Strait Islander communities

The Change the Record (CTR) Coalition expressed concern at the 2016 Federal Budget's overall lack of focus on the Indigenous sector and investment in Aboriginal and Torres Strait Islander communities.

CTR Co-Chair Shane Duffy said: "We are extremely disappointed that the Turnbull Government's Budget fails to prioritise Aboriginal and Torres Strait Islander justice issues, including the high rates of violence being experienced by Aboriginal women and children, and skyrocketing rates of incarceration of our peoples."

A high number of Aboriginal and Torres Strait Islander people in prison suffer from a mental or cognitive disability, and so we welcome the Budget's inclusion of $10.5m to provide more services for Fetal Alcohol Spectrum Disorder.

However, on the whole the 2016 Budget retains previous cuts to vital frontline services, including Aboriginal and Torres Strait Islander Legal Services. There has also been no additional funding provided to critically under-resourced organisations such as the Aboriginal Family Violence Prevention Legal Services and Aboriginal organisations in the early childhood, child and family support sectors. The peak Indigenous representative body, the National Congress of Australia's First Peoples, remains unfunded.

Our communities stand ready to work with Government, but they need to be appropriately resourced to support the development of innovative and holistic programmes

"If we are serious about changing the record of violence and imprisonment rates for our people, it is vitally important that the Government commits to long-term investment in Aboriginal community-controlled services and organisations. This includes law reform and advocacy peaks who are best placed to undertake rigorous policy development informed by evidence on the ground."

"Earlier this year the Prime Minister stated that he wanted to work to enable Aboriginal communities to provide local solutions. Our communities stand ready to work with Government, but they need to be appropriately resourced to support the development of innovative and holistic programmes," said Mr Duffy.

Aboriginal and Torres Strait Islander women are currently 34 times more likely to be hospitalised for family violence related assault than non-Indigenous women, and Aboriginal and Torres Strait Islander men are more likely to go to jail than university. This is a national crisis, and tackling these issues should be front and centre of our nation's budget priorities.

"The Federal Budget provides a roadmap of Government priorities, and we are deeply concerned that in this Budget Aboriginal justice issues appear to have been forgotten by the Turnbull Government," said Mr Duffy.

National Congress statement: The pain continues

For Indigenous Australia the 2016 Budget has delivered more of the same. There are no surprises, the policy thinking, the budgetary levers and programs remain intact.

Co-Chair Mr Rod Little, "Once again the federal government has snubbed the national representative body for Australia's first peoples and has not provided us with any financial assistance so we can effectively represent our people."

Congress still has concerns with the Indigenous Advancement Strategy (IAS) and the $500M in funding cuts rolled out in the 2014 Budget are still impacting on our people today. We encourage the government to work positively to limit the damage and devastation which resulted from the chaotic rollout of the IAS.

The continued failure to adequately fund Aboriginal Legal Service's and Family Violence Prevention Legal Services especially when incarceration rates are escalating is particularly puzzling, as is the lack of any specific response the numbers of Indigenous children going into care.

National Congress applauds initiatives which focus on providing a hand up to Indigenous people, the employment programs being rolled out are commendable, as are the focus on children and safety, the announcements and projections if realised will greatly assist the many Aboriginal and Torres Strait Islander peoples who have the opportunity to do so.

The government approach to welfare reform for Aboriginal and Torres Strait Islander people needs innovation. The Try, Test and Learn Program announced in the budget as a new initiative, deserves merit. National Congress considers that this type of innovation needs to apply to the Indigenous Affairs arena. The program is the type of thinking that we need not a continuation of the punitive, coercive, palliative care approach currently in place.

The Close the Gap strategy is not working, the Northern territory Intervention is now nearing its tenth anniversary and is not working, and incarceration and child removal rates are escalating.

We must depart from the combative approach to Indigenous Affairs and create an environment based on respect and trust. We owe this to the many Indigenous people who continue to be unable to take up the opportunities that this country can provide.

The budget includes a specific allocation of $14.6m to the Recognition of Indigenous People in the Constitution which includes another $5M to the Recognise campaign. But while the government fails to recognise the representative voice of Aboriginal and Torres Strait Islander people, the National Congress, this initiative lacks substance. Without a relationship with Indigenous peoples Constitutional Recognition will remain problematic.

Recognition must be predicated on a respectful and harmonious relationship.

"We met Prime Minister Turnbull recently and offered our support to his government in engaging with Aboriginal and Torres Strait Islander people, even though this government hasn't recognised the National Congress in this Budget, the offer is still there so we can help stop the devastation that is occurring on a daily basis to our people," Mr Little said.

Oxfam Australia statement: Turnbull Government snubs Indigenous affairs

Oxfam Australia Chief Executive Dr Helen Szoke said:

"The Turnbull Government has provided no new money to improve the health and wellbeing of Aboriginal and Torres Strait Islander Australians faced with shorter life expectancy and dramatically higher incarceration rates.

> *Aboriginal and Torres Strait Islander people have the solutions but they need the funding to implement those solutions*

"Despite the ongoing crisis in incarceration rates, child removal rates and the overall slow progress towards closing the gap in health and wellbeing outcomes for Aboriginal and Torres Strait Islander peoples, the Turnbull Government has failed in its first opportunity to restore the cuts made by the Abbott Government in the 2014 Federal Budget to Aboriginal and Torres Strait Islander Affairs funding.

"Remarkably, the Treasurer failed to even mention Aboriginal and Torres Strait Islander Affairs in his budget speech. It appears that the Prime Minister's promise in his Closing the Gap speech in February of a closer relationship between government and Aboriginal and Torres Strait Islander peak bodies and leaders remains a rhetorical flourish rather than a policy and resource commitment.

"While we welcome the previously announced $40 million to the Australian Institute of Aboriginal and Torres Strait Islander Studies for cultural preservation and promotion over the next four years – there is little else."

Other announced spending measures are within the previously announced budget parameters.

Dr Szoke said the National Congress of Australia's First Peoples remains unfunded and the cuts to Aboriginal and Torres Strait Islander Legal Services remain.

"Aboriginal and Torres Strait Islander people still represent a quarter of the prison population and are 10 times more likely to be removed from their families. Aboriginal and Torres Strait Islander people have the solutions but they need the funding to implement those solutions," Dr Szoke said.

Indigenous Allied Health Australia statement: Equity not a priority in Budget

Indigenous Allied Health Australia (IAHA) asserts that a strong and visible commitment by governments to building a culturally safe and responsive health system that provides equitable access for Aboriginal and Torres Strait Islander peoples to allied health services is required in order to really make a difference.

This was not evident in the National Budget 2016-2017, where the focus was unapologetically on ensuring 'Australia continues to successfully transition from the mining investment boom to a stronger, more diversified, new economy'.

IAHA welcomes the Government's announcement of the Child and Adult Public Dental Scheme – which aims to provide public dental services to all children and adult concession card holders, as well as the Taking More Action to Prevent Fetal Alcohol Spectrum Disorders. The Government has promised the $10.5 million over four years from 2016-2017 to reduce the occurrence of the Fetal Alcohol Spectrum Disorder (FASD), focusing on prevention of FASD in high risk, remote and rural communities. IAHA further welcomes the Government's commitment to spending $2.9 billion in additional funding to state and territory's public hospitals.

"Investing in schemes that aim to improve oral health and reduce the occurrence of Fetal Alcohol Spectrum Disorders (FASD) is positive, however the impact of these upon the lives of Aboriginal and Torres Strait Islander peoples must be not be ignored," said IAHA Chief Executive Officer Ms Donna Murray. "Particular attention to the specific needs of Aboriginal and Torres Strait Islander people must be an essential component of the implementation of such schemes."

The Government also announced $21.3 million will be allocated to the trial of the Health Care Homes model which was recommended by the Primary Health Care Advisory Group's Report — Better Outcomes for People with Chronic and Complex Health Conditions.

"Given the proportionately high population of Aboriginal and Torres Strait Islander peoples with chronic conditions and complex care needs, the outcomes of trialling the Health Care Homes model will have implications for their long term care," said Ms Murray.

"We encourage engagement with Aboriginal and Torres Strait Islander peoples to increase participation and advocate a coordinated interdisciplinary approach to chronic disease management where allied health plays a critical role."

The Government also announced the intent to increase efficiencies in the Health Flexible Funds, aimed over three years from 2017-2018. The Government plans to achieve this by reducing uncommitted funds and continuing the current pause in indexation of funds for a further two years, among other methods.

"IAHA agrees there is a need to increase efficiencies across the health system as a whole," said Ms Murray. "However it is essential that these efficiencies are not achieved at the expense of valuable programs and initiatives that build an Aboriginal and Torres Strait Islander health workforce and contribute to achieving health equality more broadly."

Although existing and new health initiatives stated in this years' budget will indirectly benefit Aboriginal and Torres Strait Islander peoples, it remains to be seen how Aboriginal and Torres Strait Islander peoples will access these mainstream services, and how relevant they will be to the unique needs and experiences of Aboriginal and Torres Strait Islander peoples.

National Family Violence Prevention Legal Services (NFVPLS) statement: inaction on violence

Targeted action to address the specific needs of Aboriginal and Torres Strait Islander victim/survivors of family violence is invisible in the Federal Budget.

"Aboriginal and Torres Strait Islander women are at the epicentre of the national family violence crisis, yet specific initiatives to confront this crisis and invest in services for safety are invisible in the Budget," said Antoinette Braybrook, Convenor of the National FVPLS Forum.

"This is yet another missed opportunity for the Government to better resource Family Violence Prevention Legal Services (FVPLS) who provide legal services and supports to Aboriginal and Torres Strait Islander victims/survivors of family violence, with more than 90% of our clients nationally being Aboriginal and Torres Strait Islander women and children."

Aboriginal and Torres Strait Islander women are 34 times more likely to be hospitalised from family violence and 10 times more likely to die of violent assault than other women. The question must be asked why there is no targeted action to address this crisis.

The Budget includes $100 million over three years on initiatives to reduce violence against women and their children. This is inadequate to meet the needs of women fleeing violence for their safety. It is also silent on a specific allocation of funding on programs for Aboriginal and Torres Strait Islander women. Without targeted investment in services like FVPLSs the horrific disproportionate impact of violence against Aboriginal and Torres Strait Islander women will only get worse. The Budget also fails to reverse the cuts to Community Legal Centres and Aboriginal and Torrs Strait Islander Legal Services.

"Violence against Aboriginal and Torres Strait Islander women and children is at epidemic levels. It will cost the nation $2.2 billion by 2021-22. Its moral cost – which sees lives lost and communities destroyed – is unquantifiable. Yet tragically a response to this violence is invisible in the Budget Papers."

"FVPLSs provide essential services for safety of Aboriginal and Torres Strait Islander victims/survivors of family violence and deliver early intervention prevention programs to break the vicious cycle of violence. Further investment is needed to build the capacity of existing services and address service gaps to ensure all Aboriginal and Torres Strait Islander women can access these services for safety."

"Budgets set out the priorities of Government. Ending the disproportionate impact of violence against Aboriginal and Torres Strait Islander women should have been front and centre of this Budget."

Memo to WA Government: how you can help to stop Aboriginal people dying in custody

Author: Change the Record campaign

Published: March 22, 2016

More than 20 Aboriginal and Torres Strait Islander and human rights organisations have signed an open letter released today by the **Change the Record campaign**, calling on Western Australian Premier Colin Barnett to stop locking up vulnerable people for unpaid fines.

The open letter, republished below, comes in the wake of the ongoing inquest into the tragic death of Ms Dhu, a 22-year old Aboriginal woman who died in police custody after being imprisoned for unpaid fines.

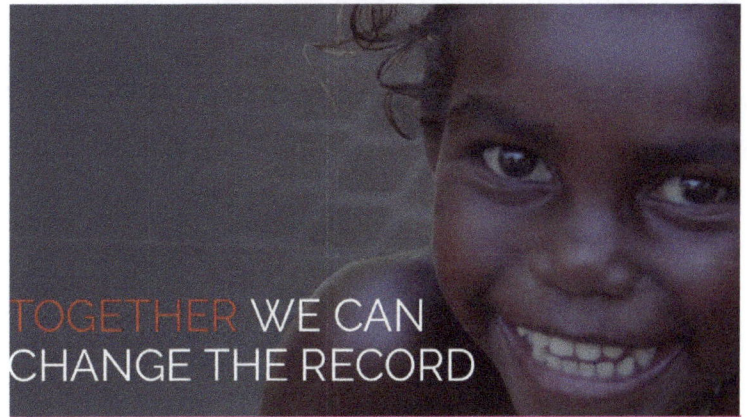

TOGETHER WE CAN CHANGE THE RECORD

The featured image is from the Change the Record campaign website

Open Letter: Stop locking up vulnerable people for unpaid fines

Dear Premier Barnett,

The coronial inquest into the death in custody of Ms Dhu, a 22-year-old Yamatji Aboriginal woman, has shone a light on Western Australia's concerning practice of locking people up for unpaid fines.

Ms Dhu tragically died just three days after she was locked up in a South Hedland police station for failing to pay her fines. At the time of her arrest, Ms Dhu was in a domestic violence situation.

We the undersigned organisations are deeply concerned by the escalating numbers of people being imprisoned in Western Australia (WA) for fine default.

We are particularly concerned at the impact of this policy on vulnerable communities, including Aboriginal and Torres Strait Islander men and in particular women, who are already significantly over-represented in the prison population.

The most effective way to prevent another death in custody, like Ms Dhu's, from occurring is to ensure that vulnerable people aren't being imprisoned for unpaid fines in the first place. A fine system which supports vulnerable and disadvantaged people to address complex underlying issues, would be far more effective for the safety and wellbeing of those persons and the community in general.

Further, there is also evidence that domestic violence victims may be reluctant to report violence or seek help for fear of arrest or other repercussions.

Governments should therefore ensure that such barriers to reporting violence are removed.

We, the undersigned organisations, call on the Government of Western Australia to immediately commit to:

- Stop locking people up for unpaid fines, by amending the Fines, Penalties and Infringement Notices Act and introducing a Work and Development Order scheme, modelled on the effective NSW approach;

- Retract any plans to introduce a compulsory scheme whereby outstanding fines may be deducted from social security payments because such a scheme will further seriously disadvantage vulnerable Aboriginal people;

- Ensure the adequate provision of gender and culturally relevant early intervention and diversion programs, to address the current over-imprisonment of Aboriginal women and girls in Western Australia; and

- Establish a legislative presumption against arresting victims of domestic violence at time of police intervention for outstanding unrelated charges.

Since 2010, one in every six Aboriginal people going to prison in WA was there to pay off fines and these figures are even more striking for women. In 2013 almost one-third of all women entering prison in WA were there for unpaid fines, and almost two-thirds of these women were Aboriginal.

Staggeringly, between 2008 and 2013 the number of Aboriginal women locked up for fine default in WA increased by almost 600 percent.

More broadly, to avoid any further tragic deaths in custody the undersigned organisations also urge the Western Australian Government to immediately commit to the following safeguard measures, including:

- Funding the Aboriginal Legal Service of Western Australia to provide a Custody Notification Service;

- Providing for a 24hour oncall nurse in all police watch houses;

- Expanding the role of the Inspector of Custodial Services to cover police watch houses; and

- Independent investigations of police- related deaths.

Yours sincerely,

Aboriginal Alcohol and Drug Services

Aboriginal Legal Service NSW/ACT

Aboriginal Legal Rights Movement

Amnesty International Australia

ANTaR

Australian Council of Social Service (ACOSS)

Binaal Billa Family Violence Prevention Legal Service

Deaths in Custody Watch Committee (WA) Inc.

Federation of Community Legal Centres (VIC)

First Peoples Disability Network (FPDN)

FVPLS (Vic)

Human Rights Law Centre

Just Reinvest NSW

Justice Connect Homeless Law

Moorditch Gurlongga Association Inc (MGA)

National Aboriginal and Torres Strait Islander Legal Services (NATSILS)

National Association of Community Legal Centres (NACLC)

National Congress of Australia's First Peoples

National FVPLS Forum

Oxfam Australia

Save the Children Australia

Sisters Inside

Southern Aboriginal Corporation

Secretariat of National Aboriginal and Islander Child Care (SNAICC)

Art project puts a powerful spotlight on Aboriginal deaths in custody

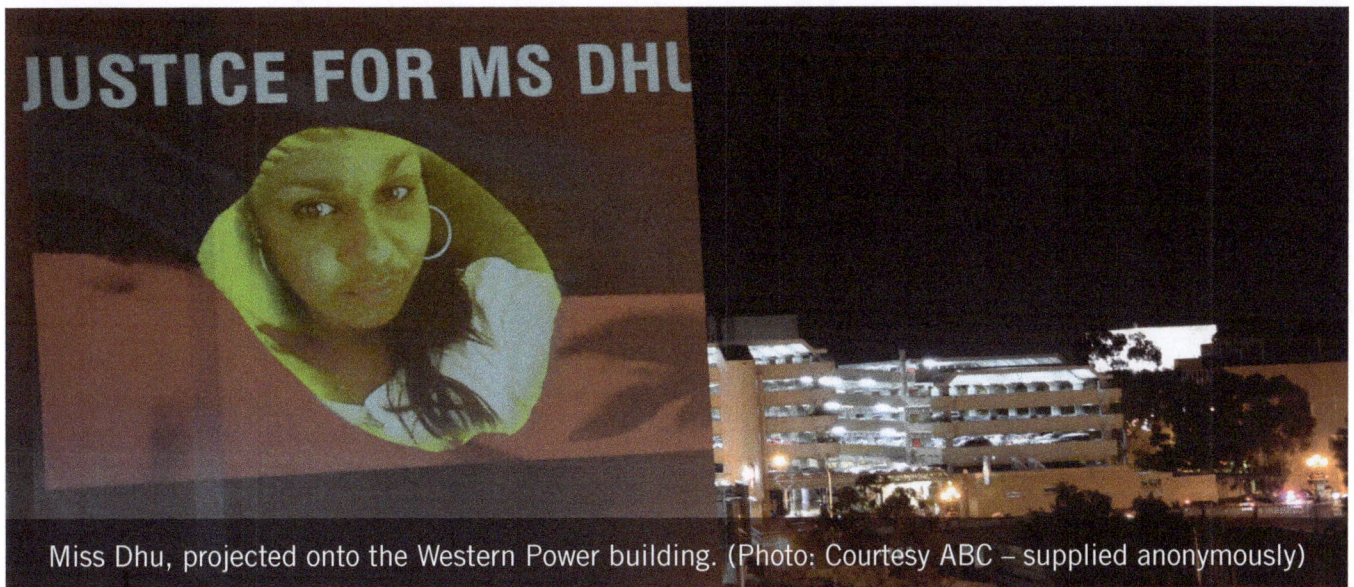

Miss Dhu, projected onto the Western Power building. (Photo: Courtesy ABC – supplied anonymously)

Author:	Ethan Blue	Published:	March 17, 2016

At an event marking the 10th anniversary today of the community-driven **Close the Gap** campaign, Social Justice commissioner Mick Gooda vowed to **continue pushing** for justice targets, as essential to improving health and social outcomes.

The focus is firmly on the need for reform in WA in particular, as a coronial inquest resumed in Perth this week into the death of Ms Dhu, a 22-year-old Yamatji Aboriginal woman (whose first name is not used for cultural reasons).

Human rights lawyers have called on the WA Government **to stop the practice** of locking people up for unpaid fines, and a public forum in Perth last night (as per the feature image above) heard detailed recommendations for change to policing and justice systems in WA.

In the article below, cross-posted with permission from **ABC Religion and Ethics**, history lecturer Ethan Blue writes that governments must stop seeing punishment as the solution to social problems.

His argument that prisons are central to maintaining modern inequality, suggests that efforts to address the social determinants of Indigenous health must have a strong focus on policing and justice systems.

Seeing Miss Dhu: Time to Turn a Light on Aboriginal Deaths in Custody

Ethan Blue writes:

Miss Dhu, a 22 year old Yamatji woman, died in police custody in South Hedland, Western Australia, on 4 August 2014. She was arrested for fine default.

She arrived at the lockup with broken ribs and a developing case of pneumonia. She complained of worsening pain and suffering, but attending medical staff and police officers dismissed her as a druggie with "**behavioural issues**," faking illness to escape punishment.

They could not see that her pain was real. They **saw a black woman**, a criminal, whose suffering could be dismissed in the workaday administration of what passes for justice.

Like many Australian women of all ethnicities, Miss Dhu was – according to her family – in a violent relationship. The justice system should have provided her with an opportunity for protection.

It didn't.

Because we live in a society that criminalises Aboriginal people, the officers were more interested in punishing Miss Dhu for her unpaid fines than in protecting her rights, let alone listening to her medical complaints.

The consequences of our society's preoccupation with seeing black women like Miss Dhu as problems rather than as human beings ought to be the focus of the inquest into her death.

Miss Dhu's tragic death has led to the highest profile death in custody case since Aboriginal elder Mr Ward's gruesome 2008 death in the back of an overheated prison van. Despite being such a high-profile case, Miss Dhu's family is frustrated by the direction and delays of the inquest, which they have called a "betrayal" and "an insult to the family."

As a result of this frustration, starting in February 2016, allies of Miss Dhu's family began projecting images of Miss Dhu on prominent buildings across Perth to raise awareness of her death and the importance of her inquest.

Each evening, a small group of people load into their car with a projector and laptop, and travel Perth's streets.

They find prominent or symbolically resonant buildings – the East Perth lockup, the Western Power building, the Telstra Building, among others. They stop and point the projector, and giant, haunting images of Miss Dhu light the walls and overlook the city.

The projections of Miss Dhu, her family and supporters, are an aesthetic and political attempt – modest, incomplete, mournful, angry – to return her to the world from which she was taken too young.

They help return Miss Dhu's memory into the night-time cityscape, shifting it into a space of hope and opposition, of mourning and care, a space of survival

They attempt to reclaim, at least on some level, a space and a presence for Aboriginal women, so long maligned by mainstream Australian society, and among those most profoundly victimised by the ongoing process of colonisation.

By shining a light on places where human rights violations have taken place and on the city's centres of business, finance and communication, the projections re-claim the surfaces of a city that has grown rich from mining and real estate. Aboriginal people have been locked out of much of this growth, despite the fact that the mineral resources come from Aboriginal lands.

For many, the city is hostile and unwelcoming. It is the seat of a brand of settler colonialism that has overseen the removal of Indigenous peoples from the land to bolster regional mining claims or to facilitate urban shopping and consumer culture.

The projections tell a different story. They help return Miss Dhu's memory into the night-time cityscape, shifting it into a space of hope and opposition, of mourning and care, a space of survival.

Moreover, the images and associated texts and hashtags – which include #BlackLivesMatter, #IdleNoMore and #SayHerName – connect the Australian struggle for justice to global movements against racism, state violence and neglect in North America and beyond.

They highlight the tragedy that Perth was and remains a deeply segregated city, in a deeply segregated state, in a radically unequal society. And a society in which rates of Aboriginal women jailed for fine default grew by 576% since 2008.

As scholars in North America and Australia alike have argued, prisons and policing are central to maintaining inequality at the turn of the twenty-first century.

The images speak to global movements against governments that see more punishment as the answer to every social problem.

The images of Miss Dhu's family, which loved her deeply and loves her still, speak to an ethic of care rather than control, of community building instead of community imprisonment. Of calls for sovereignty of the body and spirit, as well as sovereignty over political futures – a sovereignty that, as Perth's Nyoongar and other Aboriginal and Torres Straits activists remind us, was never ceded, and in which Aboriginal women, young and old, play a central part.

After her family and supporters marched in protest to Parliament House in Perth, Premier Colin Barnett claimed a special interest in Miss Dhu's case. His promise to seek justice in her case and address the over-imprisonment of Aboriginal peoples is laudable.

Yet the suite of proposed reforms – from Custody Notification Services to addressing the number of women imprisoned on remand or for fine default, especially at the grossly overcrowded and woefully inadequate Bandyup Women's Prison – have all fallen short of the mark.

It is possible that the inquest will address the structural racism, sexism and dispossession that continue to animate our history and which led to Miss Dhu's death.

Nearly 25 years ago, the Royal Commission Investigation into Aboriginal Deaths in Custody issued 339 recommendations addressing the political and material conditions that lead to deaths in custody. Relatively few of these have been implemented.

Martin Luther King, Jr., suggested that the moral arc of the universe is long, but that it bends toward justice. But King also knew that it didn't bend by itself, that grassroots and social movements for justice led the change.

The inquest into Miss Dhu's death resumed on 14 March, at the Central Law Court in Perth. It is open to the public. The optics of the court, and of this government, around racism, justice, prisons and policing, remains to be seen.

Ethan Blue is Senior Lecturer in History at the University of Western Australia, specialising in the history of punishment, immigration history and labour history. He is the author of Doing Time in the Depression: Everyday Life in Texas and California Prisons.

Croakey extends our warm thanks to ABC Religion and Ethics for permission to cross-post this article.

Government not on track to meet Closing the Gap targets because of course they aren't

Author:	Luke Pearson	Published:	December 04, 2015

The Productivity Commission this week released the **sixth report** in the series of performance assessments for Australia's '**Closing the Gap**' targets (previous assessments were prepared by the COAG Reform Council). It **concludes** that "it is becoming increasingly clear that a number of the 'Closing the Gap' targets will not be met" and says there is a strong case for rationalising the current framework for reporting on Indigenous outcomes and disadvantage.

In this article below, republished from **IndigenousX** with permission, **Luke Pearson** says the news comes as no surprise, given the massive chaos and uncertainty in Indigenous affairs policy and funding, and the ongoing failure to implement crucial recommendations from a host of previous work, including the **Royal Commission into Aboriginal Deaths in Custody**.

He says he is infuriated when someone asks him what they can do to help close the gap, because that question is prefaced on the idea that that is what is actually happening:

"A better question would be 'How can I help prevent the government from widening the gap?'"

His article also highlights this must-read article – **Gesture Politics** – by **Professor Megan Davis** in the latest The Monthly. On the desperate state of Indigenous policy in Australia, she writes:

"Cut-and-paste government press releases routinely masquerade as analysis; "bipartisanship" is the technical term for "move away, nothing to see here"; and a prime minister visiting an Aboriginal community for a few days – a seriously unremarkable thing for a prime minister in days gone by – is conflated with policy."

There was some good news this week, with the **announcement** that the Federal Government will continue to fund the Custody Notification Service, a 24-hour legal advice and phone line for Aboriginal people taken into police custody in NSW and the ACT that was recommended by the Royal Commission. However, the **disruption and distress** around its initial defunding, and the fact that similar services are **still undelivered** in other juridictions, underscore the powerful points made by both Davis and Pearson.

Luke Pearson writes:

A Productivity Commission **report** has found that the government will probably not meet 5 of the 6 Closing the Gap targets, leaving many astounded to hear that they might actually achieve one of them.

(It should be noted at the outset that the government's 'Closing the Gap' is not the same as '**Close the Gap**', which is a coalition of Indigenous and non-Indigenous health and community organisations.)

Massive cuts to Indigenous Affairs, the defunding of essential services, a highly criticised funding process in the name of the 'Indigenous Advancement Strategy', superficial slogans and punitive approaches, along with a non-Indigenous mining magnate held up as the champion of Indigenous employment were but a few of the signals that things were not going well on the road to closing the gap.

And with all of this going on, one could be excused for wondering how anyone ever thought it was going to be any different. It's a bit like Ned Flanders' parents in The Simpsons complaining 'We've tried nothing and we're all out of ideas!'

Except with many of the things that have been tried, 'nothing' would probably have been preferable. Even more preferable would have been to listen to, and act upon, what the evidence and the experts say.

The recommendations from the Royal Commission into Aboriginal Deaths in Custody have for the most part never been implemented, and the number of Aboriginal people in custody has steadily risen, as has the rate of deaths in custody.

The recommendations of the National Report into the Separation of Aboriginal & Torres Strait Islander Children from their Families have similarly been ignored and the rate of child removal is now higher than it was at the peak of the Stolen Generations.

The rights of Indigenous peoples as laid out in the UN Declaration on the Rights of Indigenous Peoples are not even on our radar.

The *Little Children Are Sacred* report was held up to justify the Northern Territory Intervention despite there being nothing in the report to justify the NT Intervention.

These are some of the most commonly known examples, but the list is near endless. Reports are frequently ignored regardless of where they originate, from universities, independent organisations, community members, or even from within the government itself. This is true within all major areas – health, education, employment, incarceration, and housing.

Despite all of this, the only Indigenous issues that have been discussed by governments in the past few years have been Constitutional Recognition, meaningless week-long visits to remote communities, and countless ignorant and racist comments from our former Prime Minister. The only change in this situation has been that Malcolm is a bit more savvy at not saying horrible stuff on record, hardly a fact for celebration.

There have also been more deaths in custody than we like to think about, community closures, defunded services, deregistered sacred sites, and a variety of one-off feel-good moments.

Professor Megan Davis recently wrote, quite brilliantly I might add, about 'gesture politics' and this basically sums up government attitudes towards Indigenous Affairs. Except of course for the more extreme rightwing members of the government, emboldened by their counterparts in the media, who actually argue that Indigenous peoples receive a kind of 'special treatment' that borders on segregation, and that places white Australia as a disadvantaged group by comparison.

These arguments are not helped by the fact that the organisations responsible for implementing Indigenous specific services rarely have the scope or capacity to address the racist misinformation that has arisen since the 1970s when many of these services were first introduced. So much so that it is a commonly held belief that Indigenous people get all sorts of

'free' stuff from governments. Free houses, cars, education, loans, dog food, funerals, and all sorts of nonsense.

This gross misrepresentation of the nature of, and need for, Indigenous specific programs and services, the demonisation of Aboriginal parents, families and communities en masse, coupled with framing of Indigenous issues as a 'wicked problem' has provided an atmosphere that allows and justifies gross breaches of human rights, the dismantling of Indigenous services, and the defunding of Indigenous affairs – all while patronisingly claiming it to be 'in our best interests'.

The three-point slogans of the previous PM (kids must go to school, adults must go to work, and communities need to be safe) translated to little more than truancy officers for some schools, attempts to close remote communities and the championing of Andrew Forrest as the saviour of Indigenous employment, and the defunding of family support services and women's refuges.

This is why I always get infuriated when someone asks me what they can do to help close the gap, because that question is prefaced on the idea that that is what is actually happening. A better question would be 'How can I help prevent the government from widening the gap?'

And I wish I knew the answer to that question.

We look for grand gestures like the apology, the bridge walk for reconciliation, or Constitutional Recognition to be cure alls that will somehow magically make all of these other issues disappear. Even former PM Kevin Rudd recently said that 'Even what some might call symbolic change can usher in a further era of substantive policy change', completely ignoring that we could just implement an era of policy change if we actually wanted to. It does not require a grand gesture to do that. He also said: 'Let us for a moment lift up our eyes from the trenches of political battle and gaze for a moment upon the mountains, unleashing our imagination on the new possibilities that might just lie beyond constitutional recognition, towards an Australia that is utterly, wonderfully, magnificently racially blind.'

It is hard to imagine substantive Indigenous rights in a country that is utterly racially blind, and it doesn't sound particularly wonderful or magnificent either. (I was tempted to tangent here into the problems of the 'racially blind'/'I don't see race' arguments here but you can google that on your time. I've got a point to make, probably.)

These arguments are not helped by the fact that the organisations responsible for implementing Indigenous specific services rarely have the scope or capacity to address the racist misinformation that has arisen since the 1970s when many of these services were first introduced

Herein lies much of the problem. We wait for grand moments that will 'usher in an era of change' like a problem drinker in the middle of February saying they are waiting until next January so they can make sobriety their New Year's Resolution. Grand claims like these buy time, but after year after year of failing to make good on the promise, people grow weary of them.

That is why so many people have grown tired of claims, of promises, and of gestures. The only thing that is required to usher in these changes is the will to do so. Nothing more.

So even if you support the apology, or reconciliation, or changing the Constitution, or even a treaty, it is important to understand that these gestures are not the societal equivalent of throwing a giant 'racism is over, we're good white people now, so please shut up and get over the past already' party. Racism in all its forms, institutional and personal, well intentioned and malicious; and its impacts, ongoing and intergenerational, will not be something 'in the past' that people can have any hope of 'getting over' until it stops, and until assurances that it will not start again have been secured. And it won't stop until we realise that it is not simply a matter of educating people about how bad it is, but a matter of power and profit, and a matter of ending the constant barrage of misinformation that protects it. It is a matter of ensuring that the institutions which were not so long ago purposefully built to ensure the exclusion of Indigenous peoples start to live up to their claims of equality, and are held to account when they fail to do anything less.

As I am known to mention, it is not simply what happened 200 years ago that most people are concerned about, rather it is what has happened every day since, and the heartbreaking knowledge that it will still be happening tomorrow, and the next day, and to the next generation, unless something changes.

I mentioned earlier that I do not have all the answers for what this change looks like but I do think it might be worth trying some of the things that experts from across all areas have been calling for for decades... seems like it might be worth a shot at this stage?

Luke Pearson is a consultant, digital strategist, keynote speaker, social commentator, educator and trainer, and the founder of @IndigenousX – a ground-breaking Twitter account which has a different Aboriginal or Torres Strait Islander person tweeting each week, and which now has its own website. *It works in partnership with Guardian Australia: each week, the site presents an online profile and* Q&A *with the latest host. You can also subscribe to the IndigenousX* newsletter. *Luke also tweets at @LukeLPearson.*

Campaign to save the NSW Custody Notification Service: 'lifeline' for Indigenous people in custody

Author:	Eugene Schofield-Georgeson	Published:	June 16, 2015

There's deep concern about the **looming threat** to the landmark Custody Notification Service (CNS) in New South Wales – which is set to lose its federal funding from July 1.

As PhD candidate **Eugene Schofield-Georgeson** writes in the post below (originally **published** at The Conversation) the CNS provides NSW with one of the most effective strategies in curbing Indigenous deaths in police custody.

There's a strong #savetheCNS campaign on Twitter, nearly 14,000 have signed this **change.org petition**, and much lobbying elsewhere from others who know how important is the service that provides Indigenous prisoners in police custody with personal and legal advice. It also ensures that they receive adequate health care while monitoring their treatment by police. See **more info and appeals** for support from the NSW Aboriginal legal Service.

The New South Wales Council of Civil Liberties has this week **written** to Indigenous Affairs Minister Nigel Scullion and the Prime Minister Tony Abbott calling for the Federal Government to continue its funding of the CNS, saying:

"The CNS has proved a vital, effective and low-cost service, acting as a lifeline for advice and support for Indigenous people in custody. We understand there have been no Aboriginal deaths in custody in NSW/ACT since the service began in 2000....

It would be a severe indictment on this Government's commitment to Closing the Gap and reversing Indigenous incarceration rates if the CNS was to cease under its tenure."

Eugene Schofield-Georgeson writes:

The federal government is **poised** to abolish the Custody Notification Service in New South Wales through a funding cut on July 1 – for the sake of saving A$526,000 a year. For that modest amount, the service provides NSW with one of the most effective strategies in curbing Indigenous deaths in police custody.

The service is a telephone hotline that provides Indigenous prisoners in police custody with personal and legal advice. It also ensures that they receive adequate health care while monitoring their treatment by police.

NSW Aboriginal Legal Services CEO Kane Ellis has told me that the service is a "transparency measure" that "increases the professionalism of police". It provides Indigenous people with assistance that is often:

> *... as simple as getting a person essential medication that can save a life.*

Why the service is essential

At **last count in 2013**, Indigenous deaths in custody had spiked to all-time highs in other states and territories where the service has not been implemented, as well as among Indigenous prison populations.

However, since the service was implemented in NSW in 2007, the state has had **no Indigenous deaths** in its police cells, watch-houses and during transport procedures. In that time, other states and territories have recorded 11 Indigenous deaths in police custody.

The **Royal Commission into Aboriginal Deaths in Custody** in 1991 recommended the establishment of the Custody Notification Service. The reasons why the service must continue reflect the commission's major findings. These are reasons that state and federal governments have mostly ignored since 1991.

The royal commission found that Indigenous people die in custody at much higher rates than non-Indigenous people. This is primarily because they are taken into custody at much higher rates than non-Indigenous people.

In NSW, **rates of Indigenous imprisonment** are currently 24%. However, Indigenous people make up less than 2.9% of the **population**. This is a higher per capita rate than in the **Northern Territory**, where 86% of inmates are Indigenous. Indigenous people comprise 29.8% of the **population**.

Put differently, in NSW, Indigenous people are more than eight times more likely to be imprisoned than non-Indigenous people. In the Northern Territory, they are less than three times as likely to be imprisoned.

The Custody Notification Service helps prevent Indigenous deaths in both police and prison custody by addressing the problem of over-representation of Indigenous offenders in prison through the provision of legal advice. Such advice usually informs an Indigenous person in custody of their right to silence. This prevents false confessions and unreliable evidence, thereby reducing unfair and unsafe convictions.

The right to silence for Indigenous people remains intact despite recent legislative amendments in NSW restricting the use of this legal right.

Background to its abolition

The Carr government implemented the Custody Notification Service as a compulsory custody right in NSW across a range of criminal legislation. Section 33 of the Law Enforcement (Powers and Responsibilities) Regulation provides that when an Aboriginal or Torres Strait Islander person is detained in police custody, a custody manager must immediately notify a representative of the Aboriginal Legal Service and inform the prisoner accordingly.

In one case, Justice Hidden of the NSW Supreme Court found confessional evidence from four Indigenous men was inadmissible as evidence in court because police failed to comply with the Custody Notification Service requirements under the legislation.

In 2013, former NSW attorney-general Greg Smith announced the O'Farrell government's commitment to these laws. Accordingly, if the service is abolished in practice by funding cuts but remains on the statute books – as it almost certainly will – the NSW government will be faced with the absurd but very real proposition that most confessional evidence from Indigenous people in custody will be rendered inadmissible because police cannot contact an Aboriginal Legal Service representative.

The federal government has regularly contested funding to the Custody Notification Service since 2012. In that year, funding to the service was cut and Aboriginal Legal Service staff were forced to perform unpaid work. They continued to operate the service on a voluntary basis. In 2013, funding to the phone line resumed.

However, requiring the service to operate through the charitable goodwill of its already overworked skeleton staff is an unreasonable and untenable demand.

Rather than abolishing this successful program, governments both state and federal should be implementing and funding more like it nationwide. Without the Custody Notification Service in NSW, deaths of Indigenous people in police custody will almost certainly increase, along with their over-representation in prison.

Eugene Schofield-Georgeson has worked as a Solicitor-Advocate for the North Australian Aboriginal Justice Agency (NAAJA) and is affiliated with the New South Wales Council for Civil Liberties (NSWCCL). Since the article was published, the author's details have changed: Lecturer, UTS Law School.

Q: What impact did the publication of your article have? Publication of my article led to a radio interview on Radio National that saw my message catapulted into broadsheet news and into discussions at the highest levels of government. It seemed that no-one had thought of the one specific consequence of this punitive Abbott Government policy, that I raised in my article, in relation to law and policing. That is, that because the Custody Notification System (CNS) is built into NSW criminal procedure law, its removal would effectively render the arrest of Indigenous people illegal. The article became an important part of the tremendous media campaign waged by the Aboriginal Legal Service (NSW) to save the CNS from funding cuts. Some months later, the campaign was ultimately successful.

Q: What would you like to see happen as a result of the #JustJustice series? I would like to see one copy of this edition provided to every State and Federal Attorney-General in the country.

Q: Would you like to provide a one-sentence quote about the #JustJustice project? 'Colonialism is thriving in contemporary Australia and nowhere more so than in our prisons and courts. This edition of #JustJustice forces us to rethink the punitive consequences of "whitefella" justice and calls for lawmakers to take immediate action across the country'.

Dying to be free: Where is the #JustJustice focus on the post-prison Indigenous deaths?

Author:	Megan Williams	Published:	November 03, 2016

Last week the Federal Government announced it would ask the Australian Law Reform Commission to examine the factors leading to the over-representation of Aboriginal and Torres Strait Islander people in our prison system, and consider what reforms to the law could "ameliorate this national tragedy".

In the post below, published as part of Croakey's #JustJustice series, Dr Megan Williams says any inquiry must urge better health care for Indigenous people while they are in prison – including the right to Medicare – and intensive support when they are first released.

Dr Megan Williams writes:

Amid calls for a new federal inquiry into the over-imprisonment of Aboriginal and Torres Strait Islander people to result in concrete actions, a more profound concern has rated barely a mention.

Many people may not realise that Aboriginal and Torres Strait Islander people are more likely to die in the days and weeks after release from prison than they are in custody, according to University of Melbourne researchers.

Where non-Indigenous people are more likely to be at risk of post-release death from accidental drug overdose, particularly opioids, Aboriginal and Torres Strait Islander people are more likely to die from alcohol-related harms, preventable health conditions and suicide. Opioid substation therapy has become more available for those who are drug dependent, and continuous from prison to the community as an effective way to reduce risk of post-release death. However, the same research attention to understanding and preventing Aboriginal and Torres Strait Islander peoples' post-release risks has not occurred, with few, if any, trials of alcohol or other interventions.

The majority of Aboriginal and Torres Strait Islander people in prison have been there before, often multiple times. High rates of re-incarceration and post-release death signal that they do not receive enough assistance under current programs and policies.

Jack Bulman, CEO of the well-recognised health promotion charity, Mibbinbah, recently collaborated on the design of health promotion program *Be the Best You Can Be* which accompanies the film *Mad Bastards*. He has worked with many men post-prison release and says "many get out of prison with very little support, money, plans, or hope."

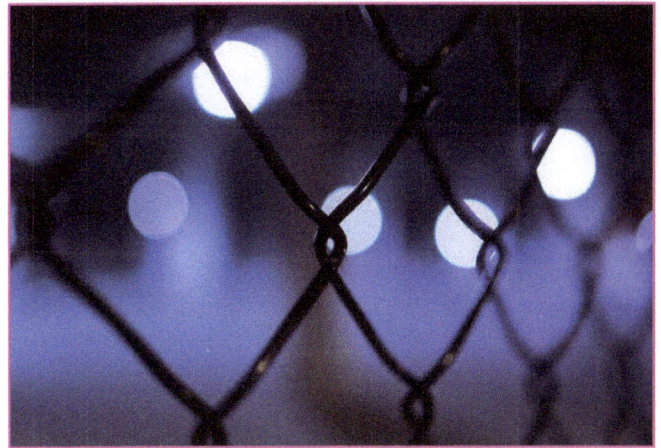

In-prison programs fail to address the disadvantage that many Aboriginal and Torres Strait Islander prisoners face, such as addiction, intergenerational and historical traumas, grief and loss. Programs have long waiting lists, and exclude those who spend many months on remand or serve short sentences – as Aboriginal and Torres Strait Islander people often do.

Instead, evidence shows that prison worsens mental health and wellbeing, damages relationships and families, and generates stigma which reduces employment and housing opportunities .

Some European countries, however, have achieved a dramatic reduction in prisoner numbers and harms.

To prevent post-release deaths, diversion from prison to alcohol and drug rehabilitation is recommended, which has proven more cost-effective and beneficial than prison. International evidence also recommends preparing families for the post-prison release phase.

Mibbinbah's work also shows that men's groups are a low-cost measure for prison-to-community continuity of care, and Elder engagement in prison programs has received overwhelmingly positive feedback.

The place where public health and criminal justice policies meet

Locally, evaluation of three *Returning Home* post-prison release pilot programs delivered by Aboriginal and Torres Strait Islander community-controlled health organisations found that intensive, coordinated care in the first hours, days, and weeks after release is required, along with strategies to better identify newly-released prisoners in clinical and program settings, to provide them with appropriate care.

However, for these improvements to occur, better integration between prisons and community-based services is required.

International human rights instruments assert that people in prison have the right to the same care in prison as they do in the community.

Prisons should be places where public health and criminal justice policies meet, particularly given that the overwhelming majority of people in prisons have addiction and mental health issues.

But because prisoners have no right to Medicare, Aboriginal and Torres Strait Islander people in prison have reduced access to the types of comprehensive primary healthcare available in the community, including health assessments, care plans and social and emotional wellbeing programs.

Instead, providing such healthcare in prisons comes at an additional cost to community organisations, if it is done at all.

The Public Health Association of Australia and the Australian Medical Association have called on the Australian Government for prisoners to retain their right to Medicare.

Renewed attention to bring about this change will enable continuity of care between prison and the community, which is vital for preventing post-release deaths.

Waiting until after prison is too late.

Dr Megan Williams is a member of the #JustJustice team, a Senior Research Fellow at the Aboriginal Health and Wellbeing Research team at Western Sydney University, a Mibbinbah research collaborator, and a descendant of the Wiradjuri people of the NSW Riverine.

4. Indigenous leadership

" We need a national conversation that recognises and celebrates the strengths of Aboriginal and Torres Strait Islander peoples and communities

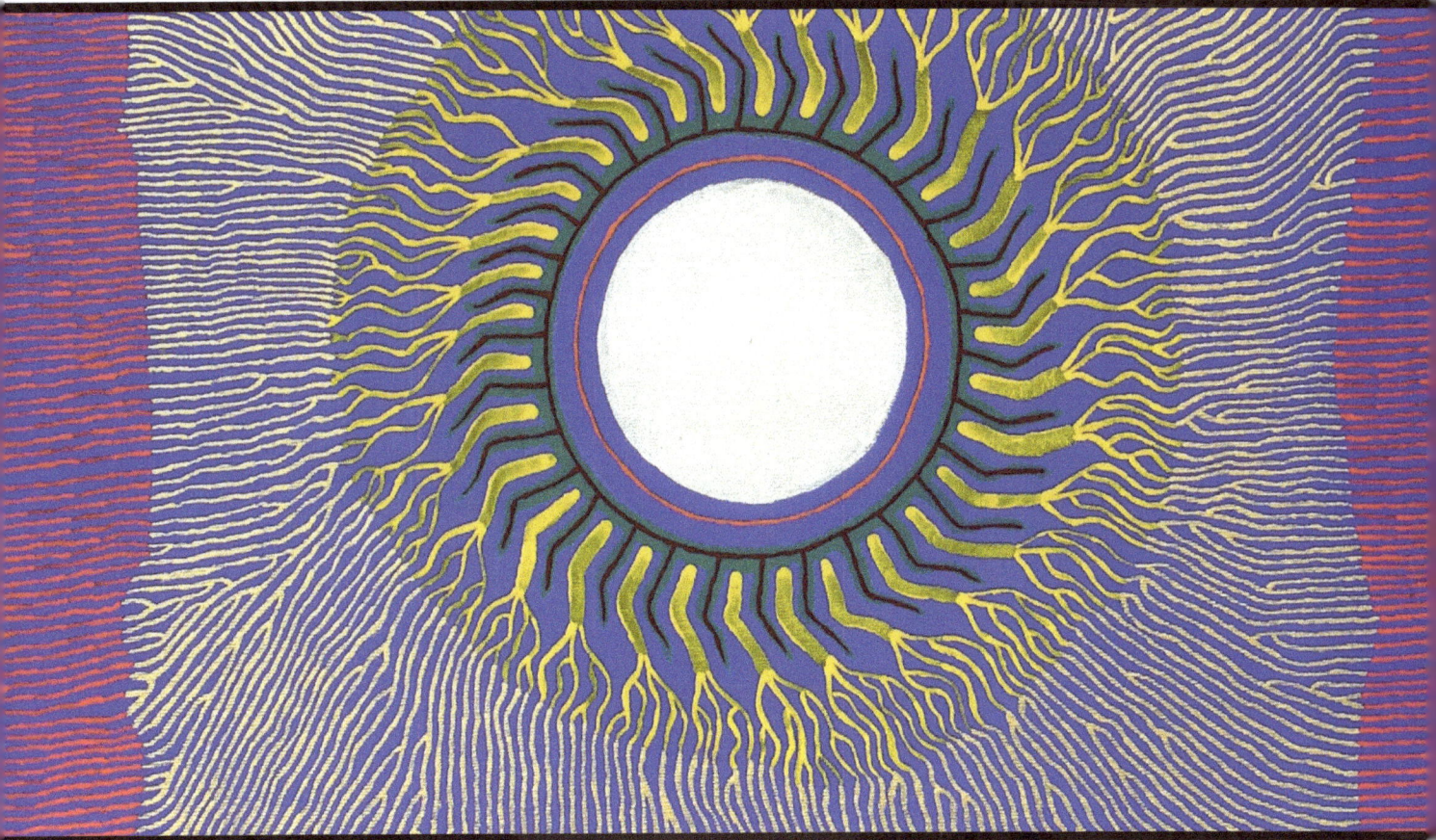

Let's work together to Change the Record on Indigenous prison, violence rates

Author:	Shane Duffy and Kirstie Parker	Published:	July 20, 2015

'Smarter justice, safer communities' is the headline objective for the Change the Record campaign, launched earlier this year by the National Justice Coalition, a group of leading Aboriginal and Torres Strait Islander, community and human rights organisations.

In this article below, the Coalition's **Shane Duffy and Kirstie Parker** outline the Change the Record blueprint for addressing over-imprisonment rates for Aboriginal and Torres Strait Islander people – arguing that the solutions lie in building communities, not prisons, and in smarter criminal justice policies that treat the causes of over-incarceration, not just the symptoms.

An early goal is to convince the Federal Government to commit to measurable justice targets in the Closing of the Gap Strategy and plans on how to achieve them.

Shane Duffy and Kirstie Parker write:

Earlier this month was NAIDOC week, a time in which we celebrate Aboriginal and Torres Strait Islander history, culture and achievement. The week was filled with powerful events honouring the many Aboriginal and Torres Strait Islander people who make important contributions to our communities and Australian society as a whole. We have much to celebrate in the resilience and diversity of Aboriginal and Torres Strait Islander people and culture. There was, however, a heavy shadow for us during the week: the imprisonment and violence rates that are growing exponentially and which are devastating our communities.

Much has been written recently about the over-representation of Aboriginal and Torres Strait Islander people as both offenders and victims/survivors in the criminal justice system. Social Justice Commissioner Mick Gooda has said it is "one of the most urgent human rights issues facing Australia". But while the issue is well known, less attention has been paid to addressing the underlying causes.

Earlier this year the National Justice Coalition, a group of leading Aboriginal and Torres Strait Islander, community and human rights organisations came together to launch a blueprint for changing the record. We argued that the solutions lie in building communities, not prisons, and in smarter criminal justice policies that treat the causes, not just the symptoms.

Prisons have been shown to be extremely costly, damaging and ultimately ineffective at reducing crime. Underlying socio-economic disadvantage such as poverty, poor education, drug and alcohol abuse, and disability are the hallmark of crime and imprisonment. In recent years, state governments have **compounded these issues through the use of tough 'law and order' policies, such as the expansion of mandatory sentencing which has contributed to unacceptable prison numbers and violence in communities. We believe the solutions lie in addressing this disadvantage and developing smarter criminal justice policies**.

At the time of the Royal Commission into Aboriginal Deaths in Custody, Aboriginal and Torres Strait Islander people were being imprisoned at a rate 7 times higher than the non-Indigenous population. Today, almost 25 years later, that figure has increased to 13 times. At the same time, Aboriginal and Torres Strait Islander women are currently being hospitalised for family violence related assault at 34 times the rate of non-Indigenous women. It is long past time that we took action to change our country's record on this issue.

It's time for us to take a different approach to crime and public safety and how it is best achieved.

Evidence clearly demonstrates that strong, healthy communities are the most effective way to prevent crime and make communities safe. Every dollar spent on prisons is one less dollar available to invest in reducing social and economic disadvantage through education, health, disability, housing, employment and other programs.

Government funding should instead be reinvested into early intervention, prevention and diversion initiatives that address the underlying root causes of crime, and can break the cycle of imprisonment and violence. It is also vital that government works in partnership with Aboriginal and

Torres Strait Islander people, communities, services and their representatives, to develop and implement solutions. Directly affected people are best placed to identify local issues in their communities, and develop and implement localised, tailored solutions.

Reducing Aboriginal and Torres Strait Islander peoples' rates of imprisonment and experience of violence will take a joint effort by communities, organisations and governments. However, there is reason for optimism. The strength of the National Justice Coalition is that it consists of a broad range of organisations that have the experience and expertise to identify what the solutions are and work with the public, Aboriginal and Torres Strait Islander communities and government to implement them.

The National Justice Coalition's 'Change the Record' campaign is calling on all levels of government to work together to address this issue. We have two overarching aims – to close the gap in rates of imprisonment by 2040; and to cut the disproportionate rates of violence to at least close the gap by 2040, with priority strategies for women and children. A welcome first step would be for the federal government to exercise critical leadership by committing to measurable justice targets in the Closing of the Gap Strategy and plans on how these will targets be achieved.

We are asking all Australians to stand with us. We know the issues and we know the solutions. We all want to live in safe and strong communities. Work with us and together we can Change the Record.

Every dollar spent on prisons is one less dollar available to invest in reducing social and economic disadvantage through education, health, disability, housing, employment and other programs

Shane Duffy is chair of the National Aboriginal and Torres Strait Islander Legal Services. At the time of writing this article, Kirstie Parker was co-chair of the National Congress of Australia's First Peoples.

To find out more about the National Justice Coalition's 'Change the Record' campaign go to: www.changetherecord.org.au

Aboriginal and Torres Strait Islander research leadership is critical for #JustJustice

Author:	Megan Williams	Published:	May 10, 2016

Aboriginal and Torres Strait Islander research leadership is fundamental to breaking the cycle of the over-incarceration of Aboriginal and Torres Strait Islander people, according to Dr Megan Williams, a Senior Research Fellow at the Aboriginal Health and Wellbeing Research team at Western Sydney University and a descendant of the Wiradjuri people of the NSW Riverine.

Governments will become more accountable to communities and taxpayers when Aboriginal and Torres Strait Islander researchers help to lead governments' evaluations of their legislation, policies and programs, and help to undertake continuous quality improvements within services, she says.

Williams says that prisoners, victims of crime and taxpayers will benefit from reduced incarceration rates when governments implement the evidence on Aboriginal and Torres Strait Islander peoples' approaches to holistic health care, develop collective healing programs and address the underlying determinants of incarceration, such as poverty.

Megan Williams writes:

Mounting international evidence now shows that incarceration contributes to still more incarceration. Incarceration causes poor health and wellbeing, which erodes an individual's social and economic capacity to integrate into the community post-prison release.

Evidence also suggests that whole communities are damaged when their members are incarcerated, and that one of the biggest risk factors for incarceration is juvenile detention, which itself is influenced by parental history of incarceration. In Australia, the underlying reasons for incarceration can be prevented and addressed such as through community-based support programs.

Countless times Aboriginal and Torres Strait Islander people have shed light on 'what works' to reduce 'acts intended to cause injury', 'unlawful entry with intent', sexual assault, driver licence offences, and breaches of state orders for which Aboriginal and Torres Strait Islander people are often imprisoned. Aboriginal and Torres Strait Islander people have participated in program design and delivery, policy development and critique, research, advocacy and government advisory committee roles to address these issues.

The types of strategies and evidence that Aboriginal and Torres Strait Islander people believe work seem to have been selectively ignored by successive Australian federal and state governments over the past decades.

Gaps in evidence and action

Overwhelmingly missing too are governments' own contributions to an evidence base. Very little evaluation has occurred of their legislative, policy and program directives in the criminal justice system. The doubling in prison rates of Aboriginal and Torres Strait Islander peoples over 10 years is sure evidence of the failure of current approaches.

Data about prison populations and re-incarceration rates are poorly reported, and information about post-prison release outcomes is almost entirely missing – despite data on all these issues being routinely collected through criminal justice system administration processes. Intersectoral collaboration is often called for to prevent crime and promote the well-being of Aboriginal and Torres Strait Islander people, however very little reporting on intersections between government departments to improve justice outcomes has occurred.

Instead of governments indicating how they are improving the implementation and evaluation of their own legal and policy responsibilities, they again ask Aboriginal and Torres Strait Islander leaders and service providers, "What do you think should be done?"

But the implementation of Aboriginal and Torres Strait Islander people's solutions has been extremely limited. Bureaucrats argue they need more evidence to support what Aboriginal and Torres Strait Islander people recommend, stating 'Our hands are tied until you can do so'.

The desired 'gold standard' evidence, gathered through assessment instruments, 'Indigenised' surveys and one-off intervention testing might elsewhere be revered as objective and reliable, but often inadequately represent Aboriginal and Torres Strait Islander peoples' worldviews, experiences and knowledge about 'what works'.

What works for Aboriginal and Torres Strait Islander peoples has been available since the origins of the new Australian nation. Founding leaders of Australia's legal, health and welfare systems had an opportunity to build on Indigenous knowledges about how they had maintained individual and collective well-being, without prisons or intergenerational poverty.

Instead, the perception of Aboriginal and Torres Strait Islander peoples as inferior humans seems to have prevailed, perpetuated by government policies of segregation from and later assimilation into Western culture within the last 100 years.

Racism is a daily experience for many Aboriginal and Torres Strait Islander people. The lack of parity with the mainstream population in education, employment, income or parliamentary representation clearly signals that discriminatory policies persist.

While the federal Parliament may have formally apologised to the Stolen Generations for past policies of forced child removal, no obvious amendments have been made. Instead, evidence now shows higher child removal rates than ever before, thus perpetuating a cycle of disadvantage and trauma. These are the types of root causes of incarceration that require addressing, which often underscore the reasons for which individual Aboriginal and Torres Strait Islander people are arrested and sentenced.

Perhaps the most extreme example of evidence being ignored relates to socio-economic disadvantage, with the key underlying factor for over-incarceration of Aboriginal and Torres Strait Islander people being poverty. Regardless of cultural identity as Indigenous, similar rates of incarceration are seen among other impoverished people around the world.

Addressing the accountability gap

Selective use of evidence, overlooking the root causes of incarceration, and ignoring Aboriginal and Torres Strait Islander people's evidence all contribute to lack of accountability, and lack of progress.

To make progress, investment in Aboriginal and Torres Strait Islander research leadership to establish a more robust evidence base is urgently required.

Australia's National Aboriginal and Torres Strait Islander Health Research Institute, the Lowitja Institute, privileges Indigenous research approaches, and draws on a wide range of research tools necessary to understand complex health issues and determinants of health, including criminal justice system engagement.

Aboriginal and Torres Strait Islander researchers can help lead governments' evaluations of their legislation, policies and programs, to improve accountability.

They can also undertake continuous quality improvements within services, partner with non-Indigenous organisations, and build the capacity of other researchers and policy makers to more respectfully take into account cultural protocols, values and perspectives.

Expanding the evidence on Aboriginal and Torres Strait Islander peoples' approaches to holistic health care, developing collective healing programs and addressing underlying determinants will be benefit anyone in the criminal justice system – prisoners, victims and taxpayers included.

Founding leaders of Australia's legal, health and welfare systems had an opportunity to build on Indigenous knowledges about how they had maintained individual and collective well-being, without prisons or intergenerational poverty

Dr Megan Williams is a Senior Research Fellow at the Aboriginal Health and Wellbeing Research team at Western Sydney University. Through her father's family she is a descendent of the Wiradjuri people of the NSW riverine. She has worked for 20 years in community health, evaluation and research, and completed a PhD investigating the role of social support to prevent re-incarceration among urban Aboriginal people.

Help change the conversations around Aboriginal health, with some #JustJustice

| Author: | Summer May Finlay | Published: | April 16, 2015 |

The over-incarceration of Aboriginal and Torres Strait Islander Peoples is a profound threat to the health and wellbeing of communities, families and individuals, according to Summer May Finlay, a Yorta Yorta woman who works in Aboriginal health and is a PhD candidate.

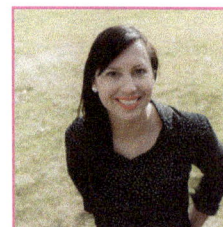

In the article below, Finlay encourages Croakey readers to engage with the #JustJustice crowdfunding campaign.

Summer May Finlay writes:

The majority of Aboriginal and Torres Strait Islander people never end up coming in contact with the law; however, for those who do, the justice system can start a vicious cycle of incarceration.

This is a critical public health issue that is causing great harm to individuals, their families and their communities.

To create a fairer justice system, we need governments and policymakers to work much harder at preventing people from becoming part of the cycle of incarceration.

We need some policies to stop, like mandatory detention now in place in the Northern Territory and Western Australia, and we need to support the wider use of programs like Justice Reinvestment and the Koori Courts.

We need strong national action, through measures like Justice Targets under Closing the Gap, and an end to the piecemeal approach that now prevails across the different jurisdictions.

We need politicians and people who work in the justice system to have a better understanding of the role that social issues like racism, poverty and disadvantage play in contributing to over-incarceration.

Change the conversation

And we also need to shift our public conversations about Aboriginal and Torres Strait Islander peoples.

I really want to make sure that when we're actually talking about justice, that we're actually talking about it from our perspective, and we're actually looking at what's really happening

I know from my own experience there is a profound disconnect from the way the media describes Aboriginal and Torres Strait Islander people to my own lived experience of our strengths.

Whenever I read about Aboriginal and Torres Strait Islander people, it's almost like it's a bad thing. I'm a proud Aboriginal person, I love being Aboriginal, and I couldn't imagine ever being anything but an Aboriginal person.

We need a national conversation that recognises and celebrates the strengths of Aboriginal and Torres Strait Islander peoples and communities.

I've had the luxury of travelling to communities around Australia, and I see these strong, passionate, caring, generous peoples. I don't see that reality reflected in the way we're described in the media.

If people actually got to know Aboriginal Peoples as a collective, they'd realise that we're a hell of a lot more than what you see in the media.

I hope the #JustJustice series will help the wider Australian community to understand the wide-ranging impacts of over-incarceration, which is fracturing our peoples, our cultures, our communities.

The story I want to see told is how over-incarceration is hurting us as Peoples. We've had so much that is being stolen or lost already. I don't want to see people having to have more taken from them than they already have.

I hope this series will help encourage a better informed conversation. A lot of people don't really understand the issues, don't really understand the history, don't really understand what Aboriginal and Torres Strait people are going through, and have gone through.

A series of articles at Croakey is a significant opportunity to help change attitudes and beliefs.

Think of the young people

One of the reasons why I'm passionate about this issue is that I used to be a youth and children's worker. I used to watch people treat these amazingly beautiful children like they weren't worth very much because they came from significantly disadvantaged backgrounds.

I'd really like to see these children growing up and doing whatever it is they want to do. But at the moment, they often don't feel like they can achieve what it is they want to achieve.

We are supposedly a lucky country but for a lot of these kids, it's not a lucky country. That's what motivates me, these young ones, they're so intelligent and they're so beautiful, and yet you know they never think they can do what they want to do.

I'm excited by the potential for the #JustJustice series to help tell the wider community about the stories that I see, the stories that actually reflect the true reality of what it is to be Aboriginal and to be part of an Aboriginal community.

I really want to make sure that when we're actually talking about justice, that we're actually talking about it from our perspective, and we're actually looking at what's really happening.

I came up with the hashtag for this series, #JustJustice, because it encapsulates where we need to be aiming.

If you would like to contribute to #JustJustice, please visit our Pozible campaign and consider supporting it – whether by donating or helping to spread the word.

See Summer May Finlay talk more about her passion for #JustJustice here.

Summer May Finlay is a Yorta Yorta woman who grew up on Lake Macquarie near Newcastle. She has worked in Aboriginal affairs for over 10 years and currently works in Aboriginal Health. Summer has a Bachelor of Social Science with a Linguistic Major, Master of Public Health with a Social Marketing Major and is just about to embark on a PhD. She has a passion for Aboriginal affairs and social justice.

Hearing from communities and experts with solutions for #JustJustice

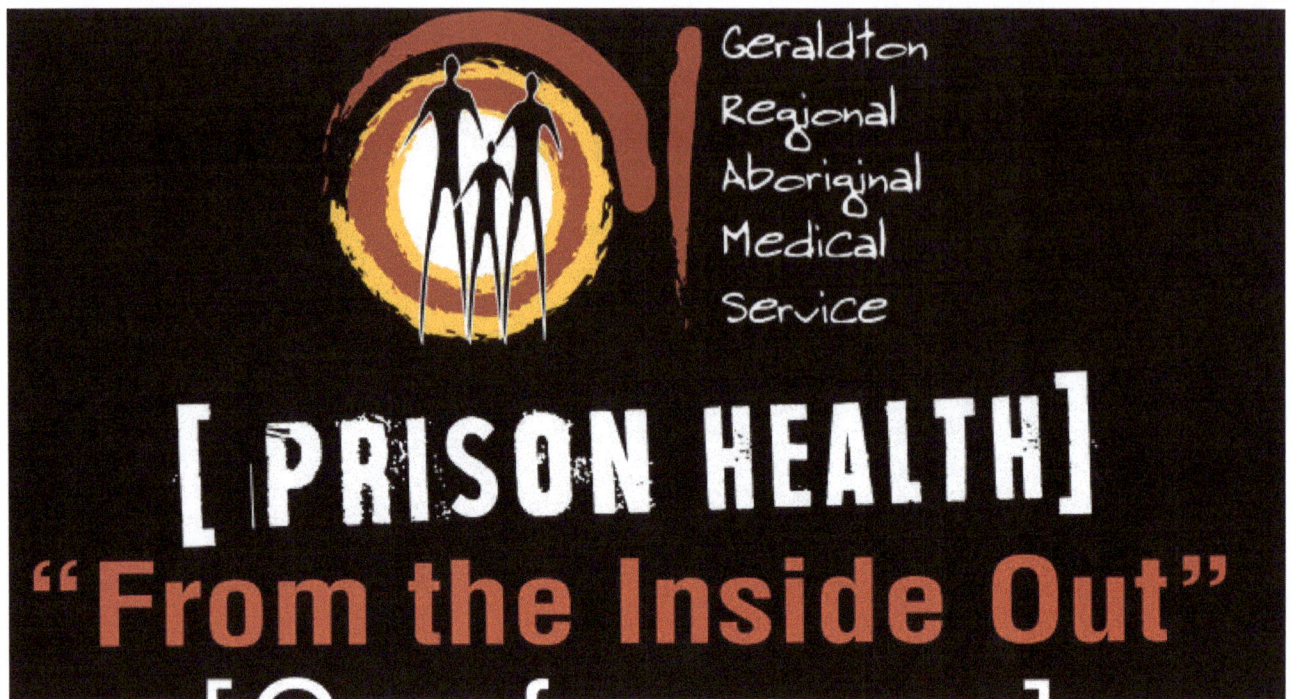

| Author: | Marie McInerney | Published: | April 10, 2015 |

The need for effective solutions to the "**public health catastrophe**" of the over-incarceration of Aboriginal and Torres Strait Islander people was highlighted at a conference held this week in Geraldton, WA.

Marie McInerney reports:

Below are some of the ideas generated by nearly 100 policy and frontline experts in Indigenous health and justice who met this week at the **Prison Health: From the Inside Out** conference in Geraldton.

- Stop jailing Aboriginal people with cognitive disabilities.

- Add justice to the national Close the Gap targets.

- Keep offenders in their own communities, close to ties.

- Reform visiting times. Make sure all prisoners are able to contact their families and communities at least once a month.

- Shut down the drug dealers in regional areas.

- Evaluate what we do. Listen to what we say.

- Set up a community fund to pay fines and let offenders pay them off in cultural ways – empowering not punitive.

- Improve the quality of justice data available.

- No one-size-fits-all solutions: local responses to local issues.

The two day event, staged by the Geraldton Regional Aboriginal Medical Service (GRAMS), brought together delegates from Broome to Albany, as well as high profile speakers like Aboriginal and Torres Strait Islander Social Justice Commissioner Mick Gooda and National Aboriginal Community Controlled Health Organisation CEO Lisa Briggs and chair Matthew Cooke.

The conference looked at the health issues for Aboriginal and Torres Strait Islander people before, during and after prison, and at disadvantage and racism within the justice system that not only affects health but, as Gooda put it, "makes us sick".

The speakers laid out the statistics:

- Indigenous people, who make up 2.5 per cent of the total population, make up 25 per cent of the prisoner population (80 per cent in the Northern Territory) and are 14 times more likely to end up in jail.

- Indigenous women are the fastest growing prison population group in Australia, having risen 58 per cent over the ten years to 2010.

- 90 per cent of young people in out of home care in the Northern Territory are Aboriginal.

- Aboriginal and Torres Strait Islander people are over-represented at the 'lower end' of the crime scale, most often jailed for fines, on 'three strike' policies, and for public order offences. In WA, up to 60 per cent of Aboriginal people are in jail for driving offences.

There are, as the conference heard, complex reasons behind these statistics, from colonisation and intergenerational trauma to inappropriate policing, family breakdown and drug and alcohol abuse.

But too often our justice responses are too shallow and/or blunt.

"We have to change the way we do justice"

For example, criminologist Professor Harry Blagg outlined his research from the Northern Territory between 2010 and 2013, in the wake of the NT Intervention, looking at the impact of tougher legislation and increased police numbers.

"Despite heavy rhetoric about saving Aboriginal women and children from sexual violence, paedophile rings, all this emotive language, we found no increase whatsoever in the rate of arrest for family violence or notifications of child abuse, despite in some cases a tripling of the number of police," he said.

"What we did find was a 250 per cent increase in the rate of arrests for driving offences. (Police would) go into communities, and do what they do elsewhere: check the cars, check the drivers. So a lot of people were ending up in prison (for those)."

Blagg also warned that the recent case of Rosie Fulton – a young women with foetal alcohol syndrome disorder (FASD) who was held in a WA prison for 21 months with no conviction after a magistrate found her unfit to stand trial – was not unique.

Failure to deal with mounting evidence that young Aboriginal people are more likely to be affected by disorders such as FASD and Acquired Brain Injury (ABI) risked "undermining our justice system," he said. Blagg said he knew of magistrates and prosecutors who were "encouraging people with FASD to plead guilty because otherwise they would be considered unfit to plead."

He said:

" Our system of justice is based on the premise that we understand what we're doing, we can make rational decisions, so we can be deterred by the prospect of being punished. In court, if you're on the FASD spectrum or have another cognitive impairment, you can't make those rational judgments.

We have to change the way we do justice, integrating health, mental health and disability services at the front end of the criminal justice system.

In his keynote speech, Gooda said he had run out of adjectives to describe the rate and impact of Indigenous incarceration – "disaster, emergency, a catastrophe in the making" – and he would make it, and the issue of community violence, particularly against women, his priority for this, his last two-year term.

So too, he said, should the Federal Government, given its Budget concern: getting Indigenous incarceration rates down to population level would mean an $800 million saving per year in prison costs.

Texas, and other US states, had shifted away from 'tough on crime' policies because they could no longer afford the prison costs, and adopted Justice Reinvestment approaches, he said.

Gooda said there were plenty of examples of success across the country – not least in the inner-Sydney suburb of Redfern where good dialogue between police and the local community had seen an 80 per cent drop in robberies committed by Aboriginal youth, helping to make it "the safest inner city suburb in Sydney".

Barriers to fairer justice

But the Prison Health conference also heard of many barriers and backward steps, at national and local levels including:

- Moves to establish accommodation for young offenders in Geraldton who would otherwise be held far from family and country in Perth were opposed on "real estate values" by the local non-Indigenous community.

- Conditions are still "appalling" at the Roebourne prison, with prisoners sleeping in unventilated tin sheds in fierce heat more than 15 years after concerns were first raised by the WA Office of the Inspector of Custodial Services. There is no local housing for them when they are released, and the local health services are overloaded (one health worker had a caseload of 300) and struggle to get ex-prisoners to engage. "Help me make it better," she pleaded.

- With $10 for a bottle of milk in some areas, food security is expected to loom as a justice issue.

- Plans to close remote WA communities will put further pressure on the justice system, if communities end up living on fringes of existing towns.

- Geraldton's Barndimalgu Court – Australia's first specialist Indigenous family violence court – was defunded this year for not showing "statistically significant" improvement on mainstream court outcomes, in a decision that overlooked other aims of the project.

Where to from here?

GRAMS chair Sandy Davies was insistent throughout the conference that it was aimed at producing action and solutions, and had to come up with at least half a dozen trials he could put on the ground locally by end June.

Those ideas are still to be finessed, but the meeting explored a range of broader potential directions too:

- Gooda agreed with one delegate that the conference may not have been necessary had governments implemented all the findings of the Royal Commission into Aboriginal Deaths in Custody. He said exploring accountability on that could also be one of his final pieces of work as Commissioner.

- Blagg said he would follow up the concern by delegates for research into the "knock-on effect" on families and communities from growing imprisonment of Indigenous women prisoners – and no doubt on Federal Government "safe community" priorities.

- University of Western Australia researcher Craig Cumming asked for stronger input from frontline organisations in the Health In Prisoners in Australia (HIP-Aus) Project, which will aim to diminish recidivism through health policy and expects to have the largest ever prisoner health cohort ever, globally. "We are always looking for collaboration to inform baseline statistics on health issues, we need culturally appropriate interventions as well," he said.

- And, after some heated debate on how to structure such a body, the meeting agreed to set up a taskforce to progress the issues, with deep local roots but focused also on national change.

Croakey thanks Sandy Davies and the staff and management at the Geraldton Regional Aboriginal Medical Service for inviting Croakey to attend, and covering flight and accommodation costs. Croakey also thanks GRAMS for supporting our #JustJustice crowdfunding campaign.

Why won't Australian leaders embrace Aboriginal and Torres Strait Islander solutions to the criminal justice crisis?

| Author: | Megan Williams | Published: | October 20, 2016 |

The breadth and depth of work being done by Aboriginal and Torres Strait Islander people and organisations to address incarceration and related issues was profiled at a recent conference, reports Dr Megan Williams for the #JustJustice project.

Megan Williams writes:

Aboriginal and Torres Strait Islander peoples' actions to address disproportionately high rates of criminal justice system contact and incarceration were profiled during the inaugural Closing the Prison Gap: Cultural Resilience Conference, recently held in northern NSW.

A majority of presenters were First Peoples, guided by Bundjalung woman Rebecca Couch as MC, and Dr Meg Perkins as conference initiator and coordinator.

Conference attendance was at capacity, with 150 registrants from around Australia meeting at Kingscliff on Cudjingburra country within the Bundjalung Nation. The welcome on both days by Traditional Owners included leader Kyle Slabb reflecting on his mob's vision for a healthy future, with dancers connecting their stories to the local landscape.

Children and families

The first conference theme on children and families was opened by Professor Muriel Bamblett, Yorta Yorta woman and CEO of the Victorian Aboriginal Child Care Agency, who described *Alternatives to Child Removal* including leadership, healing and diversionary programs.

Kaiyu Moura Bayles, a Wonnarua, Wirri and Wakka Wakka woman spoke about *Learning the Old Ways*, and Inspiring Positive Change and contributed also through her family presence and poetry.

Michelle Laurie, a Gummbaingirr woman and Rebecca Blore, Anaiwan woman discussed their *Brighter Futures, Supporting Families* work, and Natasha Mace shared her powerful story and the *Hymba Yumba Community Hub*.

Professor Ross Homel, from the Griffith Criminology Institute, explained the decade-long *Creating Pathways to Prevention* program, and sparked discussion on the need for strong partnerships in programs and research to privilege the voices of local people.

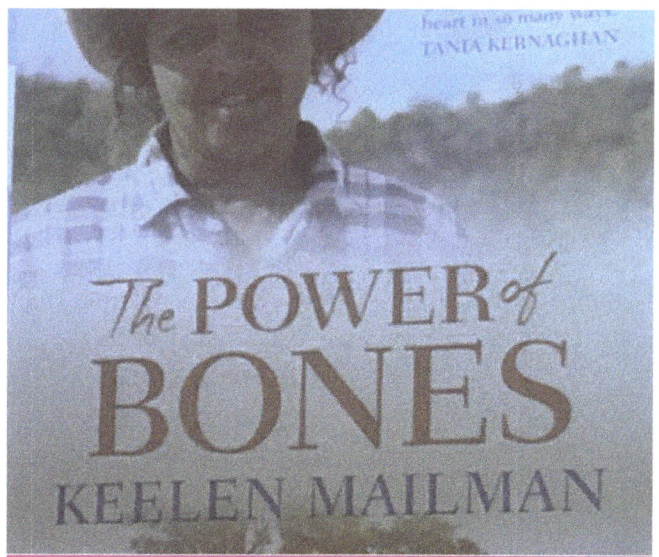

Profiling cultural resilience

Prisons and post release

The second session focussed on prisons and post-release community reintegration. Therese Ellis-Smith, a Bond University PhD candidate, overviewed *Offender Programs*, and Professor Joe Graffam of Deakin University discussed *Enhancing Employment Opportunities* post-incarceration.

Mervyn Eades, Nyoongar man and Eddie Mabo Social Justice Award winner, explained successful features of the *Ngalla Maya* prison-to-work program, including developing trusting relationships with ex-prisoners.

Focussing on children, Bond University researcher Dr Bruce Watt noted that very few in Queensland are assessed for *Fitness to Stand Trial*, despite high proportions thought to have intellectual disabilities or other issues impeding understanding of charges and trials.

Dr Janet Hammill, Gamilaraay woman from the University of Queensland, provided compelling information connecting *Foetal Alcohol Spectrum Disorder* with risks for criminal justice system contact.

Dadirri and healing

We began the second day with Ken Zulumovski and Carolyn Minchin from Gamarada Indigenous Healing and Life Training leading singing and mindful, deep listening – Dadirri.

Catherine Jackson Gidgup, from Gamarada, Yarn Australia and Grandmothers Against Removals spoke about her healing journey, and also supporting others.

Lara Bennett, a Wiradjuri woman and Deirdre Currie, Minjungbal/Nunduwal woman, International Women's Day Award Winners, outlined their well-evaluated *Kids Caring for Country and Learning our Way* Program.

Gayle Munn, Gunggari woman and Robert Lacey, Waka Waka man spoke about their *Lateral Peace Project* including healing from intergenerational trauma and strengthening connections to identity and country.

Our connection to country was deepened by beautiful images and stories of the *Mount Tabor Station Healing and Rehabilitation Centre* planned by Keelen Mailman, Bidjara woman, author of The Power of Bones and Mother of the Year winner, and Keith Hamburger, ex-Director of the Queensland Corrective Services Commission.

Underlying factors

The final session sharpened its focus on underlying factors for incarceration. Beginning with Chris Lee, the innovative *University of Southern Queensland's Education in a Box Program* overcomes complex system barriers to connect prisoners to tertiary education preparation and qualifications.

Gerry Georgatos from the Institute for *Social Justice and Human Rights* in WA received a standing ovation for his analysis of data revealing far greater rates of suicide among Australia's First Peoples compared to other countries, and for his research supporting prisoners to complete education qualifications and prevent re-incarceration.

Professor Harry Blagg from the University of WA presented on *Colonial Dispossession: Postcolonial Perspectives on the Criminal Justice System*, tracing how incarceration can be seen as extending colonial oppression, including through lack of action to rectify inequity.

Following this, my own presentation on *Aboriginal and Torres Strait Islander Peoples' Research Leadership* ended with a call for investigations into governments' own accountability to meet policy commitments.

NAIDOC Lifetime Achievement Award Winner Tauto Sansbury linked all the themes together, explaining his own journey and how barriers to Self-determination and Treaty contribute to incarceration.

The Aboriginal and Torres Strait Islander-led programs all reported high levels of engagement, access, capacity building and retention of Aboriginal and Torres Strait Islander peoples, as well as integration with other services, cultural-sensitivity and high numbers of Aboriginal and Torres Strait Islander staff.

In contrast, mainstream government and community agencies instead report struggling to achieve these, despite their funding and targets. These shortcomings seem essentially to occur because of a lack of trust for Aboriginal and Torres Strait Islander peoples, manifested by government control of programming, funding, data management and relationships.

Treaty

We talked about Treaty and how it would demand a new relationship with First Peoples, with accountabilities in law.

Mainstream Australia could benefit; it is itself suffering high rates of obesity, suicide, loneliness and alcohol-related harm.

A Treaty envisions all that Aboriginal and Torres Strait Islander cultures have to offer – holistic, integrated care, collective family and community healing, and a responsible orientation toward multiculturalism and environmental protection for future generations.

Cultural resilience was never in question.

But the question remains: **Why won't Australian leaders embrace Aboriginal and Torres Strait Islander solutions to the criminal justice crisis, and demand better efforts to address racism?**

Perhaps this will be the theme of the 2017 Closing the Prison Gap gathering?

Dr Megan Williams is a member of the #JustJustice team, a Senior Research Fellow at the Aboriginal Health and Wellbeing Research team at Western Sydney University, and a descendant of the Wiradjuri people of the NSW Riverine.

> *Why won't Australian leaders embrace Aboriginal and Torres Strait Islander solutions to the criminal justice crisis, and demand better efforts to address racism?*

An honest examination of our history could help heal the wounds contributing to over-incarceration

University of Sydney @Sydney_Uni · Nov 2
Charles Perkins started the fire in the belly: we need to reignite it.
#50back50forward bit.ly/2fgTXF0

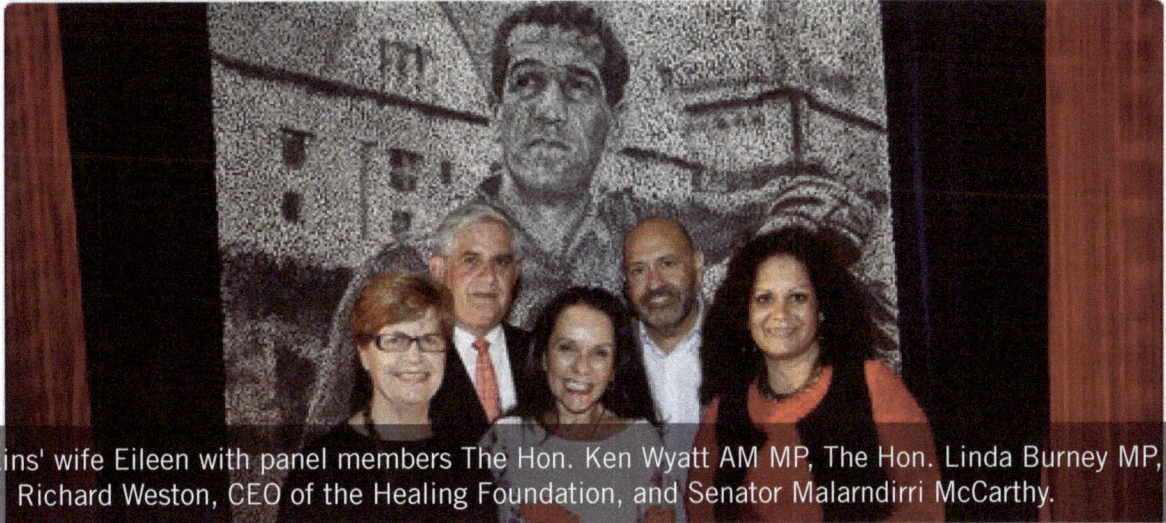

Dr Perkins' wife Eileen with panel members The Hon. Ken Wyatt AM MP, The Hon. Linda Burney MP, Richard Weston, CEO of the Healing Foundation, and Senator Malarndirri McCarthy.

| Author: | Richard Weston | Published: | November 04, 2016 |

Australia must deal with the unfinished business of the Stolen Generations through telling the truth of our history, according to Richard Weston, CEO of the Healing Foundation, and a descendant of the Meriam people of the Torres Strait.

It is only through a honest and honourable examination of Australia's history that we can heal the wounds that are contributing to the over-incarceration of Aboriginal and Torres Strait Islander people, he writes in this contribution to Croakey's #JustJustice series.

This process can start with revisiting the recommendations of the Bringing Them Home report in the context of the current policy landscape, particularly given ongoing concerns around high suicide rates, over-incarceration and removal of children, he says.

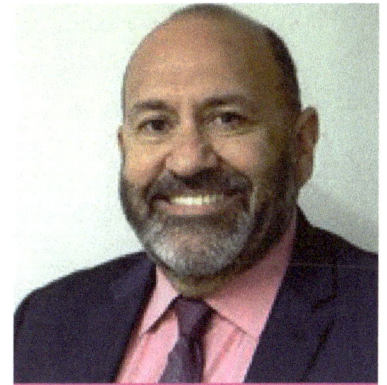

Richard Weston

Richard Weston writes:

The last 50 years have seen some amazing gains – the 1967 Referendum, land rights, better access to education.

We are seeing improved employment outcomes and many of our people are working across a range of industries and public services. We see emerging Aboriginal and Torres Strait Islander businesses and entrepreneurs.

We excel in many sports and increasingly our voices are heard in Parliaments in Australia and our own media organisations and journalists producing stories and current affairs of concern to us. Our arts community tell our stories and our experiences in dance, song, film, theatre and art. There is so much to be positive about.

On the other hand, as the 4 Corners Don Dale story showed, we still have a long way to go in areas of juvenile justice, out of home care and adult justice systems. We are over-represented in these systems.

In many of our families and communities there is a crisis of suicide, with some jurisdictions and regions reporting rates comparable to the highest in the world.

Aboriginal and Torres Strait Islander young people aged 15-24 years are 5 times more likely to suicide than their non-Indigenous peers; efforts to close the gap in life expectancy are not proceeding at a pace that will meet the 2030 target date.

Creating great futures

To create a great future for Aboriginal and Torres Strait Islanders 50 years hence, we cannot knowingly overlook the unfinished business of our Stolen Generations today.

If we overlook the Stolen Generations experience, we ignore the legacy of trauma that drives so much of our peoples' over-representation in the criminal justice systems, the levels of violence in our communities, child abuse and the ever-increasing crises of suicide.

In spite of the challenges we face, we do have an opportunity to imagine and create a great future for Aboriginal and Torres Strait Islander people.

But it has to be founded on a bedrock of truth and just action.

We need to act now. If we do not revisit the Bringing Them Home Report – reassess and address the recommendations in that report in the contemporary Aboriginal and Torres Strait Islander affairs landscape, I shudder to think of the wound we will inflict on the spirit and soul of this nation's future.

I believe that the progress we have made can be the springboard for us to address current challenges and tackle unfinished business. This is not just a job for Aboriginal and Torres Strait Islander families and communities alone. It needs the engagement of all Australians.

We have the opportunity to collectively address the truth of Australia's history and the impact on Aboriginal and Torres Strait Islanders.

A proper national healing process that engages all Australians could unfold and draw us together into a process of truth telling and reconciliation.

We can think of it as it was recently described by Professor Shane Houston, the Deputy Vice-Chancellor (Indigenous Strategy and Services) at the University of Sydney: 'There is no

one silver bullet...there is no substitute for a comprehensive, embedded strategy backed up by real commitment and the hard work that follows in implementation.'

We have to be inspired to believe that in spite of the myriad current day challenges and unfinished business, we can be optimistic and buoyant about the future.

To find this inspiration we have only to look to our own past – 60,000 years of culture and tradition – our own heroes in our own ongoing story.

We can use icons and leaders like Charlie Perkins to inspire us. We can look into our own families for inspiration. I look to my mother – Thelma – who left school after grade 7, worked all her life, raised five children, made sure they all got an education and is still working full time at 80 years of age.

> *We have to be inspired to believe that in spite of the myriad current day challenges and unfinished business, we can be optimistic and buoyant about the future*

Amazing survival

We can look to the amazing survival of our Stolen Generations to withstand a full-blown assault on their identity and their human rights as children; their ability to keep speaking their truth when the nation was in denial.

To be able to tell their heart wrenching stories to the Bringing Them Home inquiry, and then deal with the disappointment of an indifferent approach to the recommendations of that report.

Their story should serve to inspire us to make the most of the opportunities that they were denied, to honour their lives and recognise the trauma that they still live with.

Our story is a 60,000-year-old tale that still lives. It is an unfolding drama, that has an uncertainty about how it will play out, but we can honour our ancestors and recognise that we are the sum total of all who came before us.

And we can call on our non-Indigenous brothers and sisters to join us to imagine a future that deals with the unfinished business of the Stolen Generations through telling the truth of our history and to continue what the apology started.

We cannot have a healed, reconciled nation without an honest and honourable examination of the truth of Australia's history.

This is an edited version of a speech delivered by Richard Weston for the 50th anniversary of the Dr Charles Perkins AO Memorial Oration at the University of Sydney, on the country of the Gadigal people. Read more about the oration here. Follow on Twitter: @RichJWeston

5. Community-driven innovation –Justice Reinvestment

" Most failings in Indigenous affairs are not because of Aboriginal and Torres Strait Islander people but because governments and politicians are not consistent in their approach to implementing programs and applying funding

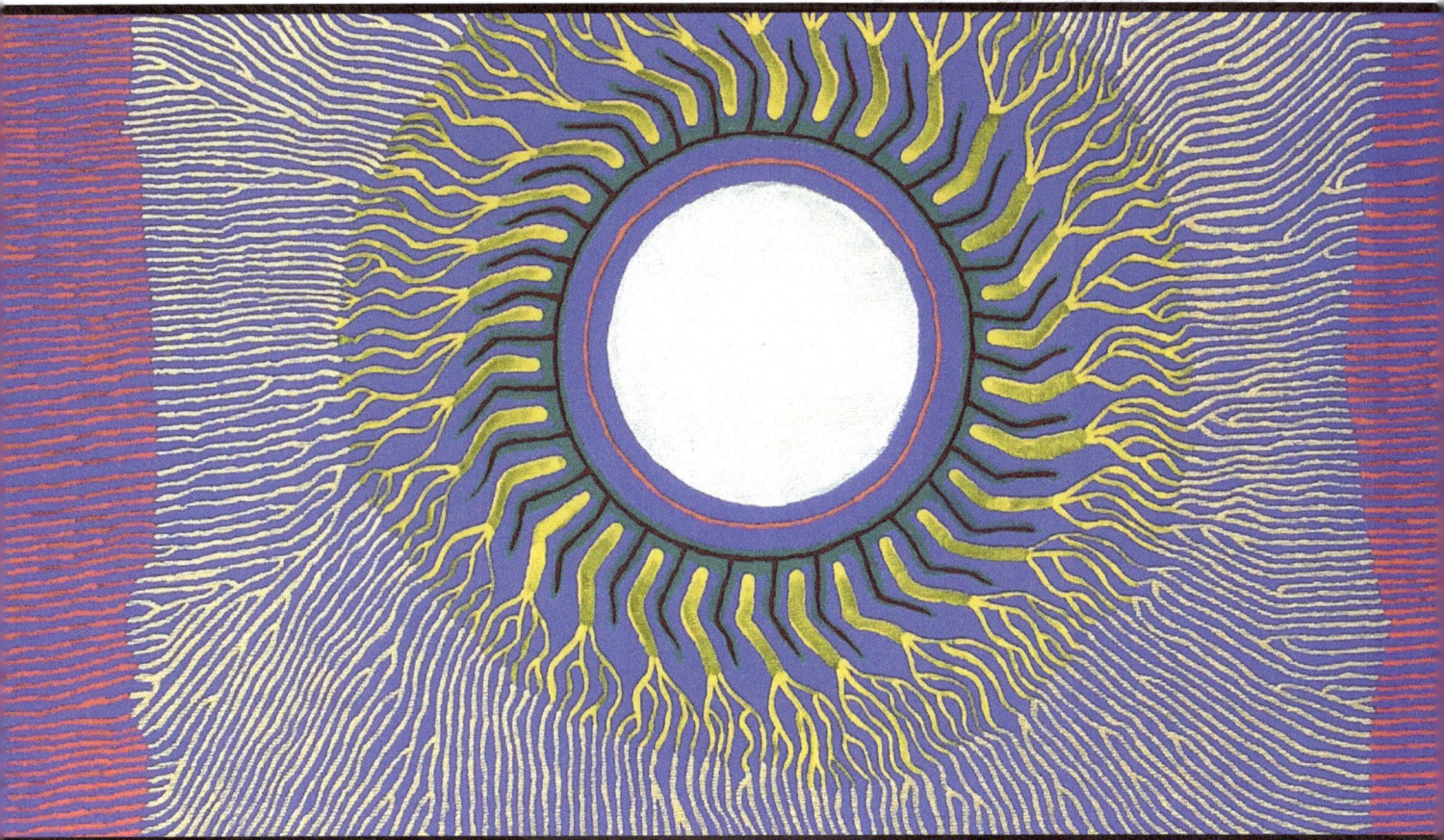

Meet "the perfect town", taking an historic step towards a fairer community

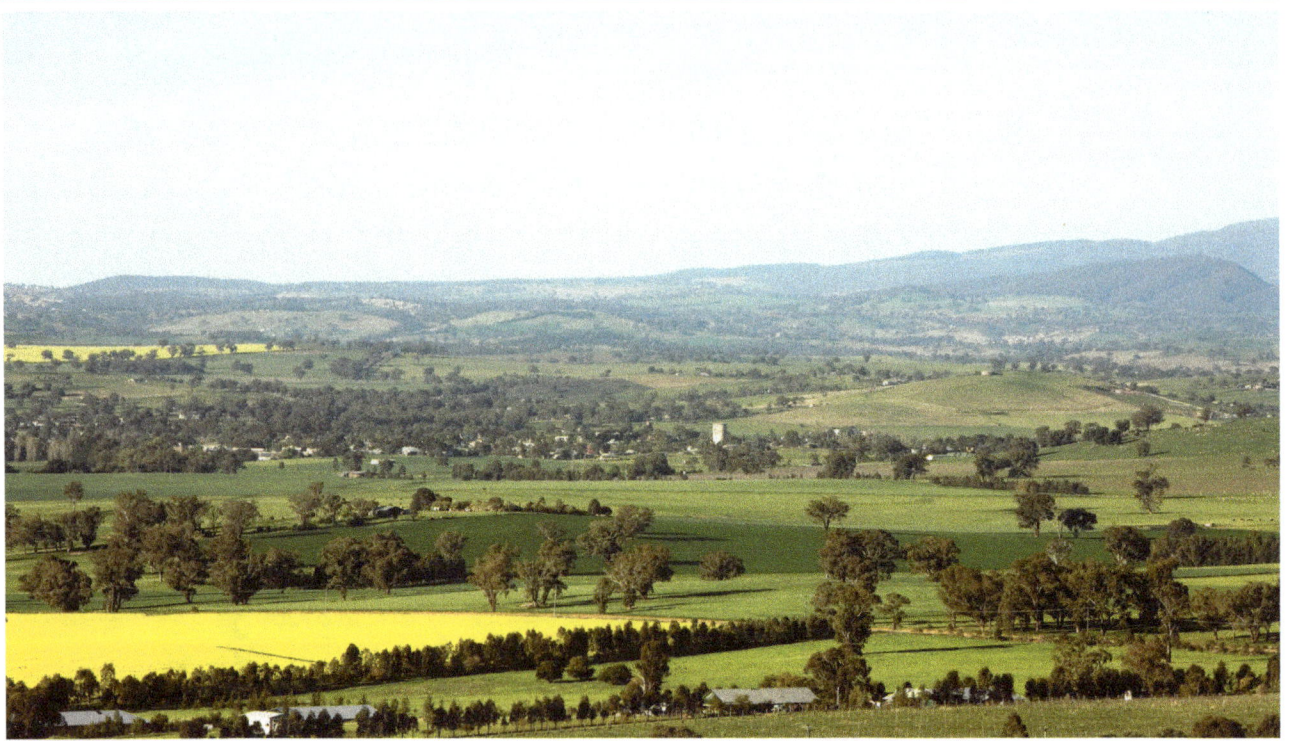

Author:	Marie McInerney	Published:	January 25, 2016

Cowra Shire Council has unanimously resolved to actively support Justice Reinvestment, and to seek to raise money and support for a pilot program in the rural New South Wales town.

Mick Dodson, Director of the National Centre for Indigenous Studies at the Australian National University and Professor of Law at the ANU College of Law, says Cowra's resolution is "historic" – the first time a community has made such a commitment in Australia.

Journalist Marie McInerney went to Cowra in the lead-up to the decision late last year, to report on the project for #JustJustice and to hear what the community hopes will emerge.

Marie McInerney writes:

A country town that votes National Party may not be the first place you would look for a justice initiative that challenges "tough on crime" approaches, but then neither is Texas, one of the US states where Justice Reinvestment originated.

Cowra lies on Wiradjuri country, stretched out along the banks of the Lachlan River in central west New South Wales.

The town is known for the Cowra Breakout, when more than 1,000 Japanese prisoners of war launched a mass escape from a detention centre on the edge of town in the dying days of World War Two. More than 200 were killed in the bloody attempt, as well as four Australian soldiers.

Now Cowra is a monument to the power of peace and reconciliation. Up a steep hill from the main street, the beauty and grace of the sculpted Japanese Gardens are testament to decades of careful, respectful work between the town, former POWs, and Japan. The town is littered with signposts, memorials and stories of the fatal 1944 breakout.

It's hard, as a first-time visitor, not to draw a comparison between that recognition and the unmarked Erambie Aboriginal mission site on the other side of the river. Only a tin shed painted with the Aboriginal flag and the Yalbillinga Boori Day Care Centre hint at its history.

"We don't have a lot," says the apologetic assistant at the town's information centre when asked for books or brochures about Erambie and its early residents, among them Mum Shirl, who later moved to Redfern and helped to found the Aboriginal medical service and the Aboriginal legal service in New South Wales.

But there is now a sense of hope that another patient, respectful process may once again transform the town, with strong Aboriginal and mainstream support for the three-year research project led by Dr Jill Guthrie. Based at ANU's National Centre for Indigenous Studies, she's been exploring the theory and methodology of Justice Reinvestment, a social justice concept that looks to shift spending on crime from punishment to prevention.

"It's been a wonderful journey," Mayor Bill West told a public forum in the town late last year when the ANU researchers presented their latest findings.

"Too often we see a problem, real or perceived, and we come up with a knee-jerk reaction that's sometimes worse than the original problem. They've taken time, done it properly, identified issues and what the community thinks."

The results, he said, were both "considerable and compelling."

Breaking the cycle

In the lead-up to last Christmas, Aunty Isobel Simpson sits in the kitchen of her Erambie home, wincing as she lowers herself into the chair.

She's long overdue for surgery on both knees but there's no date yet for the operation. In the lounge, colourfully wrapped presents lie neatly underneath the decorated tree, and framed family photos rest on every shelf or ledge.

With four children, 19 grandchildren, and eight great grandchildren, the 66-year-old Elder has a feast of family stories. There's much pride: one grandson danced with Bangarra, another is "a great little footballer".

But her focus today is on the trouble that many Aboriginal kids in the area have had with police and the broader justice system.

It's not just because she was at the Justice Reinvestment forum the night before. Police have come to her door three times in recent days after a robbery in town, checking the whereabouts of one of the grandkids. It's nothing new, she says.

"Because he has been in the system, he's done stupid things, pinching stuff, they blame him straight away," she says. "He said the detective pulled him up in the street and searched him."

Too often we see a problem, real or perceived, and we come up with a knee-jerk reaction that's sometimes worse than the original problem. They've taken time, done it properly, identified issues and what the community thinks

It's a systemic cycle for so many young Aboriginal people – early interactions with child protection and the criminal justice system that interconnect with racial profiling by police, disrupt family connections, schooling and jobs prospects, and ultimately lead to their over-representation in prison and a pattern of recidivism.

And it starts very young for many. Aunty Isobel gets me to look up a Cowra Guardian article from February 2015. It reports:

"*An 11-year-old boy who sat crying in the dock at Orange Local Court on Monday had to be taken to a juvenile correction centre on Monday night as a last resort.*

The report said the Cowra boy had spent the night in the cells at Orange Police Station after he was apprehended by police. Told by officials that his family could not be contacted, the Magistrate sent him to the Orana Juvenile Justice Centre in Dubbo – more than 200 kilometres away from home – "as a temporary measure".

While the child can't be identified for legal reasons, Aunty Isobel talks about the routine trauma involved in Aboriginal kids being taken from families, often over minor breaches of justice orders.

"It breaks your heart," she says, beginning to cry. "You tell me what child isn't naughty sometimes!"

She talks about how impossible it can be, without private transport or money for fares, for families to get to court appearances in neighbouring Orange or Dubbo, hours up the road.

Beyond quick fixes

It's a familiar problem across the nation, exacerbated by past trauma, intergenerational poverty, and health issues. Aunty Isobel says court officials are led to believe children and young people have no family support, so they are either put in care or detention, and so the cycle continues.

Go down to the Cowra Courthouse on court day, she says. "It's packed with Aboriginal people. Our kids get jumped on, always first up (to be blamed)." Then when the young ones come back to Cowra from a stint in detention or prison, they're hard to manage, they've got "a real swagger", she says. "It teaches them how to be criminals."

Aunty Isobel grew up on Erambie, on the block she lives on now. Times were often very tough. But she feels there was more respect and better prospects. Her father worked for the Shire for 37 years, her mother at the local hospital for 19 years.

Across the paddock at the end of her street is the Cowra Aboriginal Land Council, which recently organised a week's work for one of her grandsons, cutting back grass.

"He loved it," Aunty Isobel says. "Up early, dressed to go, home for lunch, off again. Motivated. Now there's nothing for him."

Land Council CEO Les Coe says he could write a book about the issues for young Aboriginal people in Cowra. Long-term unemployment is crippling, he says. It's not only a lack of work opportunities, but years of discrimination.

He says:

> *From where I sit, the education system is preparing our young people for a lifetime of incarceration. It's all about discipline, not about education.*
>
> *The kids get into trouble for acting up and it stays like that. Once you've got a name, that's it: it's passed on through the schools to the police, you become known in the community as a trouble maker, certainly well-known in the courts.*
>
> *We need to get in there early and break that cycle.*

Despite all that, Coe is optimistic about what Justice Reinvestment might bring. He's been on the Steering Committee and, like the Mayor, has been impressed with the process. He says:

> *It's not a quick fix, coming in and wanting to do things for 3, 6, 12 months and then leaving.*
>
> *Judging by what's happened in the US and Canada, we can develop something over a long period of time, rather than Band-aid treatment.*
>
> *It's long-term funding but also funding that's not extra. It already exists, it's just a matter of redirecting it.*

Economic sense

Championed originally in the United States in response to huge overcrowding in prisons, Justice Reinvestment involves the redirection of Corrections budgets to various community priorities.

Instead of spending money on keeping people in prison, it invests in prevention: in health, education, housing, employment – whatever helps.

Mick Dodson says few people realise that it costs $400,000 a year to keep a young person locked up in juvenile detention in New South Wales.

"If Cowra's got 10 of them locked up, you do the maths, " he says. "That's $4 million. Why not spend that money in the community doing good things that keep those kids out of trouble?"

He hastens to say that Justice Reinvestment is not a silver bullet or a free-for-all: "We're not talking about keeping everyone out of prison because some people who commit offences that are horrendous are a danger to society and have to be locked up. But we're talking about people who can't pay their fines, doing low level crime…"

Australia is currently spending $4 billion a year on prisons: "That's a lot of money and it's unsustainable."

But although a Senate investigation recommended a Justice Reinvestment approach three years ago, Australian governments have been slow on the uptake.

The Maranguka Justice Reinvestment Project in Bourke is the main current focus, South Australia has committed to two trials, and the Australian Capital Territory has an official policy but no active program.

One Victorian philanthropist recently told me, as part of another discussion, they wanted to support a Justice Reinvestment program but couldn't find a concrete way in. The ANU research may be the key to that.

Strengths-based approaches

There were many reasons why Cowra was "the perfect town" for the study, Jill Guthrie told the public forum in December.

Cowra is a discrete community of about 12,000 people, with a "strong and proud" Aboriginal community that makes up 7 per cent of the population, compared to 2 per cent nationally.

Another important factor for the research is that the town doesn't rely on a prison for jobs and much of its crime profile involves lower-level offences: such as traffic, public order and justice procedure offences.

It's also been important for the researchers and the town that the project wasn't precipitated by any "crime emergency" or huge media focus on justice issues. Its proximity to Canberra, where the ANU is based, was also helpful for logistics.

As it started up, the research team worked to get across some key messages, including that the project would take a strengths-based perspective.

The project's focus on all of the community, not only the Aboriginal community, was also welcomed across the board, says Guthrie.

During many consultations over the three years, the research team met with representatives from education, employment, health, community service, police, judiciary and business sectors, as well as young people, parents, grandparents and carers

"Often communities are asked to spend a bucket of money in a certain amount of time and this was the opposite of that," Guthrie says. "There was no bucket of money, no promise of funds at the end."

But there were local champions, among them the Mayor, and a local GP who works closely with the Erambie community.

In the end, Guthrie says, the project's approach freed people up to think more broadly, "to not think within the constraints of a certain amount of money".

Following due process

First up was a process to identify the town's strengths and its challenges.

Some of the protective factors that emerged were around the importance of supportive family and friends, being busy at work/school, and belonging to community groups. Two stood out: the Cowra Police Citizens Youth Club and the TAFE-based Breakaway that explores connections with culture and country. headspace was also highly valued.

Challenges included boredom and lack of prospects for young people. At a system and service level, the project heard that most local services were over-extended, often had to provide services outside their funding brief, and didn't always work well together.

Lack of jobs, particularly at the entry level, and lack of affordable or temporary housing came up again and again. Recent figures show the wait time for all types of rental housing in Cowra is between two and five years.

From there came the data crunching. The research team calculated that the cost of incarcerating Cowra citizens over the past 10 years had amounted to $42 million. Community representatives then worked through the crime categories behind that cost, and selected which crimes they believed could or should be dealt with through non-custodial sentences.

They came up with eight categories:

1. traffic offences
2. public order offences
3. justice procedure offences
4. property damage
5. drug offences
6. fraud and deception
7. theft
8. unlawful entry with intent/burglary, break and enter.

Those categories, dubbed as "JR-amenable", equated to about 50 per cent of crimes committed, offering a Justice Reinvestment 'saving' and potential funding pool of $23 million over 10 years.

The next question was, what to spend the 'saved' money on?

Priorities included emergency accommodation, homework support, community transport and service integration, a list of suggested improvements that both the Mayor and Mick Dodson found decently "modest" and would be "easily" funded at $2.3 million a year.

They included:

- service mapping (noting the difference between availability and access to services)

- keeping young people engaged in education "at all costs", through after school, suspension, homework and mentoring programs

- employment and skills development

- personal safety with an emphasis on housing (emergency, halfway houses, hostels)

- community transport.

The *Cowra Guardian* splashed the results on its front page, announcing: *"Jailing Cowra residents has cost us $46 million"*, and followed up with an editorial backing Justice Reinvestment.

At its December meeting, Council declared unanimous support for Cowra to pursue a Justice Reinvestment pilot, through the formation of a Justice Reinvestment Authority, utilising a Justice Reinvestment Accord.

It was a landmark moment for the research project, and for Justice Reinvestment in Australia, says Mick Dodson.

"It's too early to prejudge what it will look like, how long it will run, how they will fund it, but getting Council's resolution is crucial and historic," he says.

Mayor Bill West, a local farmer, admits that he didn't have a clue what Justice Reinvestment was about when he walked into the research team's first meeting.

"Mick Dodson was sitting on a bench not saying much, I was wondering where it would all go," says the Mayor. He's since spent much time with Dodson, and also met with current and former Aboriginal and Torres Strait Islander Social Justice Commissioners Mick Gooda and Professor Tom Calma as part of the process, which has been "a real eye opener".

Like Dodson, West was pleased and relieved that the process did not result in a "Taj Mahal" wish-list, but with a genuine understanding by the community of the problem and how best to deal with it: modest, practical, sensible solutions, including "a little bit of TLC (tender loving care)".

Community support

The Mayor has been pleasantly surprised by the support in the community, including from a "sympathetic" local business sector.

Still, he is conscious not to "get caught up in the euphoria of a quick fix". Council's resolution doesn't come with a budget allocation. Rather, it will need state and federal funding, as a 'down-payment' on the savings that could be reaped in years ahead.

The Senate investigation reported that, under one year of Justice Reinvestment, the Texas prison population increased by only 529 prisoners rather than the projected 5,141, contributing to a saving of $444 million, much of which was reinvested in community supports.

However, the Senate report also raised issues of concern around some projects in the US and UK, including about a lack of clarity in the definitions of Justice Reinvestment, lack of rigorous evaluation, and a focus on immediate upfront savings through basic justice reform which might skew future efforts.

In Cowra, there is agreement it will be crucial to get the right person to head the Authority, and that it should be someone who can keep the community united on the project. So too will be the need to prevent 'empire building' or competition over funds.

"This is really going to be a slow process," West cautions. But he says the premise is simple and makes sense.

He says: "We have young people out there who deserve to be looked after. You don't have to be young to make mistakes and get it wrong, so it's nice to be a caring and compassionate and civilised community, to give people a fair go."

The signs are promising, with strong support in principle from local State MP Katrina Hodgkinson.

At the very least, Guthrie says, the research has built a model for other communities to explore. However, she is hopeful that a project can be started in Cowra and that the ANU will be part of its evaluation.

"I think we'd find it quite painful to have to break the relationship now," she said. "We've built the trust both ways."

Many eyes will be on Cowra in the coming months and years to see if the town again plays a pivotal role in Australia's history and can begin to address growing levels of over-representation of Aboriginal people in our prisons.

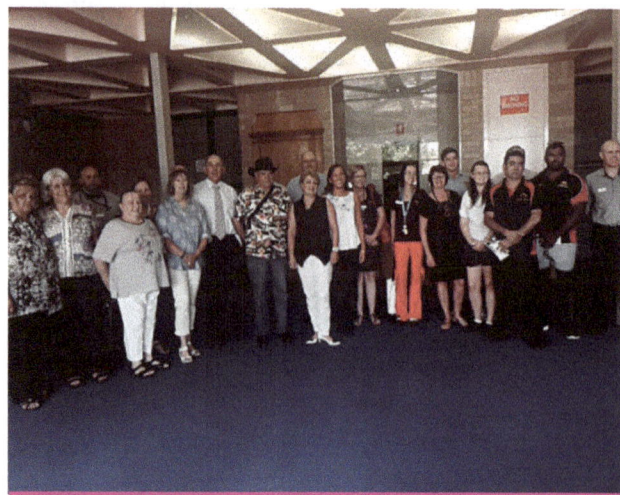

Members of the Cowra Justice Reinvestment research project & other community members at the Justice Reinvestment forum in December: Source: Cowra Shire Council.

Meanwhile, the article featured below suggests the Cowra Guardian is likely to continue keeping a close eye on the project's progress.

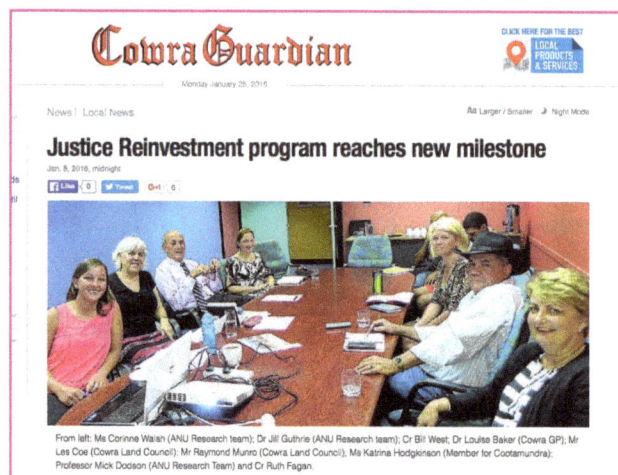

South Australia urged to trial and evaluate Justice Reinvestment pilot projects

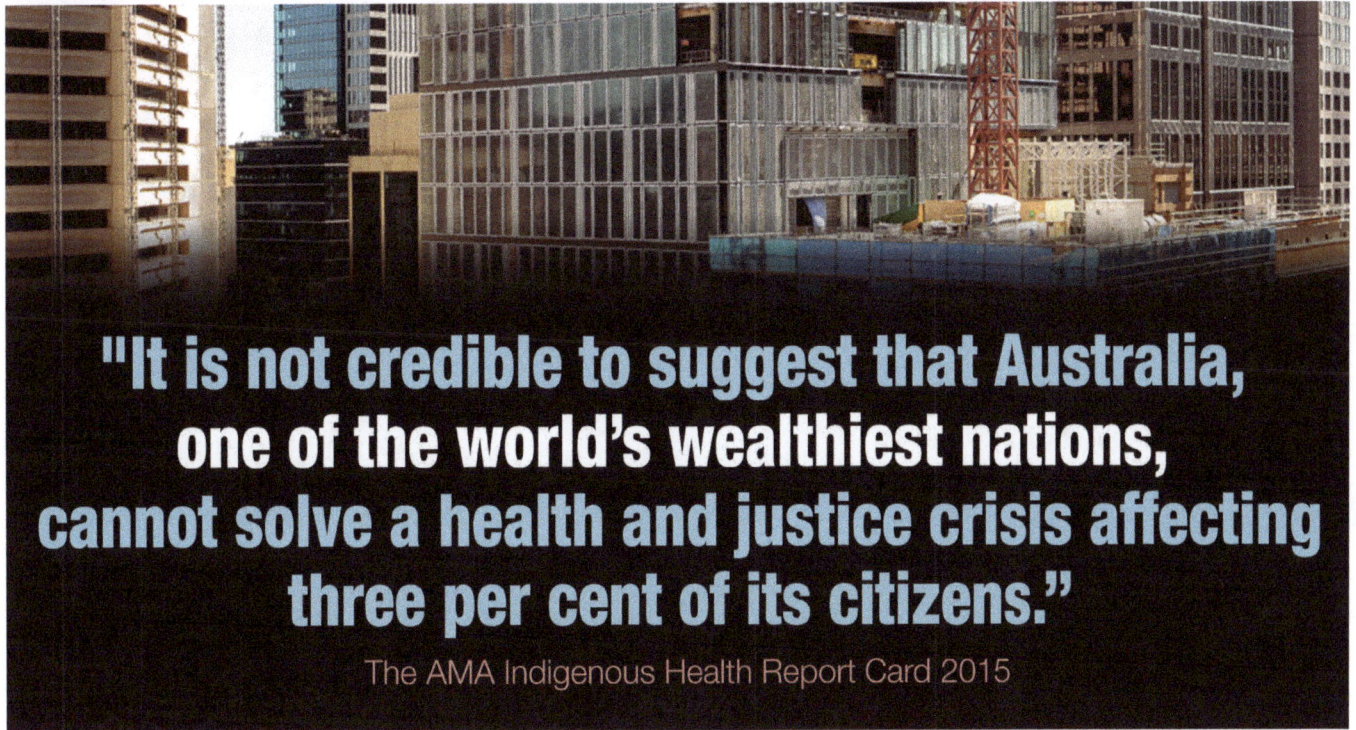

"It is not credible to suggest that Australia, one of the world's wealthiest nations, cannot solve a health and justice crisis affecting three per cent of its citizens."

The AMA Indigenous Health Report Card 2015

Author:	Robyn Layton	Published:	June 28, 2016

In South Australia, a growing community of people and organisations is calling for a smarter approach to criminal justice that may help to reduce crime and incarceration rates, reports Hon Dr Robyn Layton AO QC, Justice Reinvestment SA Chairperson.

The Justice Reinvestment SA (JRSA) group is calling on the SA Government to trial and evaluate Justice Reinvestment pilot projects in at least one metropolitan and one regional community.

Justice Reinvestment, which as previous Croakey articles have covered, involves shifting money allocated for future imprisonment costs into spending on community-based programs and services that address the underlying causes of crime in identified communities.

Robyn Layton writes:

Justice Reinvestment SA (JRSA) is a diverse community of individuals and agencies with a shared vision of strong, safe and thriving SA communities, with less crime and lower incarceration rates, according to the group's Aboriginal and Torres Strait Islander Spokesperson and CEO of the Aboriginal Legal Rights Movement, Cheryl Axleby.

"If properly implemented, Justice Reinvestment can reduce crime and imprisonment, improve public safety and strengthen our most disadvantaged communities, all without breaking the budget," says Cheryl Axleby.

The Justice Reinvestment approach is based on evidence that a significant proportion of offenders come from, and return to, a small number of disadvantaged communities.

Demographic mapping is used to identify those communities that will benefit most from targeted investment in prevention, early intervention, diversionary and rehabilitation programs.

Cheryl says that Justice Reinvestment is a not a short-term, one size fits all, top-down approach.

"It requires a collaborative partnership between government and community," she says.

"Communities chosen for Justice Reinvestment must be supported to play a central role in the design, implementation and monitoring of local Justice Reinvestment plans."

Nor is Justice Reinvestment about getting rid of prisons altogether.

Helen Connolly, JRSA Board member and Australian Red Cross Executive Director (SA), says: "Prisons will always be needed to house serious and dangerous offenders. Nor is it about stripping money away from already underfunded prison services and programs."

Why is Justice Reinvestment needed?

The continued growth of Australia's prison population is both economically and socially unsustainable.

Over the past decade, South Australia's prison population has grown by 50 percent and we now spend over $150 million a year on imprisonment. This growth has hit Aboriginal people the hardest.

Even though Aboriginal people make up just two percent of the State's population, over one in five of South Australian prisoners is Aboriginal. Of the Aboriginal men aged 20 to 39 years in SA, one in 14 is incarcerated.

Adding more prison beds and imprisoning more people does not break the cycle of crime and incarceration. Again, this is particularly so for Aboriginal prisoners, who are much more likely to report multiple periods of imprisonment than non-Aboriginal prisoners.

JRSA says special focus must be given to reducing the over-representation of Aboriginal people. If this over-representation is not addressed, SA risks losing another generation of Aboriginal Australians to the criminal justice system.

Addressing the root causes of crime

According to Professor Mark Halsey, a criminologist at the Centre for Crime Policy and Research at Flinders University and a JRSA Executive member, the best way to reduce crime rates is to prevent crime.

He says: "When people, and particularly young people offend, there are often other issues at play like homelessness,

But what is needed over the longer term is a more nuanced and culturally driven understanding of why particular communities disproportionately generate crime and disadvantage. This is the value of a Justice Reinvestment approach

cognitive disability, drug and alcohol use, poverty, family breakdown, discrimination and normalisation of violence.

"The more we spend on prisons, the less we have to spend on other essential services such as health and education to help prevent the causes of crime and the recidivism cycle of offenders. Today's young offenders are too frequently tomorrow's adult prisoners."

Mark Halsey says that, "while the Government should be praised for its Transforming Criminal Justice approach, there is much more to be done if the prison population is to be significantly reduced".

He says: "For example, the Government's current interest in allowing more prisoners to serve the remainder of their sentence under home detention might make a small inroad into prisoner numbers.

"But what is needed over the longer term is a more nuanced and culturally driven understanding of why particular communities disproportionately generate crime and disadvantage. This is the value of a Justice Reinvestment approach."

Will Justice Reinvestment work?

Justice Reinvestment was first implemented in the United States more than a decade ago, and has achieved real results in reducing imprisonment rates and dollars saved.

In 2007, Texas officials estimated they would need to spend $2 billion over 5 years on new prisons. Instead, they invested $241 million in alternatives such as treatment programs, improved probation and parole services, and nurse-family partnerships – generating savings of $444 million in just one year.

Five years on, crime rates continue to drop dramatically and growth in the prison population has slowed almost to a halt.

SA's prison population is obviously different from Texas' in scale and cost, but there is much to be learnt from the US experience.

The more recent Justice Reinvestment program implemented in New York has greater parallels with the situation facing SA. The New York initiative, which focuses specifically on assisting offenders from 'minority' backgrounds, is making slow but steady progress into the problems of crime and poverty besetting particular communities.

Every community, whether in SA or elsewhere will differ, but the overall strategy for getting communities on track will be broadly similar.

Call to action

JRSA is calling on the SA Government to trial and evaluate Justice Reinvestment pilot projects in at least one metropolitan and one regional community. These pilot projects should primarily focus on addressing the over-representation of Aboriginal young people aged 10-24 in custody.

"Focusing on Aboriginal young people is just the first step towards rolling out a comprehensive Justice Reinvestment policy across the State", says Cheryl Axleby.

"JRSA is calling on all South Australian parliamentarians to accept that adopting evidence-based criminal justice policies is more likely to improve public safety over the long-term rather than simply increasing the number of prison beds," she says.

Halsey says: "If Republicans and Democrats in the states of the United States can put aside their differences to offer bipartisan support for Justice Reinvestment, surely our South Australian politicians can do the same."

Hon Dr Robyn Layton is a former Supreme Court Judge, an adjunct Professor at the University of SA and Justice Reinvestment SA Chairperson.

Tom Calma urges Justice Reinvestment to bring #JustJustice for Indigenous people

Author:	Tom Calma	Published:	May 26, 2015

Australia needs to follow international leaders in Justice Reinvestment programs if it is to address the high rate of incarceration of Aboriginal and Torres Strait Islander people, says leading social justice and human rights advocate **Professor Tom Calma**.

Lending his support to the #JustJustice campaign, Professor Calma, former Social Justice Commissioner, said better research is also needed to understand why Aboriginal and Torres Strait Islander people are **imprisoned more often** than non-Indigenous people for lesser crimes.

He calls for justice and mental health to be added as Closing the Gap targets and says governments need to be just as accountable for their policies and programs as they demand of the Aboriginal and Torres Strait Islander communities and organisations that they fund.

Professor Tom Calma AO

Professor Calma's article is based on a **Twitter Periscope interview** he did with #JustJustice team member Summer May Finlay that attracted nearly 350 live viewers.

Tom Calma writes:

Accountability goes both ways

There are two immediate priority responses for reducing the shocking over-incarceration rate of Aboriginal and Torres Strait Islander people.

First, the time has come for a roll out of Justice Reinvestment initiatives across Australia that work with people before they offend, and provide support when they are released from prison so they don't reoffend and return to prison.

Justice reinvestment is about **shifting spending away from prisons** and juvenile detention expansion towards prevention, such as early childhood education in vulnerable communities, targeting young people at risk of school disengagement, intensive case work support with housing and employment support, and job creation.

The Justice Reinvestment model is not 'one size fits all'. It will look different in every community; for example, the current trials in New South Wales – one in **Bourke,** the other in Cowra – are being implemented by different organisations and differ in their design and focus .

I **reported** on the need for and benefits of the Justice Reinvestment approach in 2009, when I was Social Justice Commissioner and it was a relatively new public policy

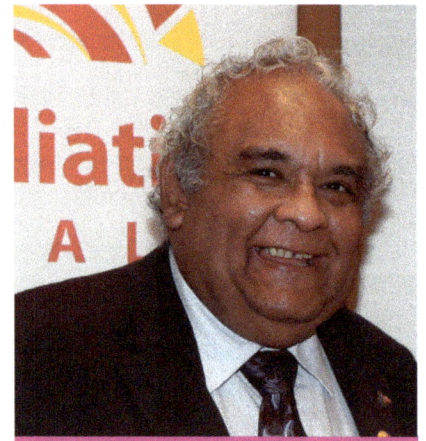

response to the out-of-control expansion of the prison population in the United States. It is now being implemented across 19 states in the US, in Canada and the UK, where evidence shows the prison rates are being reduced.

Since 2009 we have had a **Senate inquiry** that confirmed the potential value of a Justice Reinvestment approach to criminal justice in Australia, and seen the launch of **Just Reinvest NSW**. We have much support from the judiciary and from communities, but still the ideas gather dust while politicians continue to espouse a tough on crime approach.

If politicians are not moved by the social, community and personal costs of over-incarceration, then surely they are by the economics. In New South Wales, it costs more than $650 per person per day or $230,000 per year to keep a young person incarcerated. We argue that it's better to invest that $230,000 in the community, into services that help before someone commits a crime, rather than adding new prison beds or building new prisons.

The second priority is to improve the research base around why Aboriginal and Torres Strait Islander people are being incarcerated at such high rates in Australia for offences that are at the **lower end of the scale** – such as for **non-payment** of fines, breaches of community service orders, or disorderly behaviour.

That's particularly important for the groups we now identify as pressure points: young people and women whose incarceration rates are rising. We need to look hard at why that is.

Connection to culture

I come from Darwin, from the Kungarakan people on my mother's side, and the Iwaidja on my father's. We were very fortunate to have been able to get our own land back, after many years of struggle, under the Northern Territory's *Aboriginal Land Rights Act 1976*. As Aboriginal and Torres Strait Islander people, it's very important that we can maintain our relationship with our land and our culture. Yet many cannot.

This is a real issue we have to consider in relation to Indigenous over-incarceration. It's not an excuse, but we need to acknowledge that people can commit offences because of past traumas and dissociation from land and culture – whether they were forcibly removed in past days or controlled in the way they can connect. Racism also has a big influence on the way people behave, particularly in terms of discrimination in employment. If people can't get meaningful work, they are left to their own devices and sometimes will turn to crime.

We know the benefits that come from a strong relationship with land and culture, from when we feel respected and safe and secure in our own identity. A very important longitudinal study of the Utopia community demonstrates how living off the land, being secure in culture, language and law practices, has produced better mental and physical health outcomes than those experienced in regional or metropolitan areas.

These are factors we have to consider in the context of the Western Australian Government's plans to close remote Aboriginal communities; how losing connection contributes to crime and over-incarceration.

Targets and accountability

We need to continue to pressure the Federal Government to include both justice and mental health targets in the Closing the Gap framework. Once a target is set, it makes governments accountable and they have to report against those targets – that's why they shy away from them.

Governments expect us to be accountable for the money they hand out. We also expect them to be accountable, for the funding they approve and the policy directions they select. They need to recognise that they too are major contributors to the success or failures of our programs.

How we work with Aboriginal and Torres Strait Islander people in prison is vital to their future. There are very high levels of mental health problems for all prisoners, but the Indigenous burden is higher. We also know that people who are incarcerated, particularly over the longer-term, have a shorter life span on release. They don't get the treatment in prison and the support is not there on release.

One of the most positive shifts in prison health has been the move towards smoke-free prisons across Australia, with Northern Territory prisons now in their second year of smoking bans. There have been a few issues with implementation, however it's a great opportunity for our people to get healthier and stay healthier, given that smoking contributes to about 20 per cent of the burden of death for Aboriginal and Torres Strait Islander people and is a major contributor to a number of chronic diseases.

Making change

There are initiatives out there that are making a difference but we need to get the message across to a broader audience. We should promote to politicians what needs to happen at every opportunity, as well as talk to business and any other organisation or group we believe is tied to our future.

We need to keep them informed about the challenging issues we are faced with, but also talk to them about the solutions we have identified that we wish to see supported and, where we can, show them the successes.

We know most failings in Indigenous affairs are not because of Aboriginal and Torres Strait Islander people but because governments and politicians are not consistent in their approach to implementing programs and applying funding. The approach is always short-term when we need to identify a very clear long-term plan, seek bipartisan support and engage with people. That's why the Close the Gap Campaign strategy is so important: we talk about a 25 year plan.

We know that judges and magistrates are very keen to look at alternative practices. We need to make sure that politicians also understand what is driving prison numbers and make sure that alternative practices like the Koori and Nunga court systems are funded as and where they exist, or are created in other jurisdictions.

> *There are initiatives out there that are making a difference but we need to get the message across to a broader audience. We should promote to politicians what needs to happen at every opportunity, as well as talk to business and any other organisation or group we believe is tied to our future*

Support for #JustJustice

Like the National Justice Coalition's Change the Record campaign, #JustJustice aims to raise awareness about over-incarceration.

It is a very important campaign that aims to provide a platform to a range of people: those who are affected by incarceration or have been working for years at trying to keep people out of prison, those trying to keep them healthy in prison, or stop them from returning to prison after release. A platform that works with Aboriginal and Torres Strait Islander peoples to empower and educate, to curb the scourge of incarceration and reduce the number of victims. It's a chance to give these people a voice, to get them to share their experiences, their knowledge and their solutions. Please support #JustJustice.

Professor Tom Calma AO is Chancellor of the University of Canberra. He is an Elder from the Kungarakan tribal group and a member of the Iwaidja tribal group whose traditional lands are south west of Darwin and on the Coburg Peninsula in the Northern Territory of Australia, respectively. He is Co-Chair of Reconciliation Australia and a former Aboriginal and Torres Strait Islander Social Justice Commissioner.

Calling for Justice Reinvestment and safer communities: #JustJustice #ALPconf2015 #ChangeTheRecord

Author:	Tiffany Overall	Published:	July 24, 2015

The need to address the over-incarceration of Aboriginal and Torres Strait Islander people featured at the ALP National Conference in Melbourne.

The National Justice Coalition and ANTaR held a panel discussion with leading Aboriginal and Torres Strait Islander experts about a national approach to address incarceration rates and violence, particularly against women and children.

Panellists discussed the Change the Record campaign, and there were calls for greater investment in early intervention, prevention and diversion strategies, and "smarter solutions that increase safety, address the root causes of violence against women, cut reoffending and imprisonment rates, and build stronger and safer communities".

As well, Labor delegates considered a draft policy platform that supports justice reinvestment and the development of a justice target under the Closing the Gap framework. The draft platform also supports additional Closing the Gap targets in improving services for Aboriginal and Torres Strait Islander people with disability, and to increase participation in higher and further education.

Tiffany Overall writes:

Youth Justice Reinvestment: Invest in communities, not prisons

Justice reinvestment is a promising strategy to help tackle the underlying social causes of youth crime, and should be trialled in Victoria.

It also has the potential to help build stronger communities, reduce crime and relieve pressure on the soaring Corrections' budget.

At the Centre for Rural Regional Law and Justice forum in June, panel members discussed some key features of justice reinvestment, some international experiences and a couple of innovative projects in NSW that hold some lessons for Victoria.

The pressing need to explore justice reinvestment in Victoria is largely driven by prison overcrowding (prisoner numbers up 42% since 2004), disproportionately high percentage of Aboriginal people making up the youth justice and adult prison populations, record high re-offending rates of prisoners at 40%, and the rocketing expenditure (over $1 billion last year).

But it is also driven by the need to address poverty and disadvantage as an underlying cause of crime and imprisonment, and a need to focus on early intervention programs particularly for at-risk young people, as an extremely cost effective way to reduce crime.

Young people getting caught up in the criminal justice system are some of Victoria's most disadvantaged and vulnerable. For example, about a quarter of children on youth justice orders or in remand in 2010 came from between 2 and 3% of Victoria's poorer postcodes, and around 4 out of 5 children with youth justice orders are known to child protection.

Adopting a justice reinvestment approach means investing in disadvantaged communities – not prisons – to develop and implement local solutions addressing economic and social determinants and risk factors behind youth offending. It will help reduce the number of children at risk of becoming adult offenders or prisoners.

Victoria has much to learn from other jurisdictions, particularly the United States (US) and other Australian states and territories, especially NSW, which are further advanced in their exploration of and implementation of justice reinvestment approaches.

Panellist, Melanie Schwartz, Chief Investigator, of the Australian Justice Reinvestment Project shared her observations of how justice reinvestment has played out in the US. There are currently 30 states pursuing justice reinvestment at the state level, and at least 18 counties in six states undertaking justice reinvestment at the local level

Despite the promise of a place-based approach with strong community engagement, the US experience has become more focused on statewide criminal justice reforms and investment into community corrections, such as probation and parole services.

Melanie felt the lesson for Victoria is to adopt a flexible approach and make sure any justice reinvestment measures are adapted to the realities of Victoria.

Panellists agreed that the underlying power of justice reinvestment is in it being a place-based approach that invests in local communities sourcing their own answers and building their capacity to be enablers of change and to create safer communities.

Another panel member, Ben Schokman of the Human Rights Law Centre, reinforced the importance of supporting and empowering local communities to design and implement their own social programs for change, and gave some inspiring international case studies.

Even without formal justice reinvestment policy, we are seeing some very exciting initiatives across Australia at the community level.

The Bourke Justice Reinvestment Project is an innovative example of a community mobilising around a great need for change, taking control and driving positive change. Bourke is a small remote town in far western New South Wales with a population of nearly 3,000 people. It has a young population, high levels of unemployment and disengagement from education, and high imprisonment rates. Thirty percent of the population are Aboriginal and Torres Strait Islander people. Of the 223 young Aboriginal and Torres Strait Islander people in Bourke, 47 (10 to 24 year olds) were on remand or had been sentenced, representing half of the youth prison population. Annually this detention costs over $2 million.

Kerry Graham, of Just Reinvest NSW, explained how Aboriginal leaders of Bourke responded to these issues, announcing their interest in participating in a trial. Since 2012 they have been working with the Bourke Aboriginal Community Working Party (BAWP) to tackle problems around offending and incarceration, while at the same time creating alternate pathways for young people.

Kerry said a key learning was the importance of taking time to build trusted relations between participants. Bourke has used a collective impact model to guide the project, with diverse organisations from different sectors committing to a common agenda to solve their social problems through a coordinated joint plan of action.

Researchers from the Australian National University, led by Dr Jill Guthrie, are conducting an innovative community research study in Cowra, NSW to evaluate the potential use of a justice reinvestment approach to addressing crime, and particularly the imprisonment of the town's young people.

Cowra has a population of 10,000, and has been described as an ideal case study site due to its stable population and middle range crime profile.

This study is a conversation with the town to explore:

- what are the conditions, the understandings, the agreements that would need to be in place in order to return those young people who are in detention centres, to keep those young people who are at risk of incarceration from coming into contact with the criminal justice system, and

- what is it in town that works for those young people not at risk of incarceration?

Smart Justice for Young People is calling on the Victorian Government to develop a state-wide strategy for a justice reinvestment policy and to commit to trialling and evaluating justice reinvestment in selected communities.

Tiffany Overall is Convenor of Smart Justice for Young People, a Victorian campaign that brings together more than 30 legal, youth, health, welfare and community organisations, many working with young people at risk.

Australian Bar Association calls for Justice Reinvestment, shift from mandatory sentencing

Author:	Patrick O'Sullivan	Published:	April 08, 2016

The Australian Bar Association (ABA) is calling for national co-operation to tackle the alarming and disproportionate rates of Indigenous incarceration.

The ABA is proposing that mandatory sentencing laws be amended or removed and that funds saved from housing prisoners be redirected into programs that rehabilitate and reduce recidivism (known as Justice Reinvestment).

A statement from ABA President Patrick O'Sullivan QC is published here, with permission, under the #JustJustice series.

Patrick O'Sullivan writes:

Australia's Indigenous incarceration rate is one of the most challenging human rights issues facing the country today. The proportion of Indigenous prisoners has almost doubled over the 20 years since the Royal Commission into Aboriginal Deaths in Custody (RCIADIC) and is a matter of deep concern to the Australian Bar Association.

I met this week with the Federal Attorney-General George Brandis QC to discuss the ABA's proposals and to encourage the Federal Government to commit to action that will deliver better justice outcomes for all. I will also meet with other State Attorney's General throughout the year, where this issue will continue to be a high priority for the ABA.

The current situation is that:

- Incarceration rates of Indigenous Australians are at least 16 times higher than the rate for non-Aboriginal and Torres Strait Australians.

- Indigenous children between 10-14 years of age are 30 times more likely to be incarcerated than their non-Indigenous peers.

- Indigenous women are almost 20 times more likely to be incarcerated than non-Indigenous women.

Across the country, Indigenous people comprise more than a quarter of the prison population despite only accounting for almost 3 per cent of the national population. The situation is amplified in the Northern Territory where the rate of indigenous people in prison is closer to 90 per cent.

It is a shocking fact that an Indigenous young person who has served a prison sentence is more likely to return to prison than finish school. And on any given night in Australia, over half of all young people in detention are Indigenous.

A recent report by the Australian Institute of Criminology found a key factor contributing to the disproportionate Indigenous over-representation is that of State and Territory government bail and sentencing policies, particularly in jurisdictions with high populations of Indigenous people where mandatory sentencing laws operate, and individuals are often incarcerated for trivial offences.

For example, there have been numerous reported examples of anomalous or unjust cases where mandatory sentencing has applied in Australia, including in which:

- a 16-year-old with one prior conviction received a 28-day prison sentence for stealing one bottle of spring water

- a 17-year-old first time offender received a 14-day prison sentence for stealing orange juice and Minties

- an Aboriginal woman and first-time offender who received a 14-day prison sentence for stealing a can of beer

- a 15-year old Aboriginal boy received a 20-day mandatory sentence for stealing pencils and stationery. He died while in custody.

Mandatory sentencing appears a significantly attractive option to reduce crime and provide consistency in sentencing, however a lack of evidence exists as to the efficacy as a deterrent or the ability to decrease crime, particularly around minor theft, driving offences and minor assault.

We only need to look at the experience in the Northern Territory where property crime offences increased during the initial mandatory sentencing regime for such offences, and decreased after its repeal.

Mandatory sentencing contributes to a higher rate of imprisonment which often unnecessarily increases the costs in the administration of justice. Under mandatory sentencing laws, a defendant has no motivation to plead guilty as there is no chance of a reduced sentence. This means that potentially more contested cases appear before the courts requiring the use of extra resources and producing further court delays.

There are on average 30,000 prisoners in Australia at any one time, a quarter of them Indigenous, costing the country $3 billion a year. Even a 10 percent reduction in the Indigenous imprisonment rate would save more than $10 million a year.

The Australian Bar Association proposes the following:

- **Amend or remove mandatory sentencing laws** that have the biggest impact on Indigenous people but deliver minimum effects, such as minor assault, driving offences and minor theft.

- **Review fine default imprisonment:** Existing mechanisms for the enforcement of fines are unsatisfactory. Imprisonment in default of payment is unjust, unfair to poor offenders, dangerous to vulnerable offenders, expensive and disproportionate in its effect on indigenous offenders. (See the case study on Ms Dhu, below)

- **Invest in Justice Reinvestment:** channel money that would have been spent on housing prisoners into community projects aimed at keeping Indigenous offenders out of prison. Oregon (US) experienced a 72 per cent drop in juvenile incarceration after the state reinvested $241 million from prison spending to treatment programs and improved probation and parole services.

It makes moral and financial sense to reduce the number of Indigenous people in prison. The over-representation of Indigenous people incarcerated is a national disgrace. It is time to take action that addresses the problem and delivers better justice outcomes for Indigenous Australians and the country as a whole.

Case studies

Gloria – assault offences

The Territory Government increased minimum jail times for offenders while restricting judges' rights to suspend sentences for certain crimes. In 2014, a young woman and mother of four 'Gloria' faced jail. She admitted to drunkenly hitting another woman who taunted her about the death of her mother. Under the Territory's new laws, every first-time offender convicted of a violent offence faces three months in jail. It's 12 months for repeat offenders. Magistrates' hands have been tied. 'Gloria' has only appeared in court once before for a minor offence. Before the new laws were brought in, she most likely would have been released with a fine.

Driving offences

In courts across Australia, magistrates routinely issue fines and disqualifications for people charged with unlicensed driving. But for many Indigenous people, these court appearances can be the first step towards jail. In NSW alone, recent figures show more than 1,000 Indigenous people were doing prison time for offences related to unlicensed driving.

Eamonn – traffic violations

An Indigenous man first came to the attention of police when he was young for driving without a licence. Then when he was 16 he went for his licence test and started driving around and racing cars. He was charged under his father's surname but the name on his birth certificate was different. He did not know as he could not read. He was disqualified from driving.

Years later, believing his disqualification was served, he approached the Roads and Traffic Authority and was given the all clear and passed his test. Later, the police pulled him over alleging he did not have a licence. The man showed his licence from the RTA to the police and the police refused to believe him, stating he was still disqualified under another name. He was further charged with a driving offence and, under the mandatory sentencing laws, was sent to jail and disqualified from driving until 2022.

Ms Dhu – fine default imprisonment

Ms Dhu was arrested by police to be imprisoned for four days in August 2014 for unpaid fines totally $3622. Ms Dhu died two days into her incarceration at Western Australia's South Hedland Police Station.

In 2013, 1358 people were imprisoned for fine default and for no other reason. Sixteen percent of Indigenous people who entered prison that year were there only for fine default.

Australian Red Cross joins Justice Reinvestment push

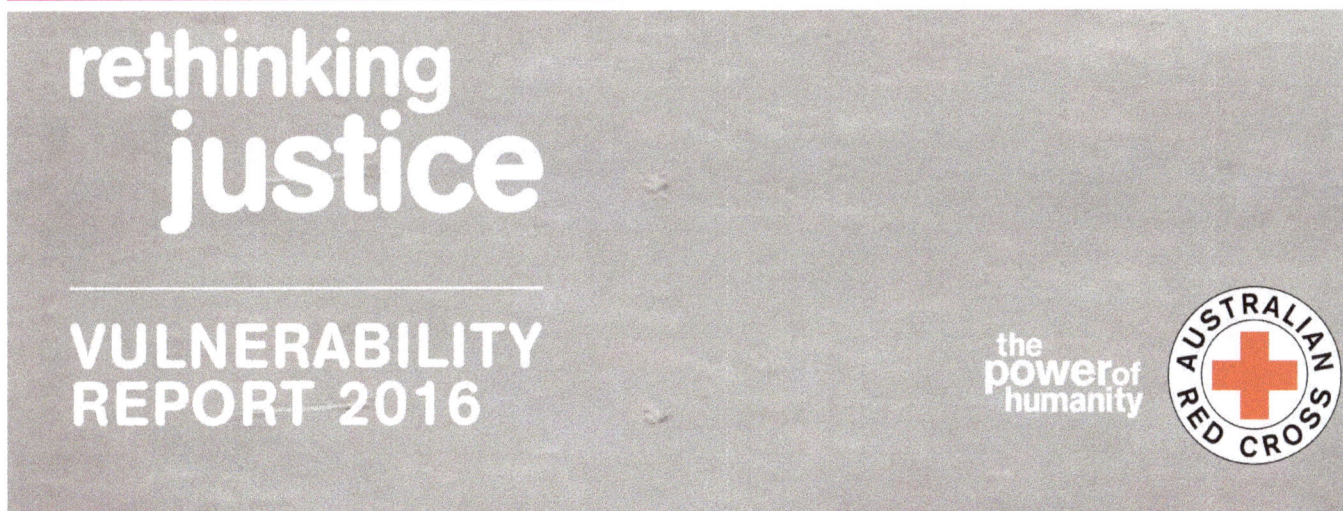

rethinking justice

VULNERABILITY REPORT 2016

the power of humanity

AUSTRALIAN RED CROSS

Author:	Amy Coopes	Published:	April 01, 2016

The Australian Red Cross has joined calls for a shift to justice reinvestment, issuing a major report urging that it be made a national priority and that trials be rolled out nationwide.

The Red Cross *Vulnerability Report: Rethinking Justice* warned that, with Australia's prison population reaching a 10-year high and Indigenous people comprising more than a third of those incarcerated, a rethink was needed.

Instead of seeing prison as the common resort to crime, the report called for it to be seen as a last resort, and urged governments to pursue justice reinvestment reforms:

"Justice reinvestment invests in people and communities to provide support, treatment and services that address the underlying issues confronting people who commit less serious offences. These issues include homelessness, mental health, deep social exclusion, and poor education and employment histories.

Evidence suggests that it is more efficient and effective to address the causes and thus reduce the need for (and greater cost of) incarceration.

Early indications from trials in Australia suggest that adopting a local justice reinvestment approach will pay bigger long-term dividends than a "tough on crime" approach."

Halting or reducing the prison population would realise savings of between $1.1 billion and $2.3 billion over five years, the Red Cross said.

The pilot program at Cowra (which you can read about in depth here) was one of four trials underway in Australia that were mentioned in the report.

Looking at the prison population, the report noted a typical background of low education, joblessness, mental health issues, cognitive impairment, drug and alcohol use, sexual abuse and family issues.

Prisoners were much more likely to come from disadvantaged or Aboriginal and Torres Strait Islander communities.

In support of its claim that incarceration was ineffective at rehabilitating people or deterring crime, the Red Cross noted:

- 59% of inmates had previously been sentenced to an adult prison

- 77% of Indigenous inmates had previously been sentenced to an adult prison (total imprisonment rate 13 times higher than the general population)

- 38% of prisoners are reincarcerated within 2 years of release

- many reoffend within their first three weeks of liberty

Outlining priorities for governments through COAG's Law Crime and Community Safety Council, the Red Cross urged:

- establishment of systems to provide more robust understanding of the financial costs of crime, justice and imprisonment

- geographic mapping of vulnerable areas where justice reinvestment may be an appropriate alternative

- national research framework and strategic agenda including longitudinal evaluation of justice reinvestment trials

- a national justice reinvestment information clearinghouse

- public education campaign to support balanced information and perceptions of crime and justice issues within the community

Implementation of the reforms — which the report acknowledged remained controversial for a number of reasons — would require bipartisanship, strong leadership, early identification of important stakeholders, substantial buy-in from all sectors, effective community engagement and ongoing commitment to implementation, the Red Cross said.

We'd encourage you to read the full report, and join the conversation online at #JustJustice or #justicereinvest.

Amy Coopes is a medical student, freelance journalist and an occasional editor for Croakey.

Recommendations

1. That all governments in Australia rethink and change their approaches to justice to achieve lower crime rates, lower incarceration rates, reduced prison costs and stronger, safer communities.

2. That all governments in Australia introduce a justice reinvestment approach and jointly support its implementation through the Law, Crime and Community Safety Council of the Council of Australian Governments.

3. That all governments in Australia establish, fund and evaluate justice reinvestment trials across Australia in specific geographic communities with high rates of crime to determine how justice reinvestment can be applied in Australian contexts.

4. That state and territory governments adopt the justice reform proposals outlined in this report to:
   - prevent crime and recidivism
   - increase non-custodial sentencing
   - improve parole and reintegration to the community.

5. That, as a first step, all governments in Australia commit to:
   - a 10% reduction in adult imprisonment rates over the next five years
   - a Closing the Gap justice target to reduce the unacceptably high adult imprisonment rates of Aboriginal and Torres Strait Islander peoples by 50% over the next five years.

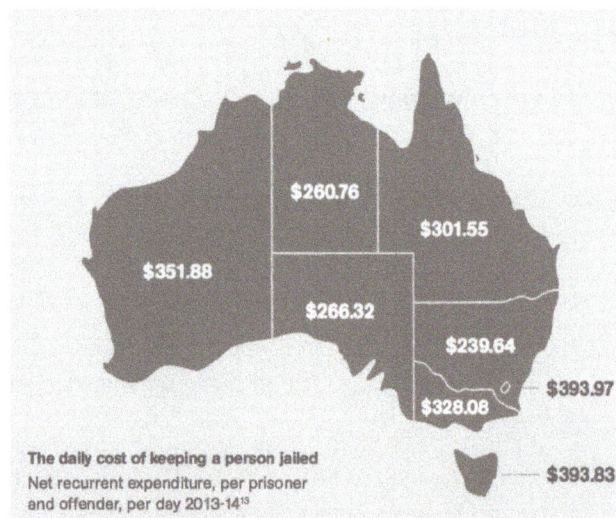

$351.88

$260.76

$301.55

$266.32

$239.64

$393.97

$328.08

$393.83

The daily cost of keeping a person jailed
Net recurrent expenditure, per prisoner and offender, per day 2013-14[13]

Bill Shorten has promised to address the "justice gap" – read his speech here

WE CAN CLOSE THE JUSTICE GAP. WE CAN. WE MUST. WE WILL.

| Author: | Bill Shorten | Published: | November 19, 2015 |

A Shorten Labor Government would support justice targets, justice reinvestment and other measures to "close the justice gap" and address the over-incarceration of Aboriginal and Torres Strait Islander people.

The promises were outlined in **a speech** by Federal Opposition leader Bill Shorten to the Melbourne Law School yesterday (published in full below).

The commitments have been welcomed by the **National Aboriginal and Torres Strait Islander Legal Services**, the **Change the Record** campaign, and **the National Family Violence Prevention Legal Services Forum**.

Bill Shorten speech:

I acknowledge the traditional owners of the land on which we meet and I pay my respects to elders past and present. Just a few weeks ago, I had the privilege of participating in the celebration of the 30th anniversary of the handback at Uluru. As part of the ceremonies, I had to provide the local Pitjantjara interpreters with a copy of my speech in advance. The lady who was interpreting my speech, Lena, had made changes to the English, because my words did not exist in Pitjantjara.

Her changes were seriously good.

Where I had written about 'dispossessing' and 'marginalising' the traditional owners, she wrote: "We took away the land from the people who knew, loved and cared for it."

I had quoted Stanner's famous reference to the 'Great Australian silence' in our history. Lena changed this to: *An empty place in our nation's heart*. I was blown away by Lena's words, ringing with truth. And it struck me as something of a metaphor for so much of what occurs in Indigenous affairs. The first Australians, knowing precisely what they have endured and exactly what it means. And the rest of us not quite speaking the same language, not capturing the same truth.

With some heroic exceptions, decades of failing to say exactly what we mean – and not always meaning what we say. This is why our efforts to close the gap, and build momentum for constitutional recognition, must always be informed by the voices of Aboriginal and Torres Strait Islander peoples and their community-controlled, representative organisations. Any proposal for change we take to the Australian people must be owned and shaped by the First Australians.

At the gathering of Indigenous leaders in July, we agreed to establish a Council to help formalise the referendum question, the timing and to lead the community conversation. I know there is a growing frustration with a lack of action in getting the Council up and running. For our part, we will continue to do as much as we can, with the Prime Minister, to progress the Council, so they can get on with their important work. Because every day of delay, every day of talk without progress, creates the risk of apathy and cynicism undercutting our goal. We can't prevaricate any longer. We need to ensure the next steps are clear – and democratic. Informed by grassroots activists and advocates, citizens and Elders in the community who know what recognition means to them – and what it must mean to Australia.

I believe a deep reservoir of national goodwill exists for success. There are those who say we should be cautious, preserving popularity by offering only minimal, symbolic change. I take a different view, I believe we draw upon this goodwill to achieve meaningful, substantive change. Change that rightly consigns the race powers in our Constitution to the same fate as the White Australia policy. Change that makes it clear there is no place for racism in modern Australia.

Recognition must be more than a new cover page of poetry we staple onto the front of the Constitution. Australians set their ambitions high – and expect their elected representatives to rise to the challenge. It's up to our generation, to all of us, to right this wrong. And yet whatever words we choose, we know recognition alone is not enough – unless it is accompanied by post-recognition action. Real action, to address the racism, injustice, poverty and disadvantage that afflict the lives of the First Australians.

When Aboriginal people die ten years' earlier than non-Indigenous Australians, we need to offer more than recognition.

When Australia is the only developed nation in the world where trachoma is endemic, we need to change more than our constitution.

When half of the young people in juvenile detention are Aboriginal and Torres Strait Islander people... When two per cent of our population makes up more than a quarter of our prison population...

When an Aboriginal man leaving school is more likely to go to jail than university... We must do more than correct historical injustice. We must strive to deliver justice.

I will never forget sitting in the Parliament in 2008 for the Apology. Kevin Rudd said sorry on behalf of a nation for the prejudice and exclusion inflicted by governments past, and the first Australians accepted that Apology in the spirit in which it was offered. That moment was a test of honesty, speaking the truth about our history. The test of this moment, of our generation, is to make sure we do not merely trade one set of mistakes for another. I don't want another Prime Minister, in another Parliament to have to deliver another apology for the failures and neglect of our generation. This is why Labor built the Closing the Gap framework – and set clear targets and timetables.

Early childhood education. Reading, writing and numeracy. Year 12 completion. Halving the employment gap by 2018. Halving the mortality gap for children under five. And closing the life expectancy gap by 2031. We are on track to halve the child mortality gap, but in other areas progress has been uneven – and there is more to do. Setting specific targets means we record our performance. It focuses national attention on closing the gap. And it keeps all of us – politicians, public servants and service providers accountable. It's why in 2013, Labor sought to create a new target, ensuring 90 per cent of Indigenous Australians with disability will be able to access NDIS support by 2020.

Labor is committed to this.

And the appalling rate of incarceration among Aboriginal and Torres Strait Islander peoples demands we create justice targets. Targets that allow us to focus on community safety, preventing crime and reducing incarceration. Less crime, and less punishment. Because nowhere is the story of unfairness and diminished opportunity more clearly defined than in the justice gap between the first Australians and the rest of us.

We must do more than correct historical injustice. We must strive to deliver justice

From family violence, to incarceration rates – the numbers are simply shocking.

If you are an Aboriginal man, you are 15 times more likely to be imprisoned than a non-Aboriginal man.

Half of all Aboriginal prisoners are under 30.

The re-imprisonment rate for Aboriginal young people is higher than the school retention rate.

The numbers are heartbreaking – and getting worse.

Imprisonment rates have more than doubled in the past decade, growing independent from changes in the crime rate.

And for Aboriginal women, the rate of imprisonment is accelerating even faster – a 74 per cent increase in the past 15 years.

Today, Aboriginal women are one-third of our female prisoners.

There are far too many people in prison with poorly-understood disability, particularly cognitive and mental disabilities. We cannot tolerate a system that just processes people, rather than a system that fairly administers justice. We cannot let it be said of modern Australia that the colour of your skin determines whether or not you end up in jail. It is devastating that jail is seen as a rite of passage for many Aboriginal and Torres Strait Islander people, part of the natural order of things.

It is an outrage that there is an attitude that this is normal. It is not normal.

It is soul-shattering that our justice system is defunct for communities in our nation. And this ongoing injustice isn't confined to outback communities, far from our gaze. We can't take the shoulder-shrugging view that this is just the tyranny of distance or a 'fact of life' in remote Australia. The injustice is just as shameful across our cities and regional towns. For individuals, an early stint in jail means you're more likely to grapple with mental health issues or develop a substance addiction... ...and less likely to finish school, learn a trade or get a job.

Children with a parent in jail are less likely to go to school. More likely to know the pain of poverty and neglect. And more likely to be part of the rapidly-growing number of Aboriginal children placed in out-of-home care. A number that has increased by a staggering 440 per cent since the Bringing them Home report was released in 1997.

Every community pays a price – with higher crime rates, reduced safety, and family violence. And it costs the taxpayer $292 a day to keep someone in prison.

It's time for Australia to face these failures. To demand an end to this grievous national shame.

The first meeting of COAG convened under a Shorten Labor Government will work on justice targets. We will work closely with State and local governments, through law enforcement agencies, corrections and community services And just as importantly, we will be guided by the people who live the reality of the justice gap: community leaders, Elders and Aboriginal representative organisations.

Crime and incarceration affects the safety of the whole community – and the solution belongs to the whole community. Two years ago the town of Bourke in the west of New South Wales topped the state for six of the eight crime categories. Including family violence, sexual assault and robbery. In February 2013, a headline in the Sydney Morning Herald reported that if Bourke was a nation, on a per capita basis, it would be 'more dangerous than any country in the world'.

The people of Bourke said 'enough is enough'. The community brought together 18 different organisations: police, magistrates, legal services, mental health experts and community groups to examine the causes of crime – and to work on preventing crime. This is not about being 'soft' on crime, or giving offenders a free pass. It's about breaking the vicious cycle of disadvantage, the demoralising treadmill of offending and incarceration. This has been baptised as a 'justice reinvestment' model: prevention, rehabilitation and diversion. An approach owned, championed by local people...informed by local knowledge, local expertise... and supported by the NSW government.

Building the capacity of communities to tackle the underlying causes of crime: substance abuse, disengagement from school and family dislocation. Similar programs are underway in Cowra, in Katherine, in the Northern Territory – where the NT Law society is helping fund a project. And the South Australian Government has offered its support to two sites. But after two

years, one of the problems confronting Bourke is a lack of co-ordinated information about what is working, and what is not. It's difficult for time-poor people on the frontline to take a step back and assess their performance. It's time for the Federal Government to step up.

A Shorten Labor Government will provide the resources for a long-term study of justice reinvestment in Bourke, to see what Australia can learn. And Labor will work with communities who are committed to this approach, and with the states and territories, to select three more launch sites: in a major city, a regional town and a remote community to roll out a local-power model for community safety.

Through COAG, we will create a national coordinating body for collecting data and measuring progress. Building safer communities, by empowering residents.

> *It's time for Australia to face these failures. To demand an end to this grievous national shame*

Of course, we can never talk about community safety, without addressing the scourge of family violence. Violence against Aboriginal women is at the very core of the national shame of family violence in Australia. An Aboriginal woman is 34 times more likely to be hospitalised as a result of family violence. And 11 times more likely to die. Family violence is the number one cause of Aboriginal children being removed from their family and their community, and all the trauma and disruption to the social fabric this entails. And too many women seeking help from family violence face significant legal, psychological and cultural barriers. Every woman living in fear must have access to safe and culturally appropriate legal support, no matter where they live. This is why Australia's 14 Family Violence Prevention Legal Services are so important. These Aboriginal community-controlled organisations work to break down the fear and isolation that affects many victims of family violence. Many Aboriginal women come to a centre after living in violent situations for many years, trusting the staff to provide support and advice – without judgment. These centres don't just provide legal advice for one day in court. They are a bridge to counselling and housing services, as well as leading community education campaigns aimed at boosting resilience and respect.

Disappointingly, Malcolm Turnbull's recent Family Violence announcement neglected to invest in these services. A decision that sits alongside a $21.5 million cut from Legal Aid Commissions. $13.4 million cut from Aboriginal and Torres Strait Islander Legal Services. And a broader $270 million cut from community support services – such as emergency relief, financial counselling and family relationships grants. Far from the front page and the nightly news, cuts like these rarely receive the media condemnation they deserve.

But I want you to know I get how much pressure these cuts place on every community legal centre. Ramping up demand on facilities already under strain, many running on their own tight budgets and absorbing cuts themselves. This is why the first funding commitment I gave as Labor leader was to restore $50 million in legal service funding – including $4.5 million specifically allocated to Aboriginal Family Violence Prevention Legal Services. I know every dollar of this money is desperately needed – and I know it will be well spent. Particularly when the presence of accessible, culturally-appropriate support can be the difference between Aboriginal women seeking help – and suffering in silence.

I know in some conservative quarters it's fashionable to say: 'money won't solve the problem on its own'. But cutting funding won't rescue family violence survivors – full stop. So, the next time you hear someone talk about the 'cost' of preventing family violence, you tell them this. By 2021, the cost of not preventing family violence among Aboriginal and Torres Strait Islander people alone...will be $2.2 billion a year. Above all, eliminating family violence from our national life, depends upon delivering equality for Australian women, regardless of who they are or where they live.

Equal opportunity for work, equal pay at work and an equal chance to lead decision-making for their communities and their country. And we cannot close the justice gap, the family violence gap – without closing the gender gap for Aboriginal women and girls. Better education for girls and young women is our best hope of promoting better health and nutrition, reducing infant and maternal mortality rates – and boosting productivity and employment. But right now, less than six in ten Aboriginal and Torres Strait Islander female students complete secondary school (as opposed to over eight in ten for non-Indigenous students). And over 50 per cent of Aboriginal mothers have their first child while they are still teenagers.

We must engage young people at school and beyond. The Clontarf academy among others has proven successful in improving school retention rate for Aboriginal and Torres Strait Islander boys. Yet while there are 28 of these various academies designed specifically for boys, there are only 13 for girls. We can't build gender equality on this shifting, uneven foundation. A Labor Government I lead will address the current inequity in programs for girls. We will partner with Stars Foundation, to build on their existing programs in schools in the Northern Territory, to engage many more Aboriginal and Torres Strait Islander girls and young women across Australia. The Stars program adopts an approach similar to the Clontarf model, but designed specifically for female Aboriginal and Torres Strait Islander students. Providing full-time mentors and using extra-curricular activities, including sport, to improve school attendance and Year 12 attainment, as well as addressing health issues and social and emotional wellbeing. Just as importantly,

We cannot close the justice gap, the family violence gap – without closing the gender gap for Aboriginal women and girls

identifying the path from school to work or further education and training. Addressing endemic poverty and disadvantage in so many Aboriginal and Torres Strait Islander families and communities... ....depends on educating and empowering the next generation of girls – the generation currently in school, the generation who will close the gap.

A Shorten Labor Government will invest $8.4 million to create 7155 new places in the Stars Program for girls across Australia. The Foundation will work with other organisations delivering school-based mentoring to girls and young women to engage and support students.

Friends, I'm not here tonight pretending to have all the answers, or that governments can resolve every issue. There's been enough of that, enough imposed solutions creating new problems. Instead, we need to recognise that the best plans and policies depend upon fundamental respect for Aboriginal and Torres Strait Islander peoples.

Empowering people has guided my whole working life. The best outcomes occur when people are empowered to make decisions about their own lives. These principles are at the heart of great campaigns like 'Change the Record' being led by Kirstie Parker and Shane Duffy...with the guidance of Mick Gooda – who has been such a strong voice for empowering communities through diversion and prevention in justice. But relying on the goodwill and generosity of an under-resourced, over-worked few is not enough. The injustice dealt to Aboriginal and Torres Strait Islander people is a stain on our whole nation, and it is a challenge to our whole nation.

The national lawmakers must lead. We should not deceive ourselves. We need new justice targets. Shared goals, shaped by the voices of all involved. Law enforcement, legal services, community sector experts, governments and – above all – Aboriginal and Torres Strait Islander peoples.

Friends, not for one minute do I underestimate the scope or the scale of the challenge before us. No generation of Australians has passed the test we face. But if we listen, if we work together, I believe we can succeed where others have failed.

We can close the justice gap.

We can. We must. We will.

Growing pressure for governments to address the over-incarceration of Aboriginal and Torres Strait Islander people

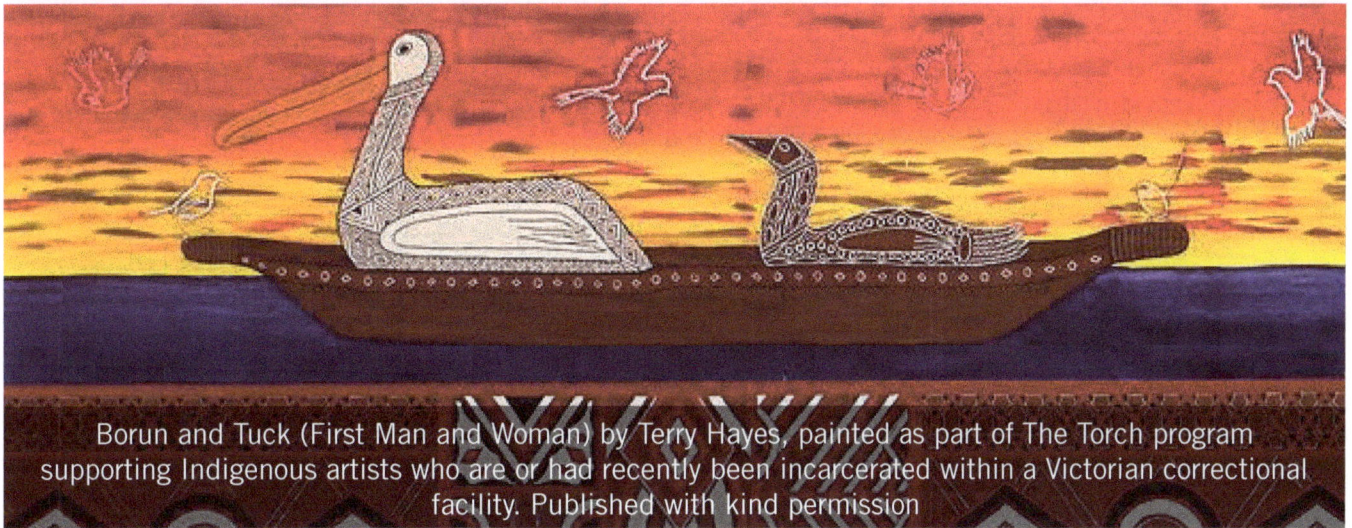

Borun and Tuck (First Man and Woman) by Terry Hayes, painted as part of The Torch program supporting Indigenous artists who are or had recently been incarcerated within a Victorian correctional facility. Published with kind permission

Author: Marie McInerney

Published: November 06, 2015

Recommendations to reduce the over-incarceration of Aboriginal and Torres Strait Islander people will be in the international spotlight when Australia's human rights record comes under scrutiny at the UN Human Rights Council.

Representatives of the Australian Government are due to appear before the Council in Geneva next Monday (November 9) as part of the Universal Periodic Review (UPR) of Australia's human rights record (follow #AusUPR for news).

A submission to the Council by a coalition of NGOs says Australia should implement justice reinvestment strategies and justice targets to address the underlying causes of over-representation of Aboriginal and Torres Strait Islanders peoples in the criminal justice system.

The submission also calls for Australia to review all mandatory sentencing laws, with a view to abolishing them. Since Australia's last UPR, the number of imprisoned disadvantaged people has increased, and the general conditions in prisons around Australia have deteriorated, it says.

A series of fact sheets prepared as part of the submission note that "overcrowding, poor conditions and substandard healthcare characterise Australian prisons", and that "there is significant under-funding of the legal system and systematic barriers to accessing justice, particularly for vulnerable and disadvantaged people".

Marie McinerneY reports on detailed recommendations to address Victoria's poor performance.

Marie McInerney writes:

The Victorian Ombudsman has found that targeted programs for Aboriginal and Torres Strait Islander prisoners in the state are "limited and constantly under pressure", contributing to high rates of imprisonment and recidivism.

Following a one-year investigation into Victoria's over-crowded prisons, Ombudsman Deborah Glass has recommended the State look at a range of different supports for Aboriginal and Torres Strait Islander prisoners, before and after they are sentenced.

Her recommendations include justice reinvestment pilots in Aboriginal communities and consideration of a New Zealand Corrections case-management initiative to cut reoffending by 25 per cent over five years.

The Ombudsman said the New Zealand initiative is centred on 'throughcare' – from a prisoner's entry into the system to their eventual release – where prisoners are assigned a non-custodial officer as their case manager, directing their prison support with programs that focus on employment, accommodation, education and training, living skills, health/well-being, whanau, family and community links.

"The position description for New Zealand case managers lists tertiary qualifications as desirable, as well as backgrounds in rehabilitative services, allied health services, psychology or social work, together with knowledge of and experience working with Maori and Pacific Peoples and their communities," she said in the report.

The NZ approach compares starkly with her findings about the lack of targeted programs and services for Aboriginal and Torres Strait Islander prisoners in Victoria. At Port Phillip prison, she found that a single Aboriginal welfare officer was responsible for supporting 99 Aboriginal and Torres Strait Islander prisoners – three times the recommended caseload – and that a number of roles had been vacant for extended periods of time.

The Ombudsman's recommendations related specifically to Aboriginal and Torres Strait Islander prison number include to:

- Pilot justice reinvestment style approaches, including in the Aboriginal community. The report says Victoria can learn from other jurisdictions in Australia which are trialling justice reinvestment (notably Bourke in New South Wales, but emerging programs in South Australia and Western Australia).

- Review the role and number of staff providing ongoing welfare, advocacy and support to Aboriginal and Torres Strait Islander prisoners.

- Expand the Koori Courts, which – along with other specialist courts – have overseen a reduction in recidivism.

- Review cultural programs for Aboriginal and Torres Strait Islander prisoners to meet demand and ensure they are as effective as possible. The report says their efficacy is "well supported" but they are not run consistently across all prisons. The Ombudsman cited the Victorian Aboriginal Legal Services submission as saying "cultural practices and observances are on par with religious observances and should be respected in a similar way".

- Provide better post-release support, particularly around housing for women who risk returning to violent or offending households.

- Continue the acclaimed art program for Aboriginal and Torres Strait Islander prisoners, and consider allowing proceeds of sale of artworks to support the prisoner's transition to the community. See this recent story on The Torch program that an evaluation found may reduce reoffending rates by up to 53 per cent.

Findings of the report

The Ombudsman's investigation into the rehabilitation and reintegration of prisoners in Victoria followed a dramatic rise in Victoria's prison numbers in the wake of tough reforms to sentencing, bail and parole measures, including the abolition of suspended sentencing, introduced by the former Coalition State Government.

She found:

" *...the rapid growth in numbers of people in the system and behind bars has overwhelmed the capacity to deliver consistent and effective rehabilitation or reintegration for prisoners.*

The investigation shows the trend is particularly a problem for Aboriginal and Torres Strait Islander prisoners: their numbers are rising the fastest in Victoria, their recidivism rates outstrip those of fellow prisoners, and they increasingly miss out on vital cultural and welfare programs in prison and supports on leaving prison.

Given the disadvantage experienced by Aboriginal and Torres Strait Islander people and their over-representation in custody, she finds a compelling case for more action to reduce both the number of prisoners in the first instance and the re-offending rate.

She quotes Social Justice Commissioner Mick Gooda as saying it is shameful that "we do better at keeping Aboriginal people in prisons than we do in schools."

"Long-term solutions do not lie within the walls of our prisons or with a single government department. Victoria needs a whole-of-government approach to focus on the causes of crime rather than its consequences," she said.

You can listen to an extended 3RRR interview with the Ombudsman here – from 19.00 minutes.

Warnings unheeded

The Ombudsman's findings have been well flagged in Victoria in recent years. Writing two years ago in the Victorian Council of Social Service's Insight magazine, Queensland academic Chris Cunneen said he was not sure that Victorians would enjoy being compared with the Northern Territory in terms of "prison policy backwardness".

But he said they certainly had one thing in common: "a dramatic race to the bottom in locking up more and more Aboriginal people."

In fact, Victoria has 'won' the race, according the Ombudsman's report. Victoria now has the fastest rate of increase in Aboriginal and Torres Strait Islander imprisonment in Australia, doubling in number to 1,435 prisoners over the ten years to 2014, an increase of 114 per cent and just ahead of the Northern Territory on 104 per cent.

Despite making up only 0.7 per cent of the population, Aboriginal people now represent nearly 8 per cent of prisoners in Victoria, and are more likely than the general prison population to return to prison, with a recidivism rate (reoffending within two years of release) of 55 per cent versus 44 per cent for non-Indigenous offenders.

According to Corrections Victoria, the recent growth in the Aboriginal and Torres Strait Islander prisoner population in Victoria has been driven largely by an increase in remand and parole cancellations. Over half the male Koori prisoners received under sentence in 2013-14 came into prison as a result of their parole being cancelled.

The Ombudsman quotes findings from the 2010 Senate Select Committee report on Indigenous incarceration that Aboriginal and Torres Strait islander people come into contact with the justice system at a much higher rates because they are "disproportionately affected by:

- policing agendas, such as zero-tolerance policing, powers to move people on and search on the spot, due to their traditional practice of gathering and socialising in public space, which increases their visibility to police, and subsequently the justice system

- increased severities in bail, where bail is often refused or, if granted, conditions make it difficult to ensure compliance

- lowering of sentencing thresholds in instances where Aboriginal and Torres Strait Islander people have a prior criminal record

- tougher crime policies in general.

The Ombudsman also looks at big gaps in post-release support for prisoners, particularly housing for vulnerable women who may return to violent or offending environments or go homeless on release. She quotes one service:

" *We're often called upon to pick up a released prisoner who has come out of prison at a late hour after public transport has finished...(or) on a Friday night. This has the impact of leaving the prisoner vulnerable from the minute they come out of prison.*

The report says only 20 per cent of prisoners get post-release support through Corrections Victoria.

Remand prisoners have doubled

A big area of concern in Victoria is the soaring number of prisoners held on remand, accounting for nearly a quarter of all prisoners and almost doubling since 2011. It is a particular issue for Aboriginal women prisoners.

An alleged offender is remanded in custody if they:

- have not applied for bail

- have been refused bail

- cannot afford to lodge bail

- are unable or unwilling to meet conditions set out in the bail bond.

Often this an issue for people who are homeless or live in rural and regional areas where they cannot access housing or mental health supports that are part of bail requirements.

High remand numbers are fuelling overcrowding, which Jesuit Social Services said recently was as much behind recent riots as the more widely reported looming smoking ban.

They are also significant in other ways. Importantly for their rehabilitation prospects, remand prisoners, who are unsentenced, have only limited opportunities to access programs to address their offending – for example, mental health or substance abuse programs. They also have very limited ability to demonstrate good conduct following an offence, such as by participating in drug treatment, compared to a person on bail.

The Ombudsman also found that growing numbers of prisoners are choosing not to apply for parole because of "onerous" new conditions. She reported they would "rather spend extra time in prison than be released on parole and risk the chance of breaching parole and being reimprisoned."

As a result, they do not have to complete programs that might have addressed offending behaviour and re-enter the community without any supervision. Others who want to participate in rehabilitation programs cannot get access (because of rising demand) and are consequently unable to obtain parole, she said.

All 25 of the Ombudsman's recommendations have been accepted in principle by the Victorian Justice and Regulation Department and the Labor Government.

It will, of course, be what happens in practice that counts.

For more information about The Torch project (see feature image): www.facebook.com/thetorchproject, www.thetorch.org.au or contact indigenousarts@thetorch.org.au

Disclaimer: Marie McInerney is a former editor of the VCOSS magazine Insight.

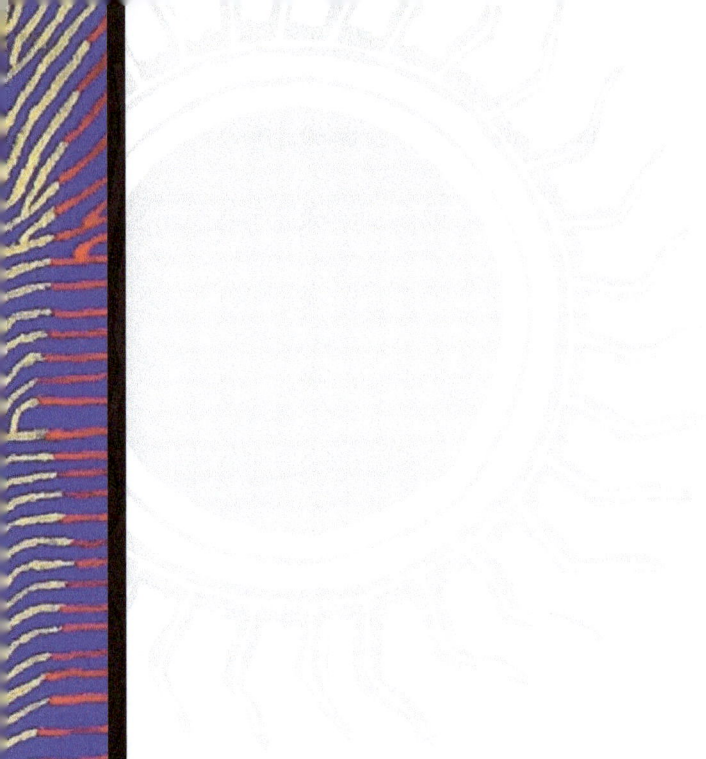

#JustJustice – Tackling the over-incarceration of Aboriginal and Torres Strait Islander peoples

6. Focus on disabilities

" It is possible to break down a big complex problem into something eminently achievable

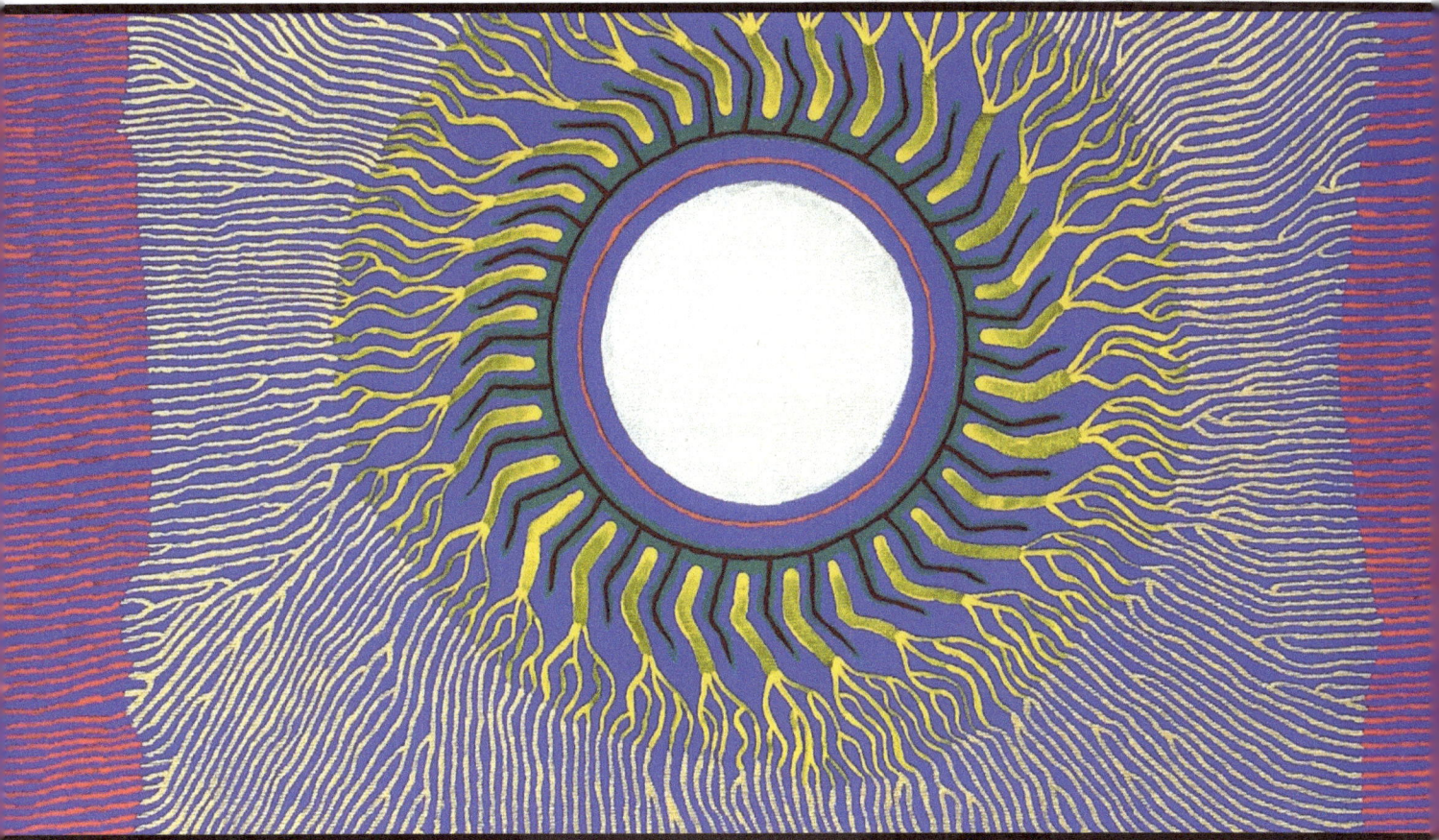

Rethinking #JustJustice for Aboriginal and Torres Strait Islander people with a disability

Author:	Scott Avery	Published:	September 04, 2015

Specific data is hard to come by, but **Scott Avery** says there are estimates that up to 80 per cent of Aboriginal and Torres Strait Islander people who come into contact with the justice system have some form of disability. The injustice of that was laid bare recently in the case of Roseanne Fulton, who was kept in custody after the West Australian court system declared her unfit to be tried on driving offences.

Avery – who is Policy and Research Director at the First Peoples Disability Network (Australia) – says the implementation of the National Disability Insurance Scheme offers a new opportunity to divert people from unwarranted incarceration to supported disability programs.

He asks: can one national-building social initiative be the catalyst for significant social change in another?

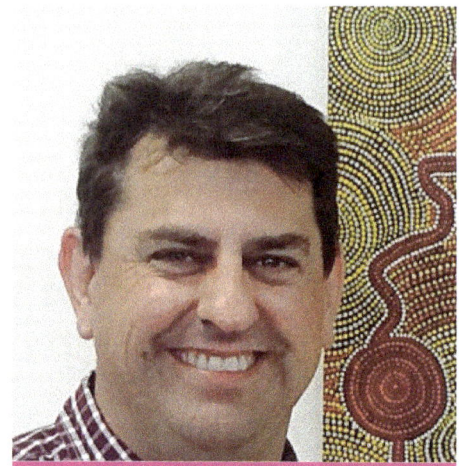

Scott Avery

Scott Avery writes:

The impact of disability on all social outcomes is not well understood, and policy responses coming from a disability perspective have largely been avoided to date, not least in the criminal justice area, where large numbers of Aboriginal and Torres Strait Islander people with disability are languishing in prison when they could be justly, and more effectively, supported on a disability program.

The Australian Human Rights Commission Report, *Equal Before the Law: Towards Disability Justice Strategies* (2014), identified a number of ways through which people with disability are inhibited in accessing their rights to a #JustJustice. These start with negative attitudes and assumptions about people with disability that affect how they are treated right through the justice system, from policing to judicial administration and conditions in prison.

Furthermore, community support programs to prevent violence and disadvantage do not necessarily exist for people with disability, and awareness and understanding of the specialist needs for people with disability to defend criminal matters are rare commodities. For Aboriginal and Torres Strait Islander people with disability, these barriers are magnified as they confront barriers related to their Aboriginality as well as their disability – in effect a 'double discrimination'.

The phrase 'game-changer' gets thrown around a bit, but the implementation of the National Disability Insurance Scheme (NDIS) would well be one when it comes to the opportunity to structurally alter the entry points of the justice system. As a national initiative to improve the rights of people with disability, the NDIS is designed to provide the social supports affecting the quality of life for a person with disability, encompassing disability services, education, employment and even social housing. This sounds very much like a social determinants approach to Indigenous Affairs. So the question is, can one national-building social initiative be the catalyst for significant social change in another?

It is estimated that one in two Aboriginal and Torres Strait Islander people have a disability or long-term health condition, with 8 per cent having a disability that is profound or severe.[1] Specific data on Aboriginal and Torres Strait Islander people with disability in prison is hard to come by. Nonetheless, many legal services advise that up to 80 per cent of Aboriginal clients could have some form of disability, once mental health conditions and trauma are taken into consideration. Even assuming a lower prevalence of 50 per cent, the capacity to divert Aboriginal and Torres Strait Islander people onto supported disability programs could significantly reduce unwarranted incarceration.

If one in five people with disability are diverted from detention and into a supported disability program, then

the overall Aboriginal and Torres Strait Islander prison population could be reduced by 10 per cent.

On the face of it, diverting 1 in 5 people away from prison and onto a supported disability programs is both significant and achievable. But there are barriers in our federal system of government which need to be thought through, with the backing of strong political leadership.

Firstly, responsibilities for the disability sector are progressively transferring from state and territory governments to the Commonwealth, principally through the establishment of the National Disability Insurance Agency (NDIA). Policing and justice on the other hand remain firmly with the states and territories. So what the diversion policy involves is not just systems mapping between sectors, it is system mapping between levels of government. Whilst this might seem complex, the good news is that, as a new scheme, there are no precedents or institutional practices within the NDIS which require un-breaking.

Second, implementing the NDIS is a massive undertaking. The temptation to prioritise what it might consider as 'core business' would be overwhelming. But start-up is when new practices and ways of doing business can be considered, and is the time to apply a broader disability perspective to the social agenda.

What is needed is a project upon which to focus.

There are about 1,000 young people currently in juvenile detention, half of whom are Aboriginal or Torres Strait Islander. [2] Assuming the opening gambit is to divert 1 in 5 young people onto supported disability program, that equates to case management for 100 young people.

It is possible to break down a big complex problem into something eminently achievable. The national initiative in disability enables us to think differently, not just about access rights to services for people with disability, but in other areas of social policy. Through collective will and ingenuity, the nation now has a National Disability Insurance Scheme, something which just a decade ago was pipe dream. We just need to cut and paste this with will and ingenuity and apply it towards a #JustJustice for First peoples.

On the face of it, diverting 1 in 5 people away from prison and onto a supported disability programs is both significant and achievable. But there are barriers in our federal system of government which need to be thought through, with the backing of strong political leadership

Scott Avery is the Policy and Research Director at the First Peoples Disability Network (Australia) and is undertaking a professional doctorate on disability in Aboriginal and Torres Strait Islander communities at the UNSW Australia. Follow on Twitter @FPDNAus

[1] Australian Institute of Health and Welfare (2011) Analysis of NATSISS 2008, Table 1.13, p. 378. At http://www.aihw.gov.au/WorkArea/DownloadAsset.aspx?id=10737420007

[2] Australian Institute of Health and Welfare (2013) Youth detention population in Australia http://www.aihw.gov.au/WorkArea/DownloadAsset.aspx?id=60129545393

What is the relationship between lifelong hearing loss and Indigenous incarceration? A powerful story to mark Hearing Awareness Week

Author:	Sam Harkus	Published:	August 23, 2016

What profound impact could be had on high rates of Aboriginal and Torres Strait Islander incarceration by ensuring better hearing for children and adults? It's an important question raised in this moving post below, to mark **Hearing Awareness Week**, from **Sam Harkus**, Principal Audiologist, Aboriginal & Torres Strait Islander Services.

It is republished here from the organisation's **Facebook page**.

See also **another moving story** from the Aboriginal Hearing Program published by the National Aboriginal Community Controlled Health Organisation (NACCHO) and, at the bottom of the post, a call from Menzies School of Health Research for more investment in the prevention and treatment of ear disease and hearing loss in Aboriginal and Torres Strait Islander children.

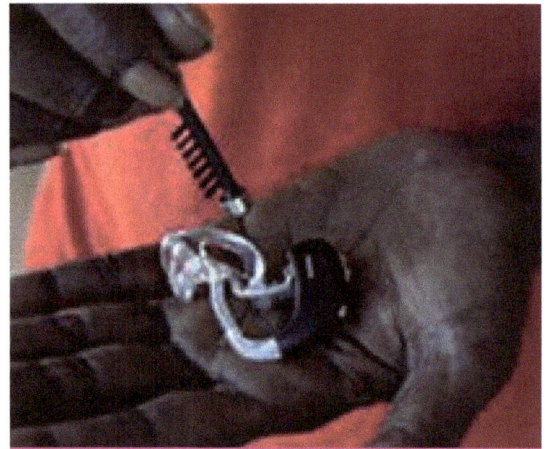

Photo by Michael Corridore

Sam Harkus writes:

It's Hearing Awareness Week. Hearing loss is over-represented among prisoners, and Aboriginal people are over-represented in our gaols. Here's a short story from the criminal justice system.

Around 15 years ago we saw a 36 year old Aboriginal woman. She had been in and out of prison 18 times: once a year since she turned 18.

She was brought in to see the Ear Specialist at an Aboriginal Medical Service, where we were working on the day. This was the first time help had been sought for her ears and hearing.

This woman had moderately severe hearing loss in her better ear and severe hearing loss in her worse ear, caused by ear infection.

When talking with this lady, she always looked tense. She watched people intently while they talked, always frowning. She sat on the edge of her seat, hunching towards me.

For someone who could only possibly hear fragments of words, she communicated well. Behind the scenes, she was working hard to do this: putting what she could hear and see together to make sense of what I was saying.

I asked her how she managed in a court room. When questions were asked, could she hear them? She said she guessed what she was being asked, and answered that.

I asked her about how she managed day to day in prison. She went regularly to rehab meetings, a round circle discussion, but couldn't hear so didn't contribute.

As she was growing up, she had wanted to be a receptionist in a doctor's surgery. One day she realised that she could never do that, because people at the counter needed to be able to speak discreetly. Raising their voices so that the receptionist could hear would never do.

She was put on the waiting list for surgery, and in the meantime the prison agreed to provide a hearing aid for her.

When we saw her after her hearing aid fitting, she was a changed woman: she was wearing the aid and smiling, not frowning. She was sitting back in her chair looking relaxed.

She talked about the difference for her: she could talk to her mum over the phone. She could take part in rehab discussions and was finding that was good. She said 'There's nothing better than being able to hear'.

Later we heard that she had become the Koori Women's Delegate at the prison: representing the interests of

Aboriginal women in prison with her. Being able to hear easily enabled her to start realising her own potential.

Then she left prison and we lost contact. I often wonder where she is and what she is doing now.

This woman and the whole experience made a huge impression on me. I had just read this article by Damien Howard and Sue Quinn on Aboriginal hearing loss and the criminal justice system, and this breathed life into it. Many of the issues dealt with in the article became real, including the challenges of the court room.

As an audiologist of ten years experience at that point, in a country with relatively good access to hearing services, I had not come across anyone before who had had such a significant level of unremediated hearing loss for so long. How many cracks had she slipped through to get this far without help? How good was our system if that was able to happen?

Because her significant hearing loss had gone on for so long, the change in her after receiving the hearing aid was dramatic, including the transformation in the way in which she physically held herself. This was the first time I had seen this.

It was also a lesson for me in the way hearing loss disempowered, and the way being able to hear well again empowered. Look at what she was able to achieve with one hearing aid, and look at how she had been limited by not being able to hear. Imagine how disappointing the realisation was that her dream job was out of her reach. What had been the relationship between her lifelong hearing loss and her incarceration?

I will never forget her statement: 'There's nothing better than being able to hear.'

Statement from Menzies School of Health Research:

"In recognition of Hearing Awareness Week (August 21-27), leading ear health experts at Menzies School of Health Research (Menzies) are calling for more investment in the prevention and treatment of ear disease and hearing loss in Aboriginal and Torres Strait Islander children.

Menzies Professor Amanda Leach says the failure to recognise the damage of prior or current ear disease and hearing loss imposes further disadvantage to Indigenous children that might already be struggling in the education and juvenile detention systems.

Indigenous children have the highest rates of otitis media – commonly known as middle ear infection – and burst eardrums in the world, Prof Leach explained.

In remote communities, otitis media and significant hearing loss establishes in almost all babies within weeks of birth. Research has revealed these ear infections are not as painful for Indigenous children compared to non-Indigenous children, so the disease progresses undetected and often results in perforated ear drums. "Hearing loss impacts on

the development of speech and language and is linked to educational disadvantage, communication and behavioural problems.

Indigenous children almost always have bilateral hearing loss which impacts on auditory processing difficulties, lead to social isolation, disengagement with the education system, their community and their peers.

Prof Leach said Hearing Awareness Week provides an opportunity to help Australians understand the difficulties Indigenous children with ear disease and hearing loss face and how hearing loss impacts everything from education outcomes, to employment opportunities, to living standards and personal safety.

A National Health and Medical Research Council (NHMRC) funded Centre of Research Excellence in Ear and Hearing Health of Indigenous children (CRE_ICHEAR), led by Prof Leach, is dedicated to improving ear and hearing health among Indigenous children and ending the disadvantage associated with hearing loss.

Indigenous leaders, researchers and other experts in our CRE_ICHEAR have worked hard to find out what works and what needs to be done in addressing potential prevention and treatment strategies, but more is needed. What we really need is a whole of government approach, Prof Leach said.

The health sector needs to invest in clinical training; clinicians need to understand the aetiology and appropriate use of antibiotics when treating ear disease; and the education system needs to allocate resources to training teachers in effective strategies for engaging and teaching children who have hearing loss.

Research Excellence in Ear and Hearing Health of Indigenous children (CRE_ICHEAR), led by Prof Leach, is dedicated to improving ear and hearing health among Indigenous children and ending the disadvantage associated with hearing loss.

Indigenous leaders, researchers and other experts in our CRE_ICHEAR have worked hard to find out what works and what needs to be done in addressing potential prevention and treatment strategies, but more is needed. What we really need is a whole of government approach, Prof Leach said.

Calling for #JustJustice for Aboriginal and Torres Strait Islander people with cognitive impairments

Author:	Julie Edwards	Published:	June 15, 2016

Aboriginal and Torres Strait Islander people with cognitive impairments are suffering terribly at the hands of discriminatory justice systems, particularly in the NT.

Julie Edwards, CEO of **Jesuit Social Services**, calls for reforms to ensure justice systems better meet the needs of people with cognitive impairments.

Julie Edwards writes:

In the Northern Territory, Aboriginal and Torres Strait Islander people with cognitive impairments are being indefinitely detained in prison despite not being charged.

In 2014 the **Australian Human Rights Commission** found that the inability of both the Commonwealth and Northern Territory Governments to provide adequate accommodation and support services for four Indigenous men with disabilities (all of whom were deemed unfit to plead and detained in a correctional facility) constituted a clear abuse of human rights.

One of the men spent more than four and a half years detained in the Alice Springs Correctional Centre before being transferred to a secure care facility; however, if he had been found guilty of the offence with which he was charged, the Court would have imposed a term of imprisonment of 12 months.

There is a chronic lack of alternative options to prison for people with cognitive impairments

While the lack of screening and diagnostic tools means there is no definitive data on the total number of Indigenous people with cognitive impairment in the criminal justice system, **expert opinion** and estimates suggest this group is significantly over-represented compared to the general population.

As part of a study about Aboriginal people with psychiatric and cognitive impairments in the NT and NSW, **University of NSW researchers** found that "police and prisons have become governments' default way of managing this vulnerable group rather than appropriately supporting them to have a life of stability and self-worth in the community".

So why is this happening?

First, current legislation does not protect people with cognitive impairment charged with lower level crime.

Although there are legislation and schemes in the lower courts (i.e. Court of Summary Jurisdiction) that "may be relevant to a person with a cognitive impairment", unfortunately most of these schemes focus on the needs of people with a mental health problem, which are generally quite different to the needs of cognitively impaired people, states **one analysis**.

The Criminal Code Act stipulates that the Supreme Court must decide whether someone found not guilty due to mental impairment must be either liable to supervision (custodial or non-custodial) or released unconditionally ('mental impairment' in the Act includes 'senility, intellectual disability, mental illness, brain damage and involuntary intoxication').

Unfortunately, **according to criminal lawyers Michelle Swift and Jonathan Hunyor**, people are rarely released unconditionally, and the lack of appropriate facilities in the NT to house people on custodial supervision orders often sees people with cognitive disabilities indefinitely detained.

In 2012, the **Aboriginal Disability Justice Campaign found** that all of the nine people who were on a supervision order due to mental impairment were Aboriginal.

This situation is compounded by mandatory sentencing in the NT, which significantly limits the court's ability to take a person's disability into account in determining an appropriate sentence.

For relevant offences, the court can no longer take account of a symptom of disability (such as poor impulse control) as a contributing factor in offending. Nor can the court consider the particular impact of imprisonment on a person with a disability.

In its paper on the indefinite detention of Aboriginal people found unfit to plead, the Aboriginal Disability Justice Campaign argues that a sentence of imprisonment imposed on a person with a cognitive impairment may be inappropriate and ineffective because the person may not fully understand the connection between the offending behaviour and the prison experience.

As well, in some cases a person with a cognitive impairment may 'do it harder' in prison because of difficulty understanding the rules of prison and the experience more generally.

In most cases prison offers a poor therapeutic environment, and fails to support the particular needs of this group.

As well, there is a key difference between mental illness (such as depression, personality disorders, psychosis and schizophrenia) and cognitive impairment (such as intellectual disability, acquired brain injury, dementia and foetal alcohol spectrum disorder).

Mental illnesses may be episodic and can be treated, whereas cognitive impairments are ongoing and permanent. They affect intellectual functioning, including comprehension, reasoning, learning and/or memory.

The model for treating mental illness is neither appropriate nor effective for people with cognitive impairments.

Too often, according to NSW researchers, support focuses on offending behaviour – rather than addressing social disadvantage, mental health, disability or alcohol and drug issues.

Lack of culturally appropriate assessment services

Exacerbating this is the lack of adequate services available for workers in the criminal justice system (lawyers, corrections officers, magistrates, etc) to support comprehensive and culturally appropriate assessments.

Cognitive impairment requires highly specialised assessments and support programs; however, current arrangements in the NT mean that these sorts of programs are sorely lacking.

In addition, Aboriginal people with cognitive disabilities have the added complexity of the impact of intergenerational trauma, grief, loss and locational disadvantage. Colonisation and discriminatory government policies have seen generations of Aboriginal people experience racism, dispossession, early deaths of family and community members and the forced removal of children.

Finally, there is a chronic lack of alternative options to prison for people with cognitive impairments. The shortage of appropriate prison-based support and post-release programs increases the likelihood this vulnerable group will return to prison.

Aboriginal people with cognitive disabilities, particularly those living in remote communities, have limited community-based support options, which can exacerbate feelings of isolation and disconnection.

In failing to offer alternative options, the system discriminates against people with cognitive impairments and sees them exposed to the justice system for longer periods of time than those who are criminally charged.

Calling for a therapeutic focus

The pathway into prison for Aboriginal people with cognitive impairments is predictable but preventable.

Steps must be taken immediately to ensure the justice system truly meets the needs of people with cognitive disabilities in culturally appropriate ways, with a focus on therapeutic responses.

In response to the Senate inquiry into the indefinite detention of people with cognitive and psychiatric impairment, Jesuit Social Services is calling for an end to indefinite detention by reforming the justice system to better meet the needs of people with cognitive impairment.

This can be achieved by improving screening tools, amending legislation, expanding specialised problem-solving courts and providing a wider variety of therapeutic, community-based alternatives to prison.

Aboriginal people with cognitive impairments are entitled to opportunities to engage meaningfully in society and to flourish as individuals. More must be done to stop this discrimination and clear abuse of human rights.

Julie Edwards joined Jesuit Social Services in 2001 and was appointed as CEO in 2004.

> *In most cases prison offers a poor therapeutic environment, and fails to support the particular needs of this group*

New project to tackle the detention of Aboriginal and Torres Strait Islander people with disabilities

Author:	Louis Andrews, Anna Arstein-Kerslake, Piers Gooding, and Bernadette McSherry	Published:	January 06, 2016

Governments are under widespread pressure to stop the indefinite detention of Aboriginal and Torres Strait Islander people with disabilities.

As University of Melbourne researchers explain below, efforts are being made to address the "system-wide" factors contributing to this ongoing violation of human rights.

Louis Andrews, Anna Arstein-Kerslake, Piers Gooding, and Bernadette McSherry write write:

Imagine being charged with driving offences and then being detained in prison for months on end without any prospect of a trial ever taking place. This is what happened to Rosie Anne Fulton.

Rosie, an Aboriginal woman with foetal alcohol spectrum disorder, was declared by a Magistrate to be 'unfit to be tried' under the Criminal Law (Mentally Impaired Accused) Act 1996 (Western Australia).

When the ABC Lateline show reported on her plight, she had been detained in a Kalgoorlie prison for 18 months and Northern Territory authorities rejected advocates' pleas to move her to supportive accommodation near her Alice Springs family.

Indigenous people with disabilities, particularly cognitive disabilities, are vastly over-represented in the Australian prison population. The term cognitive disability captures a broad range of impairments, and affects a large number of people. It includes intellectual disabilities, but also mental health conditions such as depression, schizophrenia and psychosis, as well as acquired brain injury and foetal alcohol spectrum disorder.

In all states and territories, a defendant can be found 'unfit to stand trial'. This legal process is designed to protect vulnerable defendants from miscarriages of justice — for example, where they cannot understand the case against them or follow court proceedings. The problem is that these processes can perpetuate and entrench injustice.

After a court finds an accused unfit to stand trial, the best case scenario is release into the community, most likely under the supervision of disability services. The worst-case scenario is incarceration in prison or an institution. And it can be incarceration with no end in sight — potentially for far longer than if the accused had been convicted and sentenced for the alleged crime.

Unfitness proceedings can violate a range of rights, including the right to a fair trial, the right to equal recognition before the law, and the right to be free from cruel and unusual punishment.

One of the worst cases of injustice concerned Marlon Noble, an Aboriginal man who was imprisoned for over 10 years without conviction in Western Australia. Noble has now been released into the community but remains under indefinite supervision, and is subject to severe restrictions on his freedom.

People with Disabilities Australia (PWDA) estimate that there are at least 100 people detained across Australia without conviction in prisons and psychiatric units under mental impairment legislation; and that at least 50 people from this group would be Aboriginal and Torres Strait Islander.

System-wide failings

According to the Aboriginal Disability Justice Campaign (ADJC), a community organisation campaigning on this issue, cases like that of Marlon Noble are indicative of much deeper, system-wide failings that lead to the incarceration of Indigenous people with cognitive disabilities.

Current figures suggest that Aboriginal and Torres Strait Islander people with disability are almost 14 times more likely to be imprisoned than the rest of the population.

There is a range of explanations for the over-representation of Indigenous people with disabilities in Australian prisons. Indigenous people are more likely to experience disabilities caused by structural disadvantage, including poverty and inaccessible health services.

At the same time, people with disabilities in general are more likely to experience poverty, isolation and increased interactions with the criminal justice system. Indigenous people with cognitive disabilities then experience double-disadvantage and discrimination.

The indefinite detention of people with disabilities in Australia has drawn criticism from law reform agencies, human rights bodies and non-government organisations.

Critics include United Nations human rights treaty bodies such as the Human Rights Council and the Committee overseeing the Convention on the Rights of Persons with Disabilities. Indeed, the Committee didn't just criticise indefinite detention, it unequivocally called for an end to the practice of indefinitely detaining people after finding them unfit to be tried.

In the face of this criticism, the Australian Government recently announced a Senate Committee Inquiry into the indefinite detention of 'people with cognitive and psychiatric impairment'. (Submissions to the Senate committee inquiry are due by the 8 April 2016).

A number of government and non-government reports have made recommendations to address this issue.

The First People's Disability Network, Australia's leading body representing Australia's First Peoples with disability, their families and communities, has made a detailed submission to the Western Australian government. Recommendations for national reform have come from the Australian Human Rights Commission, as well as the Aboriginal Disability Justice Campaign, among others.

A group of researchers, led by Professor Eileen Baldry from the University of New South Wales, has charted reform options to address what is described as the 'predictable and preventable path' of Indigenous Australians with cognitive disabilities in the criminal justice system.

University of Melbourne researchers – ourselves included – have recently partnered with Professor Baldry to commence a trial program to offer support to people at risk of being deemed unfit to stand trial.

The research will be undertaken in partnership with the North Australian Aboriginal Justice Agency to focus specifically on supporting Indigenous people.

Despite three State and Federal law reform agencies recommending formal support in this area, no support measures have been tested in any Australian jurisdiction.

Our research aims to address this gap, testing such measures and analysing unfitness rules against Australia's international human rights obligations.

See related news items compiled by the Aboriginal Disability Justice Campaign.

Disclosure: This project is funded by the Australian Government through a National Disability Research Development Grant.

The project is being undertaken jointly between the University of Melbourne, the University of New South Wales, the North Australian Aboriginal Justice Agency, the Intellectual Disability Rights Service, and the Victorian Aboriginal Legal Service. The researchers include Professor Bernadette McSherry, Professor Kerry Arabena, Professor Eileen Baldry, Dr Anna Arstein-Kerslake, Dr Piers Gooding, Dr Ruth McCausland, Mr Louis Andrews and Ms Sarah Mercer. This project is jointly funded by Commonwealth, state and territory governments under the National Disability Special Account, administered by the Department of Social Services on behalf of the Commonwealth, state and territory Research and Data Working Group.

Q: What impact did the publication of this article have?
Piers Gooding: This provided a way for us to share our research with government and non-government organisations, and particularly Indigenous-led organisations. This dissemination increased the likelihood that our research might inform law, policy and practice.

#JustJustice: young offenders must be screened for fetal alcohol spectrum disorders before sentencing

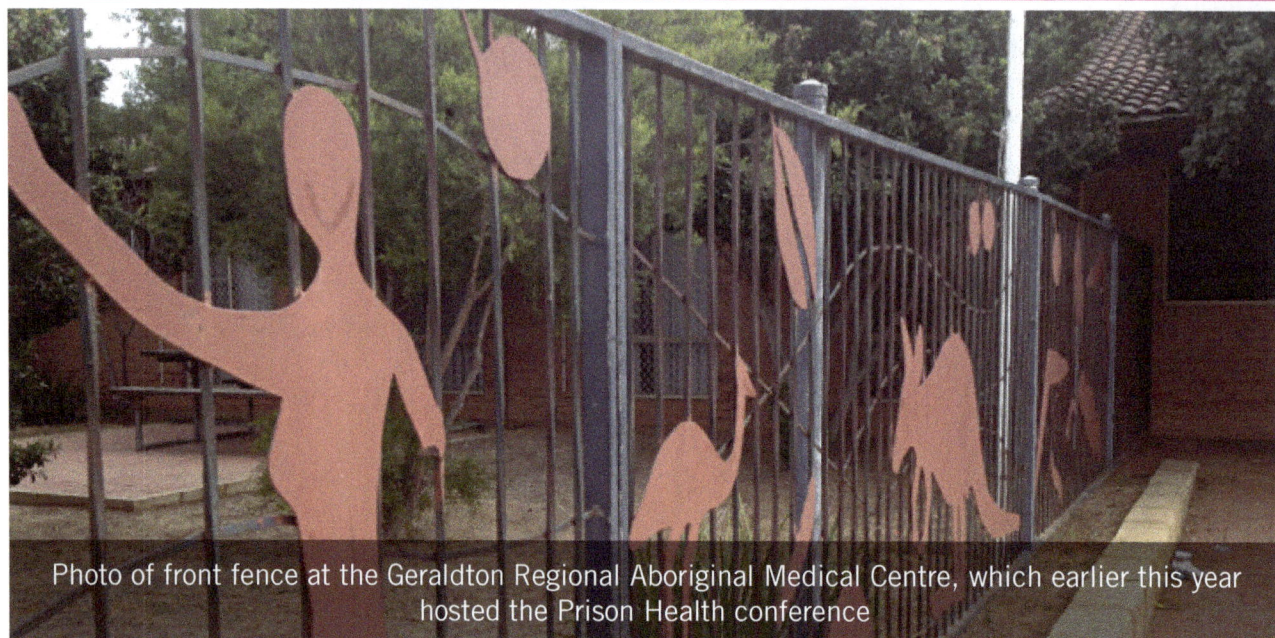

Photo of front fence at the Geraldton Regional Aboriginal Medical Centre, which earlier this year hosted the Prison Health conference

Author:	Elizabeth Elliott	Published:	October 13, 2015

The recent case of Rosie Fulton – a young women with foetal alcohol syndrome disorder (FASD) who was held in a Western Australian prison for 21 months with no conviction after a magistrate found her unfit to stand trial – showcased a terrible injustice that is particularly acute in Aboriginal and Torres Strait Islander communities.

In this article below, published originally at The Conversation, Professor Elizabeth Elliott makes an urgent call for evidence-based strategies to ensure offenders with FASD are recognised early and receive the care they deserve.

Elizabeth Elliott writes:

Australia's prison population is growing at unprecedented rates. In some states Indigenous prisoners far outnumber their non-Indigenous counterparts.

Last year in the Northern Territory, 86 per cent of those in prison and 96 per cent of those in juvenile detention were Indigenous. In Western Australia, Indigenous people account for only 3 per cent of the population, but 40 per cent of prisoners.

It is unacceptable to ignore the intellectual capacity of a person facing the court and it's vital to ensure that youth put behind bars have been properly assessed before sentencing. This is particularly important for Australians affected by fetal alcohol spectrum disorders (FASD). These occur throughout society and in high levels in some Indigenous communities.

The capacity to screen for prenatal alcohol exposure – as well as to diagnose FASD – must urgently be increased. This echoes recent calls by Perth Children's Court magistrate Catherine Crawford for clinicians to assess children and youth before sentencing, so the court understands their cognitive limitations.

Cognitive limitations

Fetal alcohol spectrum disorders are a group of preventable conditions resulting from exposure to alcohol in the womb. Alcohol readily crosses the mother's placenta, entering the circulation of the developing fetus with devastating effects.

Significantly, it can disrupt brain development and that of other organs, causing lifelong problems. These include developmental delay, intellectual and memory impairment, as well as a range of behavioural, emotional and mental health disorders.

People with FASD can suffer from attention-deficit hyperactivity disorders (ADHD), communication disorders, poor impulse control, disobedience and hostility issues, and learning difficulties.

They often struggle to distinguish right from wrong and fail to learn from mistakes. Few with FASD will live and work independently. Many have mental health and substance misuse problems.

It is no surprise that many also come in contact with the law. An adolescent living with a FASD in Canada or the United States, for instance, is estimated to have a 19 times higher risk of incarceration than someone without a FASD.

Despite this, the condition remains poorly recognised and few obtain a diagnosis prior to offending. Offenders with FASD are often poor witnesses and fail to understand why they have been detained. Unable to negotiate the justice system, they are adversely influenced by others and often enter a cycle of re-offending.

FASD and the justice system

Rosie Fulton, a 21-year-old Aboriginal woman with FASD and significant intellectual impairment, was arrested last year after stealing and crashing a car. Declared unfit to stand trial, Rosie was sent to Western Australia's Kalgoorlie Prison for lack of alternative accommodation.

She stayed in jail for 21 months with no trial or conviction. Only after her story broke, mounting pressure on the health ministers of Western Australia and the Northern Territory led to Rosie being transferred to supervised community accommodation close to her family in Alice Springs.

In Australia, we don't know how many people deemed "unfit to plead" are in prison and how many have cognitive impairment, as we lack recent data regarding rates of FASD in prisons. US studies suggest up to 60 per cent of young people with FASD will at some time enter the juvenile justice system.

Another study, conducted in a forensic mental health facility in Canada, showed 23 per cent of resident youth had one type of FASD. This figure may be higher in vulnerable Australian populations, particularly in some remote regions where alcohol use in pregnancy is prevalent.

The economic impact of incarcerating people with FASD is huge. In Canada, the direct cost to the correctional system between 2011 and 2012 was CAD$17.5 million for youth and CAD$356.2 million for adults.

Screening for FASD

Diagnosing FASD is a challenge because as children get older, a firm history of prenatal alcohol exposure may be elusive. With age, the characteristic facial features (small eye openings, a thin upper lip and flat philtrum, the area between the upper lip and base of the nose) of fetal alcohol syndrome – a subset of FASD – diminish, and growth deficits correct.

Thorough assessment by a physician, a psychologist and, if necessary, allied health professionals, can identify impairments

required for a FASD diagnosis, whether fetal alcohol syndrome or a neuro-developmental disorder associated with prenatal alcohol exposure. Such impairments can be in IQ, communication, memory, motor and executive function, and other areas.

In Canada, youth probation officers are using a tool for screening young offenders for FASD, and identifying the need for referral and assessment.

Another tool for health professionals with accompanying guidelines for assessing and diagnosing people with FASD is being developed in Australia. This will standardise the diagnostic approach.

Tools such as these are necessary to increase screening and diagnostic capacity in the justice and health systems. If a diagnosis is known, the associated behavioural and cognitive deficits can be taken into account when considering the reliability of evidence given by an offender, the supervision required in detention, and the sentence.

Appropriate care

There has been a call for better legal support for people with vulnerabilities in their journey through the criminal justice system. Consideration should be given to the defence of diminished responsibility in conditions such as FASD.

And alternative models of care need to be found to avoid imprisonment of those unable to plead. As identified in the case of Rosie Fulton, this poses a significant challenge, particularly in remote Australia where alternative accommodation is not readily available and would be costly to establish.

But prison is far more costly. In Canada, the justice system accounts for 40 per cent of the total costs of FASD (including health and education). And Australia's Senate inquiry on justice reinvestment heard that the estimated cost of detaining a juvenile offender in New South Wales in 2010–11 was much higher ($A652 per day) than the cost of supervision in the community ($A16.73 per day).

To end the cycle of re-offending, we urgently need evidence-based strategies to ensure offenders with FASD are recognised early and receive the care they deserve.

Elizabeth Elliott is Professor of Paediatrics & Child Health, University of Sydney. She receives funding from the National Health and Medical Research Council of Australia and the Australian Government for research into Fetal Alcohol Spectrum Disorders. She is a Member of the Board of charities Cure Kids Australia and the Institute for Creative Health and a member of the Medical Advisory Committee of the Steve Waugh Foundation.

This article was originally published at The Conversation and is republished with permission.

New approaches urgently needed for people living with fetal alcohol spectrum disorders (FASD)

Author:	Anne Messenger	Published:	May 19, 2015

When Croakey's #JustJustice campaign was launched by **Aboriginal and Torres Strait Islander Social Justice Commissioner Mick Gooda**, it prompted this heartfelt tweet from **Sue Miers**, the Chairperson of the **National Organisation for Fetal Alcohol Spectrum Disorders (FASD) Australia**:

"**Will never be addressed whilst #FASD continues to be ignored in Aus. A significant recognised root cause.**"

In the post below, **Anne Messenger**, Editor of *Public Health Research & Practice* at the Sax Institute, outlines what needs to be done and how we are seeing a "good start" to a different approach in New South Wales.

Anne Messenger writes:

As Sue Miers made clear in her tweet (above), government, policy makers and the community cannot continue to ignore FASD, this 'root cause' of over-incarceration. People living with fetal alcohol spectrum disorders (FASD) are **born with a brain injury** and experience great difficulties with learning, memory and cognition. That means that **in some parts of Australia** they disproportionately come into contact with the juvenile justice and corrective services systems.

Much more needs to be done, but there has been some recent movement from the New South Wales Government, which before last month's state election pledged $2.3 million to what will be Australia's **first dedicated centre** for diagnosis and treatment of fetal alcohol spectrum disorders.

The Children's Hospital Centre for the Prevention of Harm to Children and Adolescents is an expansion of a successful pilot program run out of the hospital at Westmead, Sydney. It will provide a multidisciplinary team for those affected by FASD, including a paediatrician, a psychologist, a speech therapist, occupational therapist and physiotherapist, as well as counselling for teenage mothers through a 'Teenlink' service at the hospital.

Although $2.3 million is not enough to meet the needs of all people living with FASD in New South Wales, the centre will also provide training to rural and remote community health workers; and it is hoped that other states and territories will follow the New South Wales lead. A research arm will

Although the young brain is adaptable, prenatal brain injury cannot be reversed so, for FASD, the future must be prevention

investigate the best treatment, diagnostics and counselling for the disorders.

Like the #JustJustice campaign, the centre is looking for collaborative and realistic solutions to a problem that (by extrapolation of United States prevalence data) may affect more than 100,000 Australians, a large proportion of whom are likely to be Aboriginal or Torres Strait Islander people.

Paediatrician Professor Elizabeth Elliott, from the Children's Hospital, believes there is a vital need for a focused, national prevention plan. In a **Perspective** article for *Public Health Research & Practice* (PHRP), published last month, she said the best way to address FASD and its accompanying health effects and social distress – for both those with the disorders and their families – is prevention.

FASD has "lifelong implications and may lead to significant secondary impairments, including academic failure, substance abuse, mental ill-health, contact with the justice system, and difficulties living independently and obtaining and maintaining employment," she wrote.

"Prevention requires education, adequate drug and alcohol services, support of initiatives such as community-led alcohol restrictions, and enforcement of existing legislation, as well as measures to decrease access to alcohol including pricing, and restrictions on promotion and advertising of alcohol.

"Although the young brain is adaptable, prenatal brain injury cannot be reversed so, for FASD, the future must be prevention."

Professor Elliott, who has spent seven years working in remote Aboriginal communities, said all staff working at the centre would receive cultural awareness training.

She is co-author of a working party report to the National Drug Strategy (2009), which reported on a US study of 415 adults with FASD or fetal alcohol effects (FAE), which found that 60 per cent had been in trouble with the law, half had been "confined" and 35 per cent imprisoned. Drug and alcohol problems were present in 29 per cent of adolescents and 45 per cent of adults.

In June 2014, funding of $9.3 million was announced for FASD programs, including a National FASD Technical Network, chaired by Professor Elliott, to help implement the plan.

In her PHRP article, Professor Elliott said the action plan focused attention on the need to prevent FASD, but Australia lacked FASD surveillance and a national register to measure the success of any prevention programs. In the meantime, she says, the $2.3 million from New South Wales "is a good start".

"It will allow us to fund a clinic one day per week, and we'll be able to audit our services to get an estimate of the need for services. We already get referrals from around the state and one of our remits will be training health professionals from throughout New South Wales.

"We hope there will be capacity for such a service in other states, if not a dedicated clinic then embedded in their existing services, and we hope our service will provide a model. We believe our clinic is unique nationally and we see it as a great opportunity to put some focus on this area."

Anne Messenger is Editor of Public Health Research & Practice at the Sax Institute.

Q: What impact did the publication of the article have? It was great to see, within a year of the #JustJustice campaign beginning, the federal government allocating more than $10 million to boost prevention of FASD. It would be great to see other jurisdictions follow suit (and NSW increase its contribution).

Q: What would you like to see happen as a result of the #JustJustice series? What's needed is system-wide funding, policy and implementation to reduce and prevention Indigenous incarceration, involving all Australian jurisdictions and incorporating the coordination of justice, corrective, health, education, welfare and other vital services.

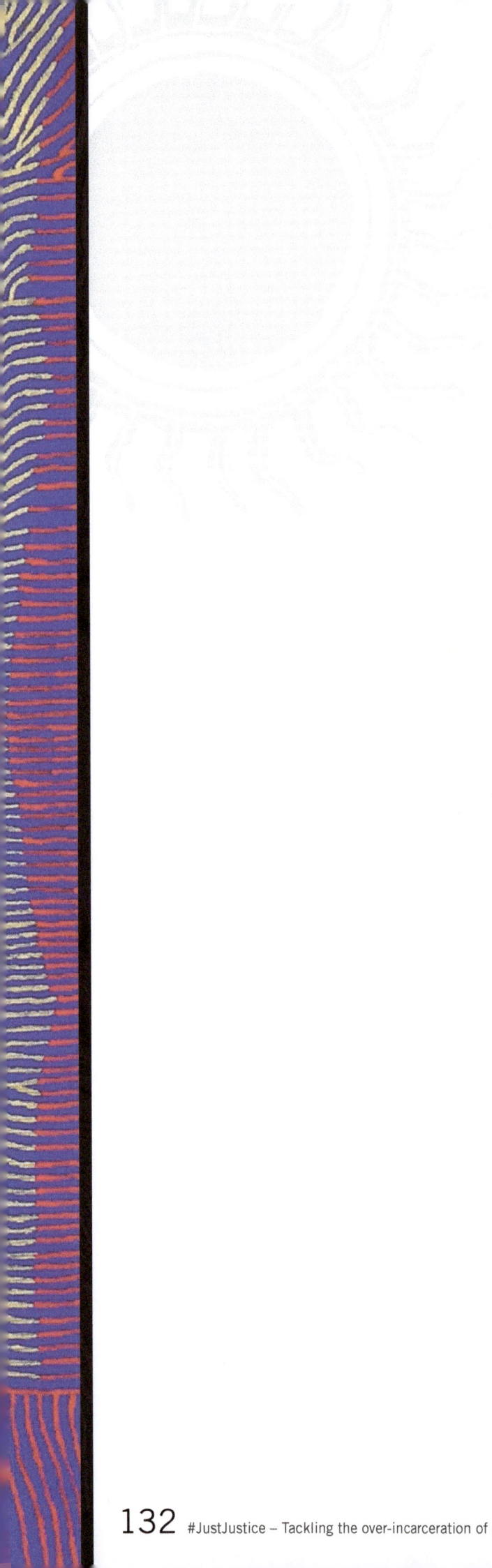

7. Trauma-informed solutions

" A good starting point would be to not put any Aboriginal women in prison because of how much that destroys family and community

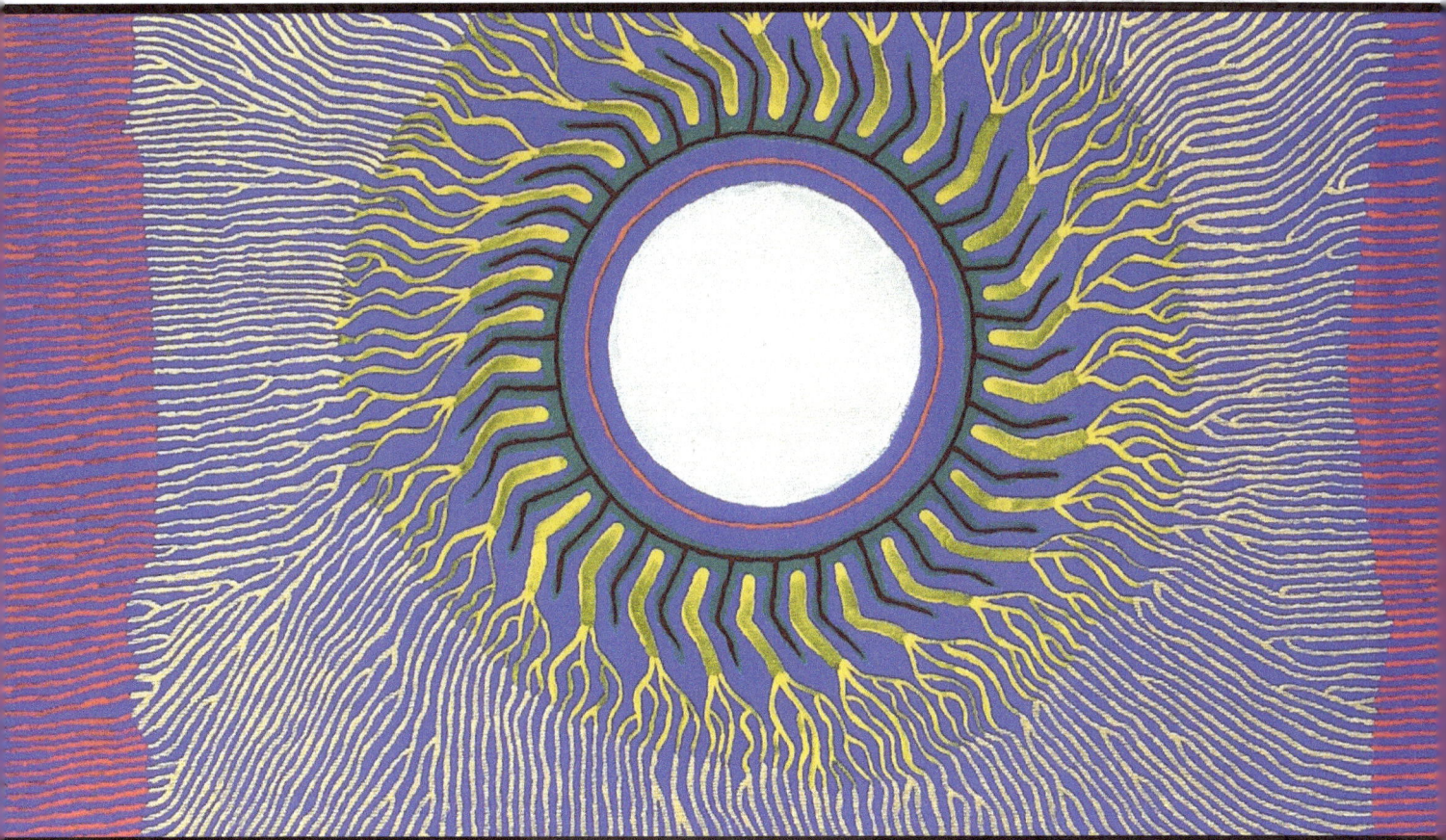

End childhood trauma and punitive policies: a call for collective responsibility and #JustJustice

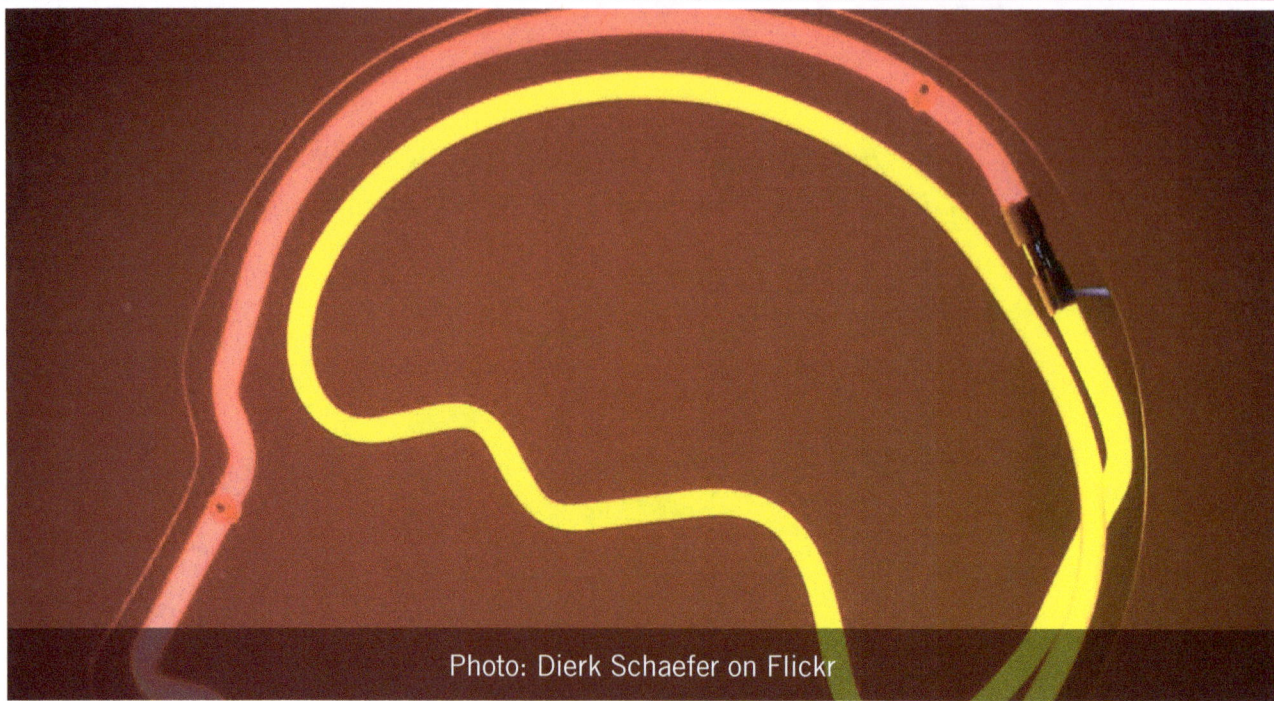

Photo: Dierk Schaefer on Flickr

| Author: | Sharon Payne | Published: | June 02, 2016 |

If we are to address the over-incarceration of Aboriginal and Torres Strait Islander people, policy-making must be more responsive to scientific evidence showing the need to reduce early childhood trauma and poverty, according to an Aboriginal lawyer and researcher, Sharon Payne.

Payne, who is planning to undertake a PhD at ANU looking at the neuroscience behind the treatment of Aboriginal people in the criminal justice system, says policymakers should also turn their attention to Portugal and other countries which have shown that huge gains can be made from investing in rehabilitation and prevention, rather than policing and punishment.

Sharon Payne writes:

When humans are under threat, our cognitive brain is "switched off" as all our resources (oxygen, glucose etc) are directed to the amygdala and muscles for immediate action (fight or flight).

The impact on developing brains constantly under threat (from abuse and/or neglect, for example) is a decrease in ability to develop the cognitive part of their brain.

Early life experiences that promote or inhibit the neural development of the immature brain mean that children who endure continual abuse and deprivation have their neurology altered in damaging ways well before they start school.

So when they first go to school, their brains aren't up to it; and it doesn't take very long for them to start identify themselves as inadequate (as contended by neuroscientist Michael Merzenich), as 'less' than their peers, and to be ashamed of themselves because of it.

And it doesn't take long before these self-identified failures (surrounded by success and connections they have no part of) begin misbehaving. A lack of self-control and aggressive bullying behaviours are all evidence of neurological inadequacy – but our societal response is to blame the child, to criticise and condemn, and finally to criminalise them.

And we also blame the parents whose inadequate parenting is likely due to their own traumatic childhood, and so we set up intergenerational self-reinforcing life trajectories that assure continued failure. We do anything but see these patterns as our collective social responsibility.

Insights from neuroscience

Thanks to neuroscientific research, we now know that (due to our evolution as life forms on this planet) human beings are bonding animals. Our brains are social organs with a basic need to connect, to be part of a community.

If we can't connect with each other, we will connect with anything we can find, from a pet or a peer group who 'understands us', to the spin of a poker machine or the prick of a syringe.

Conversely, however, we have created a society that cuts us off from connecting or bonding with each other, or offers only a parody of it via the Internet (with parents too busy 'FaceBooking' to connect with their young children, or children using the number of 'likes' they receive as proof of their worthiness).

And in response to the "problem" for which we are collectively responsible, punishing strategies have been adopted that add to the neurological burdens.

Learn from Portugal

Take the "war on drugs" as an example of how we respond to so-called addicts when they do predictably offend us. Criminalisation is the main response.

Instead of implementing approaches to rehabilitation that would enable neurological repair, our approach is based upon conviction and/or imprisonment (generating more shame) and isolation (generating more disconnection).

Indeed, the one thing we may be sure of is that if people weren't neurologically damaged before they enter the system, they will be afterwards.

There is some hope, though, that neuroscientific approaches are beginning to influence how we respond to the challenges caused by early childhood trauma.

The Portuguese drug law reforms decriminalising previously illegal substances have shown that much more successful outcomes are possible by adopting 'harm reduction strategies' which encourage people to connect (or reconnect) and by removing the fear and stigma associated with arrest/imprisonment.

As the Transform Drug Policy Institute says in its analysis of Portugal's drug laws, "The reality is that Portugal's drug situation has improved", with significant decreases in drug-induced deaths (80 to 12), heroin use (50% less) and improved mental and physical health outcomes since they were introduced.

Portugal, however, spends 90% of its budget on rehabilitation and prevention and only 10% on policing and punishment. In the United States, whose lead Australia follows, it is the opposite.

In other countries (for example, France and Scandinavian countries), a focus on early childhood development programs ensures that children are less likely to suffer neurological damage leading to and/or caused by drug abuse.

It also means that their socio-economic health gradients are flatter than in countries with the more punitive approaches (societies with flatter gradients are not only healthier but have higher literacy and educational attainment, lower poverty rates and smaller prison populations).

Steeper social gradients (for example, reflecting the inequalities faced by Aboriginal people compared to other Australians) may be modified by changing public policies, as the Portuguese strategy demonstrates.

Address the political gap

While all this is now quite well understood, it has yet to penetrate the political leadership in Australia, although it is estimated that a quarter of all children will not attain the competencies they need in a modern society (with much worse figures for children with additional disadvantages like race, gender, physical/genetic disability).

The result is increased social overhead costs, and human misery on an increasing scale, where we all pay for the lack of political will and individual effort to make those changes.

It does not have to be this way but self-interest and conservative ideology have more influence over government policy than science, and opinions carry more weight than fact. (But that's a topic for another time.)

Sharon Payne is from the Wannamutta clan of the Batjula people of K'gari (Fraser Island). Her background both educationally and professionally (and personally) has all contributed to a unique understanding of the criminal justice system and the cultural, social and now [neuro]scientific influences on how it operates. Sharon has a law degree from ANU as well as a background in psychology.

Sharon has worked extensively in law and justice including the Royal Commission into Aboriginal Deaths in Custody; the Indigenous Deaths in Custody 1989 – 96 Report; establishing the ACT Aboriginal Justice Centre and the ACT Circle Sentencing Court (where she is currently a Sentencing Panel member) and the CEO of three Aboriginal Legal Services where she witnessed the unfairness and discrimination first hand. Her most recent studies in neuroscience continue to provide even greater insight into how the system works against the most vulnerable and disadvantaged.

Meanwhile, on related matters at The Conversation, read "Emotional abuse of children is a growing problem in Australia", by Professor Aron Schlonsky, Professor Kerry Arabena and Associate Professor Robyn Mildron at the University of Melbourne. They call for services, programs and policy to focus on children's wellbeing.

"**Each** family has got a story to tell" – when it comes to #JustJustice concerns

| Author: | Rosemary Roe | | Published: | November 04, 2016 |

In discussing the current crisis of over-incarceration, it is important to acknowledge the ongoing impact of the Stolen Generations, according to Rosemary Roe, a Yamatji woman.

In this interview below conducted on Whadjuk Nyoongar country at Walyalup (Fremantle), Rosemary gives many insights into how the past of colonisation is woven into the present of incarceration.

In her own family, there is experience of Stolen Generations and imprisonment, as well as resistance and advocacy.

Rosemary's mother, whose own mother was taken as a young girl from her family in the Leonora area, was one of the first Aboriginal teachers in Western Australia.

Rosemary is now researching her mother's biography, and believes that investigating family histories can be healing, even if it is painful.

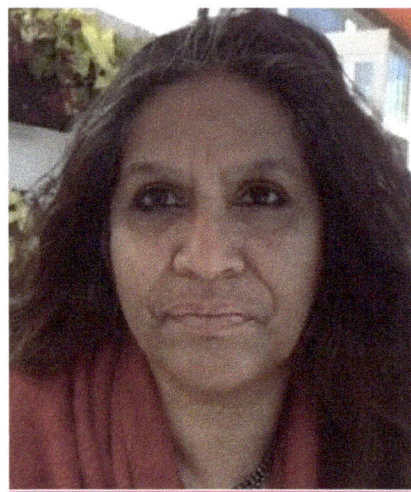

Rosemary Roe: "Sharing stories is very powerful."

"You have got to know your past for your future. It's important for our kids, so that we learn that and pass it on," she says.

"Sharing stories is very powerful. Each family has got a story to tell. It's about sharing stories, surviving and helping each other understand each other's different cultures. It's time for Australia to stop and think."

Rosemary also talks about the stress experienced by families when members are in the grips of justice and child protection systems, and urges governments and policy makers to "start listening to the Elders".

She also discusses the need for treaty and wider issues of justice and reparation. "I'm getting to the stage, your law is not my law; it's not working," she says.

Rosemary Roe is a Yamatji woman living in Fremantle, Western Australia.

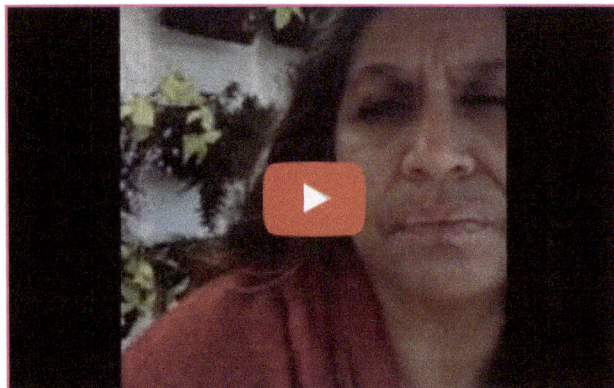

See the interview here: https://youtu.be/WvhpwJbq5TY

Prison is not the answer. Instead, address the needs of traumatised Aboriginal women

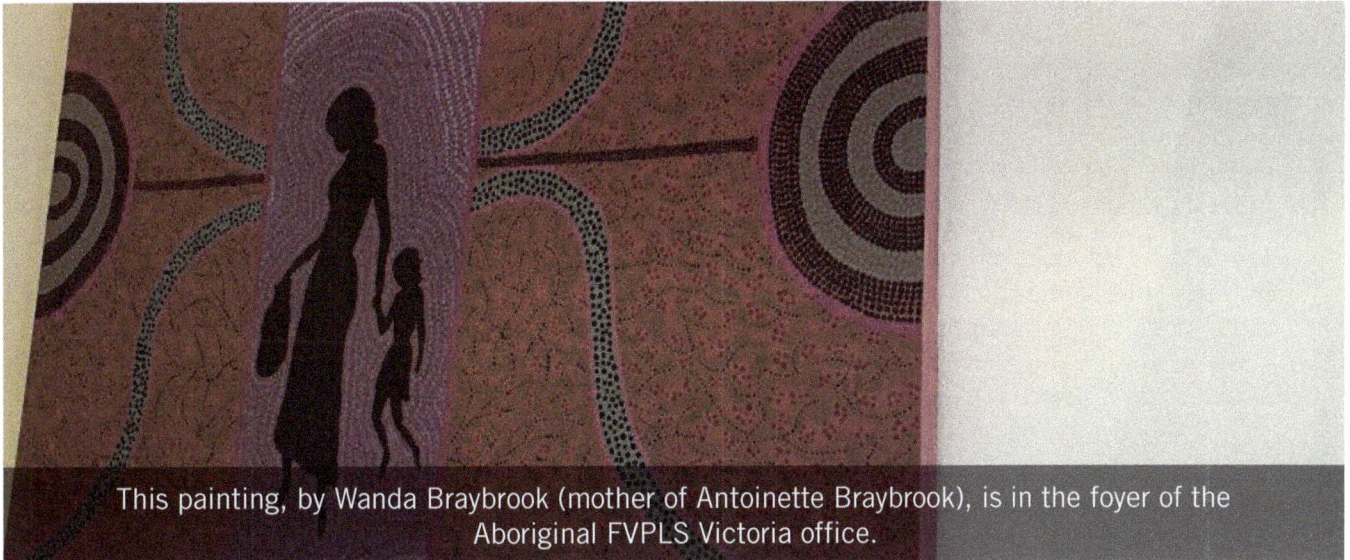

This painting, by Wanda Braybrook (mother of Antoinette Braybrook), is in the foyer of the Aboriginal FVPLS Victoria office.

Author:	Marie McInerney	Published:	October 06, 2015

Journalist Marie McInerney investigates the urgent need for action to address the rising rates of Aboriginal women going to prison, the majority of whom have experienced family violence.

Marie McInerney writes:

Aboriginal and Torres Strait Islander women should only be jailed as a matter of last resort because of the devastating impact this has on families and children, according to a leading Aboriginal advocate.

The resources spent on imprisoning Aboriginal women would be better spent on legal, cultural and community services, including safe and appropriate housing, says Antoinette Braybook, CEO of Victoria's Aboriginal Family Violence Prevention and Legal Service (FVPLS) and National Convenor for the National Family Violence Prevention Legal Services Forum.

While Aboriginal women are the fastest growing group in Australia's prisons, their numbers are actually still low enough – less than 50 in Victoria's prisons – that it should be possible to provide individually tailored alternatives to incarceration.

"A good starting point would be to not put any Aboriginal women in prison because of how much that destroys family and community; one day in prison can cost an Aboriginal woman her life, her children, her home and her family," says Braybrook.

The legal system also has to learn how to take into account the high levels of family violence experienced by Aboriginal and Torres Strait Islander women prisoners, and its connection with criminalisation and incarceration rates, she says.

Asked what mainstream organisations can do better in the #JustJustice space, Braybrook said a commitment to ongoing cultural awareness training for staff is a basic need.

But she also wants them to "work hard to build relationships with organisations like ours", rather than trying to build their own business cases. She said:

" Don't just want something from us, give us something.

A good starting point would be to just understand that all Aboriginal people have had really bad experiences with mainstream organisations and white authorities.

We always say: 'refer Aboriginal people to an Aboriginal organisation and support that organisation to provide that additional support to the woman, rather than try to get your own numbers up.'

Racism and family violence

Braybrook is an Aboriginal woman, born on Wurundjeri country in Melbourne, who was prompted to study law by the racism experienced by her family in suburban Melton as she grew up.

She was formerly an Executive Officer of one of nine Victorian Regional Aboriginal Justice Advisory Committees, formed out of the work of the Royal Commission into Aboriginal Deaths in Custody.

As a result, she has a keen understanding of the intersection between family violence and offending for Aboriginal women, and the impacts of family violence occurring within a broader context of lateral and community violence for Aboriginal people.

The FVPLS was one of a range of organisations that endorsed a submission to the Victorian Royal Commission into Family Violence by Flat Out, a statewide advocacy and support service for women who have had contact with the criminal justice and prison system.

It focuses on the experiences of criminalised women – those who have been imprisoned, in contact with police or who engage in criminalised activities such as illicit drug use or sex work, and how existing police approaches to family violence are failing them.

It says:

Research reveals that the overwhelming majority of women in prison have experienced family violence. Our case studies further suggest that family violence is a contributing factor to many women's imprisonment.

The failure of government and society to recognise this and instead to focus on women's criminalised behaviour and consequent punishment, serves to compound the trauma these women have experienced.

Imprisonment further disrupts the lives of women and children who have experienced or are experiencing family violence. The trauma of imprisonment will be endured and carried with them throughout their lives.

Braybrook says a big priority is to provide a safe place – physically and culturally – for Aboriginal women after prison, so they don't reoffend or breach parole, like the Wulgunggo Ngalu residential diversion program for Aboriginal men, which a Corrections evaluation found is "widely valued and supported throughout the justice system".

The culturally safe regional facility run by her brother Shaun Braybrook was set up to address high breach rates for Aboriginal men who are on community correction orders. It was also recommended as a model to halt high recidivism rates for Aboriginal women in Unfinished Business, the 2013 Victorian Human Rights and Equal Opportunity Commission (VHREOC) report on Koori women and the justice system.

Braybrook says:

The really important thing about Wulgunggo is the programs are around culture, identity and Aboriginal men's role in communities. And it's been so successful.

They've got different units set aside so men's families can come down, link them into stuff in communities when they've completed their order. That's the kind of thing we need for women so they can have their children with them.

Like Aboriginal men, many Aboriginal women 'cycle' in and out of prison, often for minor crimes or justice breaches, and routinely miss out on pre-prison diversionary options even when they are first-time offenders.

Many are also denied bail because of a chronic lack of safe and secure accommodation to which they can be bailed. This has led to an escalating number of Aboriginal women entering prison on remand. In 2012, of 67 Koori women on remand in Victoria, 60 per cent were released without being sentenced.

Braybrook says this is not a new issue as it is in the rest of the Victorian prison system. For Aboriginal women, it's been going on "for years" for a range of reasons, including racist attitudes in policing.

She said:

One thing we think contributes is the lack of legal representation for Aboriginal women – they haven't got an advocate.

The data tells us that Aboriginal women are the most legally disadvantaged group in Australia and that contributes to why they are the fastest growing prison population.

Funding cuts

That's only been made worse by the funding uncertainty undermining that support nationally, since Family Violence Prevention Legal Services (FVPLS) lost status as a stand-alone program – the basis on which it had operated for the last 16 years – under the Federal Government's new Indigenous Advancement Strategy.

The 14 FVPLS services across Australia won a reprieve in March this year, but some were granted only 12 months funding, and there is no CPI indexation or opportunity for increased funding across the terms of contracts.

"That puts a lot of pressure on our budgets and capacity to retain specialist staff. The uncertainty leading up to the decision also impacted strongly: we lost some staff and had to be very careful about how many clients we took on in case we couldn't support them in the longer term," Braybrook said.

Funding cuts have also hit the highly regarded Sisters Day Out and Dilly Bag initiatives, which have 'pampered' about 7,000 Aboriginal women across Victoria over the past seven years, and delivered targeted family violence information and support, including to women in Melbourne's Dame Phyllis Frost maximum security prison.

"Everyone talks about how wonderful this program is, how successful it is," Braybrook says of Sisters Day Out. "It's a proven success but we've been 'piloting' it for 7 years and now we've run out of funding."

There was further disappointment last month that the family violence package announced by new Prime Minister Malcolm Turnbull did not include a focus on improving access to frontline legal services for Aboriginal and Torres Strait Islander women.

In a statement, Braybrook outlined how family violence impacted on Aboriginal and Torres Strait islander people "at vastly disproportionate rates and has devastating impacts".

Aboriginal and Torres Strait Islander women are 34 times more likely to be hospitalised from family violence and almost 11 times more likely to be killed as a result of violent assault than other Australians. A big issue behind those figures is a fear among Aboriginal women that their children will be removed from them if they report violence.

Prison replicates violence

Braybrook said up to 90 per cent of Aboriginal women in prison have experienced family violence and many are in prison because of crimes that relate to homelessness and financial hardship.

"The connection between family violence and homelessness, the connection between financial hardship and family violence, it all goes hand in hand with rising rates of incarceration," she says.

The FVPLS submission to Victoria's Royal Commission into Family Violence says that while family violence victimisation is not a direct cause of Aboriginal women being jailed, "it is a precursor to a range of conditions that lead to imprisonment".

It says its work in Victorian Aboriginal communities for the last 12 years confirms a New South Wales study in which over 80 per cent of female Aboriginal prisoners reported that their incarceration was an indirect result of their victimisation.

Women who have been to prison also struggle to later get support not just from police, but also from the mainstream family violence sector, she said, pointing again to the submission to the Royal Commission from Flat Out, that says:

" Family violence services often have refused support for criminalised women based on the assumption that they are too difficult, pose a threat to other women, a threat to the service model of high security, or present with a complex range of support needs to which services feel unable to appropriately respond...

Criminalised women may therefore fear mainstream services because they fear discrimination.

Braybrook says that's why dedicated Aboriginal legal services and programs like Sisters Day Out are so important.

"Sisters Day Out lets us take our organisation and many others to communities, there's no expectation that women will walk through the door and report violence," she says.

"For me, being an Aboriginal woman, I'm contacted all the time on Facebook and the phone. When women come to see us they know they won't be judged; we understand why they haven't reported (violence) and why it's difficult for to leave their community."

Flat Out echoes Braybrook's call for an end to imprisonment for vulnerable women, saying prison replicates all the features of family violence and often re-traumatises women.

" The prison therefore cannot serve both punitive and therapeutic purposes because these goals are antithetical. The prison's primary focus is security, not therapy.

Prison, by its very nature, excludes normal society, promotes prison living skills and actively erodes community living skills.

Prison compounds women's systemic disadvantage.... specialist support for criminalised women should be provided in the community and there should be a targeted reduction in the numbers of women imprisoned in Victoria.

To tackle family violence affecting Indigenous women, holistic approaches are needed

Author:	Anna Olsen and Ray Lovett	Published:	January 31, 2016

Efforts to address family violence affecting Indigenous women should be holistic, focus on intergenerational trauma and family relationships, and involve cultural-based leadership and governance, according to a wide-ranging review.

Services and programs also should be funded for adequate community input, evidence-based evaluation and longer-term operational costs, the review recommends.

The findings are detailed below by the authors, Dr Anna Olsen, Visiting Fellow at the National Centre for Epidemiology and Population Health (NCEPH) at the Australian National University, and Dr Ray Lovett, Research Fellow at the Australian Institute of Aboriginal and Torres Strait Islander Studies and at the NCEPH.

Anna Olsen and Ray Lovett write:

Violence against women in Indigenous communities has been highlighted by politicians and the media as an issue of national importance, but less is known about Indigenous experiences and viewpoints on the issue.

We conducted a comprehensive review of published literature for Australia's National Research Organisation for Women's Safety (ANROWS) to present the current state of knowledge, practice and responses to violence against women in Australian Indigenous communities.

We found that Indigenous Australians see violence as a family and community issue. In general the term "family violence", rather than domestic violence, is preferred to reflect an understanding of violence being the result of a range of community and family factors, rather than one individual's problematic behaviour.

The literature reveals a wide array of theories about causes of violence against women but no evidence for one causal factor.

Instead, academics, advocates and community members describe a number of inter-related factors that contribute to the issue – including intergenerational trauma and the breakdown of traditional culture and kinship practices. These highlight the complex and cumulative nature of violence and victimisation.

Indigenous communities also want to play a more significant role in shaping program and service responses

While the evidence does suggest a higher rate of violence against Indigenous women, many authors stress that violence is not normal or customary in Indigenous communities. Instead, violence should be approached as the result of, and perpetuated by, a range of historical and contemporary social factors.

The big picture finding from this review is that the cumulative nature of socio-economic disadvantage (such as personal, family and economic related stressors) and the lasting effects of colonisation are thought to be linked to violence against women in Indigenous communities.

Holistic approaches needed

Attempts to reduce violence in Indigenous communities require a multi-faceted and holistic approach, including efforts to improve the wider social, economic and health of Indigenous communities.

Much of the grey literature contained information about Indigenous viewpoints on "what works" to prevent violence against women.

Approaches to dealing effectively with violence, and solutions that are valued by Indigenous communities include cultural based leadership and governance, and programs focused on preventing the transfer of intergenerational trauma.

Because Indigenous family violence is, in part, attributed to the breakdown of culture and kinship practice, the rebuilding of these family relationships is often seen as central to developing any type of response.

Indigenous communities also want to play a more significant role in shaping program and service responses.

Solutions developed by Indigenous people and communities are likely to focus on healing the community, restoring family cohesion, and developing processes where the victim and perpetrator can deal with their pain and suffering.

Generalised family violence services can be considered effective if they are operated in a culturally sensitive way and/or run in partnership with Indigenous organisations.

Justice system problematic

For example, family violence research suggests that Indigenous women's experiences of the justice system are often filled with misunderstanding, fear and racism.

The criminal justice system is not necessarily considered the most appropriate means for dealing with family violence. Indigenous experiences of family violence and the justice system suggest that people are interested in programs that focus on preventing the transfer of violence, not just prosecuting or punishing people for being violent.

Instead, co-designed justice initiatives, which include Indigenous leadership and values can be more appropriate.

There is currently a patchwork of responses to family violence in Indigenous communities provided by federal, state and territory governments as well as local initiatives.

Ways forward

We reviewed literature on a number of previous and current programs working to address family violence in Indigenous communities. Most of the programs assessed showed a positive impact on various aspects of behaviour, wellbeing, attitudes and skills related to addressing family violence in Indigenous communities.

There is positive progress being made in Indigenous communities; however, quality evidence and wider information sharing is needed.

The report reviews 24 programs for which there was available evidence. However, many more programs are not widely known about as they are not evaluated and do not receive sustained funding support. More data is needed on the effectiveness of these programs, as well as broader policies.

Not all Indigenous women are subjected to violence and not all Indigenous communities have high rates of violence. Family violence is an issue in Australia beyond Indigenous communities and it is important to understand that despite the disproportionate burden of violence against Indigenous women, violence against women is not normal in Indigenous culture.

The findings of this report suggest that there are some approaches to dealing with violence against women that may be more appropriate and successful in Indigenous communities.

Family violence services, both Indigenous specific and general services, should focus on intergenerational trauma and family relationships, involve local consultation or Indigenous leadership, and be funded for adequate community input, evidence-based evaluation and longer-term operational costs.

Dr Anna Olsen is Visiting Fellow at the National Centre for Epidemiology and Population Health (NCEPH) at the Australian National University, and Dr Ray Lovett is a Research Fellow at the Australian Institute of Aboriginal and Torres Strait Islander Studies and at the NCEPH.

Calling for smarter approaches that address underlying causes of crime

Author:	Antoinette Braybrook and Shane Duffy	Published:	January, 2017

Addressing violence against Aboriginal and Torres Strait Islander women and rising imprisonment rates requires a nuanced approach, according to Antoinette Braybrook and Shane Duffy, Co-Chairs of the Change the Record Coalition.

Antoinette Braybrook and Shane Duffy write:

In recent times we have seen a renewed and welcome discussion about the crisis of violence against Aboriginal and Torres Strait Islander women. These conversations are particularly pertinent given the 16 Days of Activism to End Gender-Based Violence.

What we need now is for all levels of government to start listening to peak and representative Aboriginal and Torres Strait Islander organisations, so that we can work together to address the unacceptably high rates of violence towards our women and children.

We all want to live in a safe community - with less crime and fewer victims. As a result we often default to the assumption that locking up as many people as possible will keep us safe.

But the evidence proves otherwise, with punitive approaches often compounding underlying issues. If we really want to address both rates of violence and rising imprisonment rates, we need to adopt a more nuanced approach.

Since our launch in April 2015, the Change the Record campaign has been working towards twin goals - to stop the disproportionate rates of violence against Aboriginal and Torres Strait Islander women and children, and to end the over-imprisonment of Aboriginal and Torres Strait Islander people.

These two goals are mutually reinforcing in a number of ways. Family violence is both a cause and a consequence of imprisonment. Our women are at the epicentre of the national family violence crisis. Aboriginal and Torres Strait Islander women are currently 34 times more likely to be hospitalised as a result of family violence than non-Indigenous women and 10 times more likely to be killed as a result of violent assault.

We need Governments to shift their focus away from responding after an offence has been committed, towards investing in services which build communities, reduce violence and prevent offending from occurring in the first place.

However, it is important to note that the Aboriginal and Torres Strait Islander women who access our services experience family violence at the hands of men from a range of different backgrounds and cultures.

At the same time, Aboriginal and Torres Strait Islander women also represent the fastest growing prison population in Australia and it is estimated that around 90 percent of our women in prison have previously been a victim/survivor of family violence.

The experience of women accessing our services tells us that, more often than not, the criminal justice system fails to protect women from family violence, with punitive approaches providing an incomplete response to stopping the violence.

Both violence and imprisonment rates are also driven by a range of underlying and interlinked root causes, such as mental health, substance abuse, homelessness, poverty, family violence, exposure to the child protection system and other factors.

If we want our justice system to work, we need to recognise and respond to the complex needs of the individuals involved. For instance, the resources that are currently put into imprisoning our people could be better spent on investment into holistic wrap-around family violence services that aim to build resilience and reduce offending.

This includes for example a focus on prevention and early intervention programs, such as Family Violence Prevention and Legal Service Victoria's Sisters Day Out programme or Central Australian Aboriginal Legal Aid Service's Kunga Stopping Violence Project.

We need Governments to shift their focus away from responding after an offence has been committed, towards investing in services which build communities, reduce violence and prevent offending from occurring in the first place.

An example of the complexity of these issues is the story of Ms Dhu - a young, vulnerable Aboriginal woman who tragically died in police custody after being imprisoned for unpaid fines. At the time of her arrest, she was only 22 years of age and was a victim of domestic violence. She was arrested at the same time as the perpetrator and locked up in a police cell adjoining his.

The sad reality is that Ms Dhu should never have been arrested and she certainly should not have been locked up. Instead, she should have been provided access to holistic family violence support services - such as access to safe housing, community services, legal assistance and prevention and early intervention programs.

However, chronic under-funding and budgetary cuts to services means that we currently don't have capacity to meet demand. For example, Aboriginal Family Violence Prevention Legal Services (FVPLS) around the country are currently reporting a turn away rate of 30-40 percent because they are so under-resourced.

As Aboriginal and Torres Strait Islander people we both know first-hand the pain that is caused by violence against our women and children, and we want the violence to stop. But we also know from personal experience the ongoing impact of intergenerational trauma, mental health issues and the breakdown of our communities that is caused by the escalating over-imprisonment of our people.

Talking about addressing violence and imprisonment rates in tandem is difficult but, if we are to make progress in this area, it is critical that we adopt a balanced response which tackles these dual issues head on.

We don't need more knee-jerk, ill-considered policies. It is essential that peak Aboriginal and Torres Strait Islander organisations are front and centre in the solutions. Governments must meaningfully engage with the experts in frontline service delivery rather than seeing them as an afterthought.

Continuously defaulting to a simplistic 'law and order' approach only perpetuates cycles of trauma and disadvantage, and will not make our communities safer in the long-term.

It is in all of our interests to work together to develop smarter approaches, which are targeted at addressing the underlying causes of crime. This approach will not only cut offending and imprisonment rates, but critically will also increase safety by working to address the root causes of violence against women and children in the first place.

Antoinette Braybrook and Shane Duffy are Co-Chairs of the Change the Record Coalition.

Who is talking for us? The silencing of the Aboriginal woman's voice about violence

| Author: | Marlene Longbottom, Yvette Roe and Bronwyn Fredericks | Published: | October 17, 2016 |

Aboriginal women have been speaking out and identifying solutions to violence against them for decades, despite recent reports seeking to suggest otherwise.

It's time that governments and others listened to and acted on these longstanding calls for proper funding of community-based services, according to three "assertive and passionate" Aboriginal women and researchers, Marlene Longbottom, Dr Yvette Roe and Professor Bronwyn Fredericks in their contribution below to Croakey's #JustJustice series.

It's particularly timely given that the Council of Australian Governments announced it would hold a summit on violence against women, in Brisbane on 27 and 28 October.

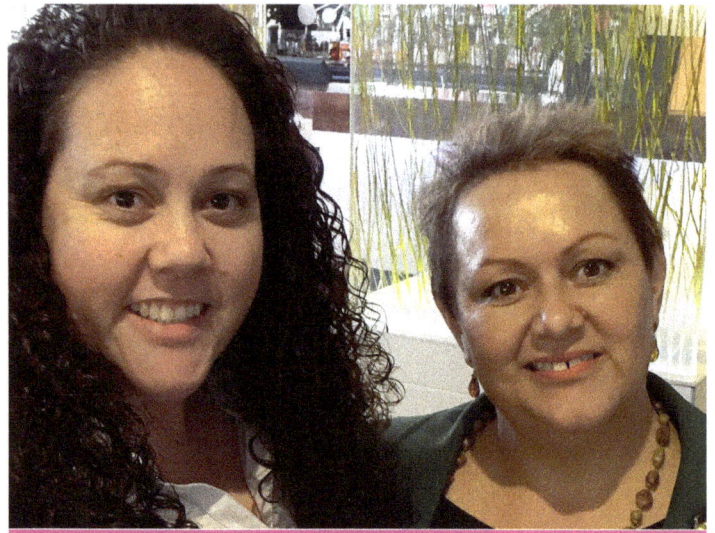

Marlene Longbottom and Professor Bronwyn Fredericks: "We are taking our power back"

Marlene Longbottom, Yvette Roe and Bronwyn Fredericks write:

" It seems that someone has claimed the space to speak on Indigenous violence and that space does not necessarily belong to Indigenous women.

Sonia Smallacombe (2004, 50)

The violence experienced by Aboriginal women in Australia is not new. Aboriginal women have experienced violence from the point of contact of colonisation (Behrendt, 1993, Moreton-Robinson, 2000).

Aboriginal women's bodies were appropriated along with the land by the Europeans from the first point of contact and through the generations (Behrendt, 1993, Moreton-Robinson, 2000). This has resulted in trauma experiences for Aboriginal women and, along with being experienced through the generations, it has also transferred across the generations.

Trauma research by First Nation scholar Renee Linklater states:

" Colonization has caused multiple injuries to Indigenous people, and therefore many Indigenous people experience trauma in a multi-traumatic context. Multigenerational trauma points to the multiple types of trauma understood as current, ancestral, historical, individual or collective experiences.

This intergenerational and multigenerational transference of trauma (Al-Yaman et al., 2006) and the associated post-traumatic stress disorder (Atkinson, 2002, Linklater, 2014) are what we now witness. The internalising of oppression and the externalising expressions of violence result from cumulative traumatic experiences over time (Al-Yaman et al., 2006, Atkinson, 2002, Linklater, 2014).

Violence towards Aboriginal women is not isolated to one particular community, State or Territory. They are disproportionately over-represented as victims

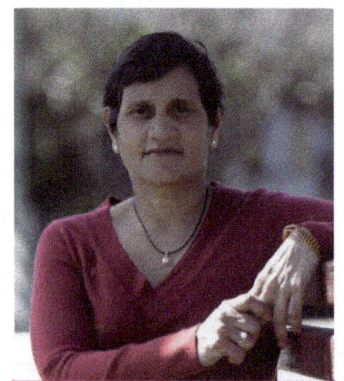

Co-author, Dr Yvette Roe

of inter-personal violence homicide in New South Wales (New South Wales Government., 2015, Sherwood and Kendall, 2013).

Significantly concerning is Aboriginal women are moving from the positioning of victim to offender, as a means to protect themselves from violent partners (New South Wales Government, 2015, Sherwood and Kendall, 2013).

Thus violence in Indigenous communities remains a key risk factor or vulnerability to the increasing incarceration rates, not only for Aboriginal men but also as more Aboriginal women are being incarcerated for violence against violent perpetrators (Sherwood J and Kendall S., 2013).

What is alarming is that the relationships of inter-personal violence in homicides in New South Wales were known to the police (New South Wales Government., 2015) prior to women's deaths. We question: *Why aren't Aboriginal women being protected?* We also question: *Why are Aboriginal women being silenced on this issue?*

We write this paper from a standpoint as Aboriginal women first and foremost, then academics, who seek to express our deep concerns and have more than a key interest in addressing violence with Aboriginal women. We intentionally assist women in sharing their stories of survival.

We, along with scores of other Aboriginal women, add our voices and support to the already published and unpublished literature of the Aboriginal women before us who have spoken up (Atkinson, 2002, Behrendt, 1993, Ingram, 2016, Moreton-Robinson, 2000, O'Shane, 2002, Smallacombe, 2004, Langton, 1988).

We are strong in our Aboriginality and are not complicit in our views about the urgency to address violence against Aboriginal women

In light of the research and media attention, it is evident that Aboriginal women's voices are not being heard, thereby raising the question: *who speaks for who? Aboriginal women are either not given the platform to speak, nor are they heard when they do.*

Often the privilege of being heard is granted to men, both Indigenous and non-Indigenous men, or white women (Moreton-Robinson, 2000). While Aboriginal women may speak, their advocacy may be misunderstood or interpreted as anger, or they may be positioned as angry and aggressive women.

Rather than being interpreted and positioned as assertive and passionate Aboriginal women, it results in Aboriginal women being defined as angry Black women and as a result dismissed as being irrelevant (Fredericks, 2010, Griffin, 2012).

The intersections of race, gender and classism are often omitted from the discussion along with the social construction of Aboriginal women who are often perceived to be the problem, passive victims, and often never as survivors (Crenshaw, 1989, Crenshaw, 1991, Moreton-Robinson, 2000, Moreton-Robinson, 2015).

So be it. We make no apology for being three passionate and assertive women who seek to advocate and who may be interpreted and understood as three angry Black women. We are strong in our Aboriginality and are not complicit in our views about the urgency to address violence against Aboriginal women.

Uninformed or Ill-informed commentators have privilege

Violence towards Aboriginal women came to the attention of the media with the recent comments of Mr Warren Mundine (Mundine, 2016). While Mr Mundine's comments are welcomed, the issue is not new. He falsely accuses feminists and progressives of not speaking up on the issue of violence.

The reality is that women, progressives and feminists have attempted to bring the issues of interpersonal violence to the forefront of Australia's narrative for a long period of time (Atkinson, 2002, Behrendt, 1993, Ingram, 2016, Moreton-Robinson, 2000, O'Shane, 2002, Smallacombe, 2004, Langton, 1988).

Amy McQuire and Celeste Liddle are two of the many Indigenous women who wrote in response to Mr Mundine's claims of complicity in Aboriginal communities (Liddle, 2016, McQuire, 2016). Further, in 2015, media reported the story of Marlene Tighe from the South Coast of NSW, who shared and continues to share her story of survival after her former partner attacked her with a hammer after learning of her intentions to leave the relationship (Bowden, 2015).

More recently, Linda Burney, who is an Aboriginal parliamentarian and self-identified survivor of intimate partner violence, challenged Mr Mundine, by reminding him that she and many others had been lobbying for years for recognition and changes about domestic and family violence (Caccetta, 2016).

Further, MP Burney asserts in her opinion piece in The Australian (dated 11 October 2016) that "the issue has been raised by communities for a very long time; however the response by governments was a shrugging of shoulders" (Burney, 2016). MP Burney says the recent media coverage provides for the opportunity to continue the discussions and calls for the funding that was removed from front line services to be reinstated.

The stance Mr Mundine takes in asserting community complicity implies there is a state of paralysis in communities to take action while also oppressing the voices of the women. The responses by these women can only be described as brave and courageous – and not complicit.

We believe that Mr Mundine's claims that community and advocates are silent about the issue adds to the silencing of these brave and courageous women. While we do agree that some sections in the community shun the discussion related to violence, there are others who do speak up and talk about the issue.

A blanket statement of community complicity denies and further silences those brave enough to speak out. The difference in all of the discourse is that Aboriginal women often are not afforded the opportunity to speak to share their stories. This is evident in the media responses to Mundine's commentary.

Over the last 30 years, there have been the *National Aboriginal Health Strategy* (National Aboriginal Health Strategy Working Party, 1989) and the *Royal Commission into Aboriginal Deaths in Custody* (Australia Royal Commission into Aboriginal Deaths in Custody and Johnston, 1998) that have actively sought to capture the voices of women and communities closest to the issue of violence.

More recently, The Little Children are Sacred report (Northern Territory Board of Inquiry into the Protection of Aboriginal Children from Sexual Abuse et al, 2007) was the catalyst for an emergency response in the Northern Territory (Australian Government, 2008).

Yet again we remain disheartened as the reports have not lead to the systematic reforms that tackle the horrendous violence inflicted upon Aboriginal women (Maddocks, 2016).

Time to start listening

A contemporary literature on Indigenous women's experiences of interpersonal violence identified, in what is a continuous discourse, that Aboriginal women's voices are absent and calls for research inclusive of their stories (Olsen and Lovett, 2016). Put quite simply, those closest to the issue are likely to know how to address it if afforded the opportunity.

The continual absence of Aboriginal women's voices remains a subject position, which has been written about time and again by Aboriginal women (Behrendt, 1993, Ingram, 2016, Moreton-Robinson, 2000, Moreton-Robinson, 2003, Smallacombe, 2004).

The fact that Aboriginal men and non-Aboriginal women and men speak for and about violence that affects Aboriginal women specifically, further perpetuates the silencing of Aboriginal women. The Bell–Huggins debate is another example (Ingram, 2016, Moreton-Robinson, 2003, Smallacombe, 2004).

We are not saying that we do not support advocacy by Aboriginal men and non-Aboriginal women and men, but we argue that it should not occur in ways which silence Aboriginal women or that maintain power over the voices of Aboriginal women.

Community-based solutions – not rhetoric

Addressing the ongoing issues in Aboriginal communities around violence cannot be approached from the one-size-fits all response. Understanding that violence is an expression of trauma and a major vulnerability to health and wellbeing is vital.

Addressing the issue of violence in Aboriginal communities will take more than a brief paper being written or a flavour of the month attempt by the government to redirect funds back to services

It must also be understood as being grounded in a history where violence was and still is experienced by Aboriginal women, not just perpetrated by Aboriginal men, but also by non-Aboriginal perpetrators.

Unlike the approach of feminism that seeks to separate Aboriginal women from Aboriginal men, we understand the need for Aboriginal men to be part of the solution; however, one voice should not take precedence over the other (Moreton-Robinson, 2000).

Additionally, there needs to be an understanding of how Aboriginal communities have adapted and adopted the patriarchy and the colonial systems which victim-shame and blame Aboriginal women for not seeking help and speaking up (Moreton-Robinson, 2000, Sherwood and Kendall, 2013).

Quite clearly, for almost thirty years, Aboriginal women have spoken about the violence in communities, have suggested solutions, yet there is little evidence that their advocacy has been taken into consideration.

Community responses to violence must be designed to invest and support the individuals, families and communities. Additionally the systemic and structural environments which maintain the silencing of Aboriginal women, such as the law and corrections systems, need to be addressed.

Investment needed

In many communities, organisations that deliver front line services to this vulnerable population are severely under resourced. We implore that community-based approaches and services must be supported by adequately funded services that are equipped to support Aboriginal women, men, their families and communities.

Addressing the issue of violence in Aboriginal communities will take more than a brief paper being written or a flavour of the month attempt by the government to redirect funds back to services. Aboriginal communities know that community-driven initiatives have been defunded by government agencies (Burney, 2016).

Addressing the issue starts with Aboriginal women being given the opportunity to share their stories of survival in a supportive and culturally safe manner without the fear of retribution by the perpetrator and the community.

Time and time again, we have seen very little action to support and protect those who are most vulnerable – Aboriginal women and children. It is time that men and women, regardless of Aboriginal status, make a space for Aboriginal women to speak about their experiences while also offering practical solutions.

We propose that the way to address the issue is to restore the power that was taken from Aboriginal women from the time of colonisation (University of Saskatchewan, 2016). We support processes that re-empower Aboriginal women (Fredericks, 2010).

We are taking our power back and if this is interpreted as us being aggressive and angry, rather than being passionate and advocating with a sense of urgency, then you need to deal with this. We have more important issues, like addressing violence in our communities, to deal with!

Marlene Longbottom is undertaking a PhD at the University of Newcastle on Aboriginal women's experiences of interpersonal violence and support mechanisms available in the Shoalhaven region. Follow on Twitter: @MLongbottom13

Dr Yvette Roe, Institute of Urban Indigenous Health (IUIH). Follow on Twitter: @YvetteRoe

Professor Bronwyn Fredericks, Central Queensland University. Follow on Twitter: @BronFredericks

Download the Reference List for this article.

"**Keep** out of prison those who should not be there"

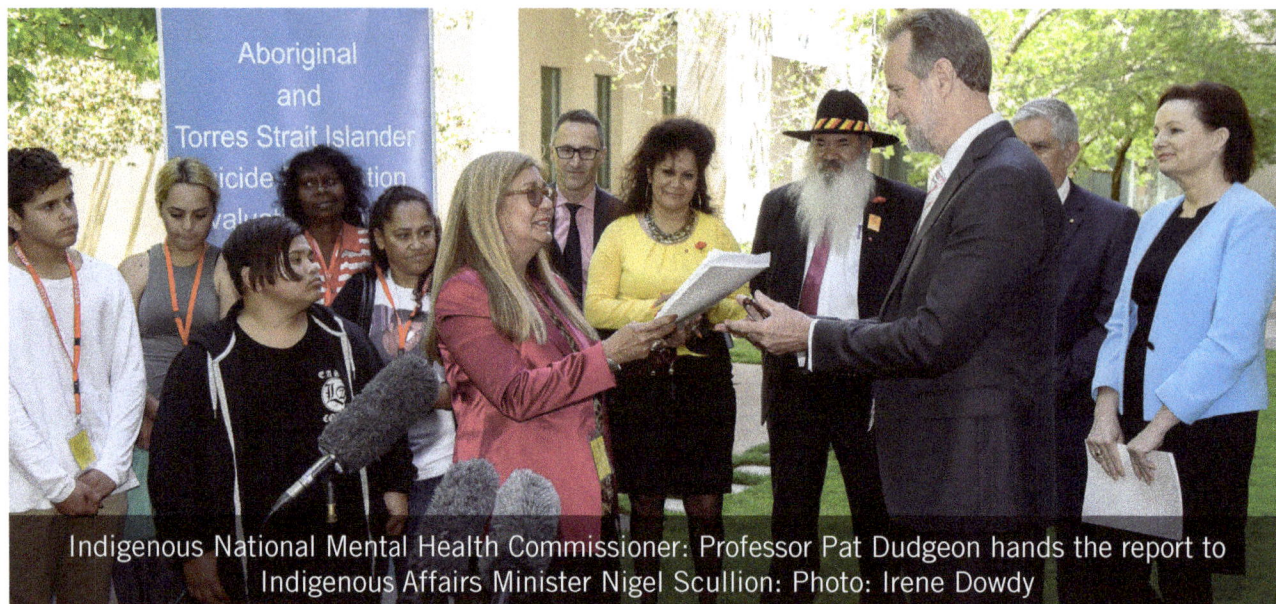

Indigenous National Mental Health Commissioner: Professor Pat Dudgeon hands the report to Indigenous Affairs Minister Nigel Scullion: Photo: Irene Dowdy

Author: Pat Dudgeon, Gerry Georgatos and Adele Cox   **Published:** January, 2017

Efforts to prevent suicides among Aboriginal and Torres Strait Islander people should include a focus on reducing over-incarceration, according to a major new report.

The Aboriginal and Torres Strait Islander Suicide Prevention Evaluation Project (ATSISPEP) report has backed Justice Reinvestment, to divert funding from prisons to communities.

Justice Reinvestment involves investing in upstream programs to support young people and families, and sport or other activities, and by enhancing access to quality education and employment.

The report also says Justice Reinvestment principles should be used to fund improvements to Indigenous mental health and alcohol and other drug services and programs.

In the article below, Professor Pat Dudgeon, Gerry Georgatos and Adele Cox, who helped to produce the ATSISPEP report, describe some of the roundtable consultations that informed their recommendations, and highlighted the importance of addressing intergenerational trauma.

Pat Dudgeon, Gerry Georgatos and Adele Cox write:

In developing the recommendations in the ATSISPEP report, a series of community-based and youth roundtable consultations were held, as well as the inaugural National Aboriginal and Torres Strait Islander Suicide Prevention Conference.

These consultations highlighted the impact of the high rates of Aboriginal and Torres Strait Islander imprisonment on suicidal behaviours.

A common observation was that imprisonment and contact with the criminal justice system was part of a matrix of factors that collectively contributed to suicidal behaviours (among other problems) in young Aboriginal and Torres Strait Islander people.

A major theme from the community consultations was to "keep out of prison those who should not be there", particularly young people with mental health and substance abuse disorders.

On March 20, 2015, the ATSISPEP facilitated a Justice Roundtable in Canberra at our partner organisation, the Healing Foundation.

A cross section of people and organisations were invited to best represent the intertwining issues affecting incarcerated

Aboriginal and Torres Strait Islanders, their families and communities.

These were some of the observations made by attendees:

"The prisons are full of people with mental health issues who should not be there. We have three psychiatrists here today that can attest to the fact prisons are full of people with undiagnosed mental health disorders."

"We need to bring our leaders together from all over the country and work more closely together to influence change. Governments are failing to respond to us because they are not working with our leaders. Governments are not close to them. They work through other voices not closely aligned with our people and communities."

"I am both Aboriginal and a Torres Strait Islander. In Cherbourg I managed a project to improve mental health and to reduce addictions. I have spent years working in the prison system as a clinician in mental health. My work has been more with the adults rather than youth. I am working with mothers and grandmothers to build support cultures. We're all very invested in the need for outcomes."

The Justice Roundtable discussions also highlighted the impact of intergenerational trauma in contributing to over-incarceration, and attendees called for policy changes to ensure the mental health assessment of detainees and prisoners, and their access to quality mental health care and other treatments, psychosocial and cultural.

Attendees said:

"The intergenerational trauma remains the biggest issue but when you get down it, no-one wants to talk about the intergenerational trauma. Governments want it swept under the carpet. If we do not deal with the intergenerational trauma then we will not be able to deal successfully with preventing suicides, we will continue to fail to lower incarceration rates."

"The intergenerational trauma is real. We have to focus on it. Healing is about dealing with trauma."

Attendees also raised concerns about the impacts of child protection authorities removing children from families.

One attendee said: *"There is also a vital period after a child or children are removed from their families where the family members are shattered and are at heightened risks of self-harm and suicide. Who is looking after them at this time?"*

Another said: *"There is so much guilt, shame, hurt, anger and distress when a child or children are removed."*

Attendees wanted to see more Aboriginal and Torres Strait Islander people working in prisons in mental and allied health services, and in wellbeing and healing programs, of which there are very few at this time.

They also called for Aboriginal and Torres Strait Islander people to be in executive management positions in these workforces, which would lead to more effective services and programs, and also help to address institutional and structural racism and discrimination.

The inaugural National Aboriginal and Torres Strait Islander Suicide Prevention Conference heard about the Western Australian-based Ngalla Maya reintegration program founded by a former inmate, CEO and founder, Mervyn Eades, a Nyoongar man.

On the smell of an oily rag, Ngalla Maya has achieved the positive reintegration into society of former inmates through training and education programs.

In the last 15 months, all 120 of its graduates – former inmates, 50 per cent females – have been supported by Ngalla Maya into employment.

"Our people in prison are damaged but most of them can be helped," said Mervyn Eades.

Professor Pat Dudgeon, from the Bardi people of the Kimberley, a psychologist and academic at the University of Western Australia, chairs the ATSISPEP project.

Gerry Georgatos is the project's community consultant and media liaison officer.

Adele Cox, a Bunuba and Gija woman from the Kimberley region, is the project's Senior Indigenous Community Research Consultant.

Overseer/Officer

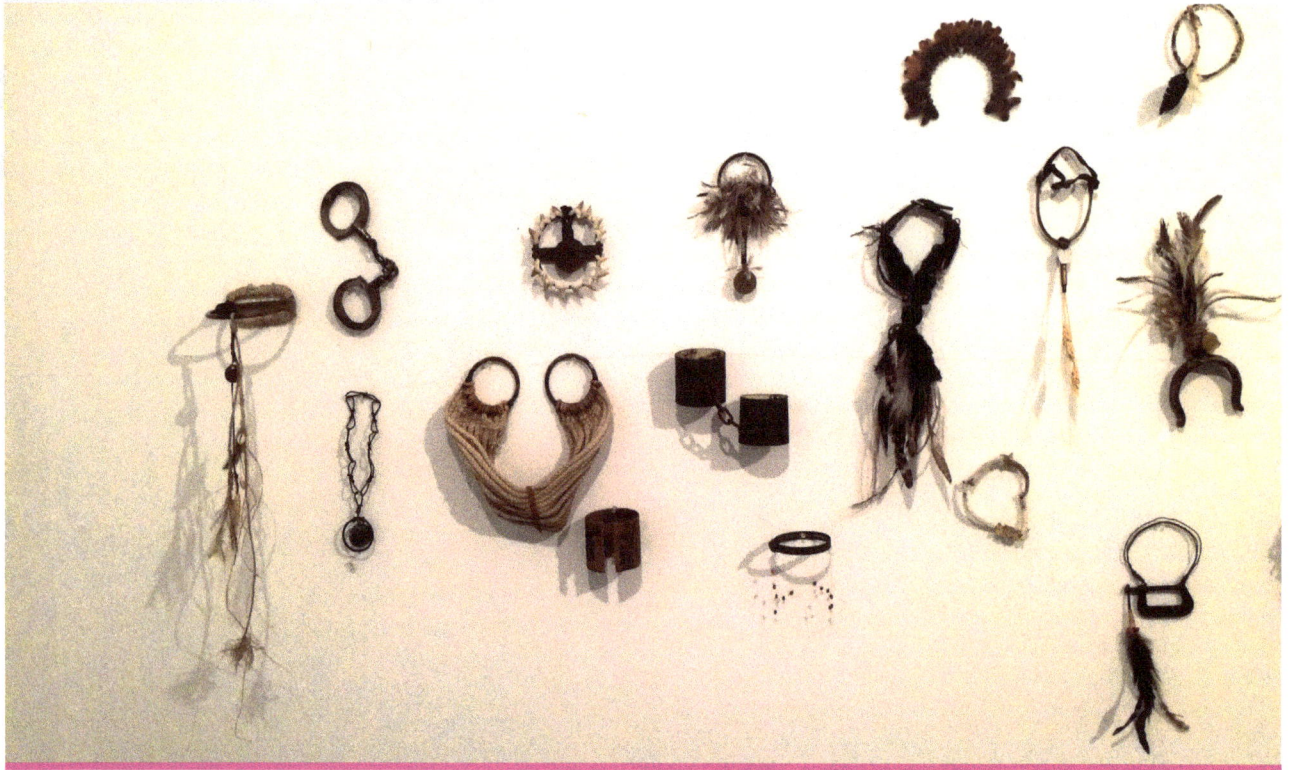

Overseer/Officer, 2015, is a mixed media installation using feathers, found objects, beads, and chains. It is a narrative about Aboriginal deaths in custody. It was created by Jason Wing, a Sydney-based artist who strongly identifies with his Chinese and Aboriginal heritage. Wing began as a street artist and has since expanded his practice to incorporate photomedia, installation and painting. Influenced by his bi-cultural upbringing, Wing explores the ongoing challenges that impact his wider community. Adopting the semantics of this 'flatline', Wing highlights in this work the institutional amnesia towards what he describes as 'systematic genocide'. Up until 2014, there had been 340 Aboriginal deaths in custody since the 1987 Royal Commission. Of the report's 339 recommendations, few have been implemented – Gina Fairley.

8. Caring for youth

" Be outraged at the Indigenous youth imprisonment rate!

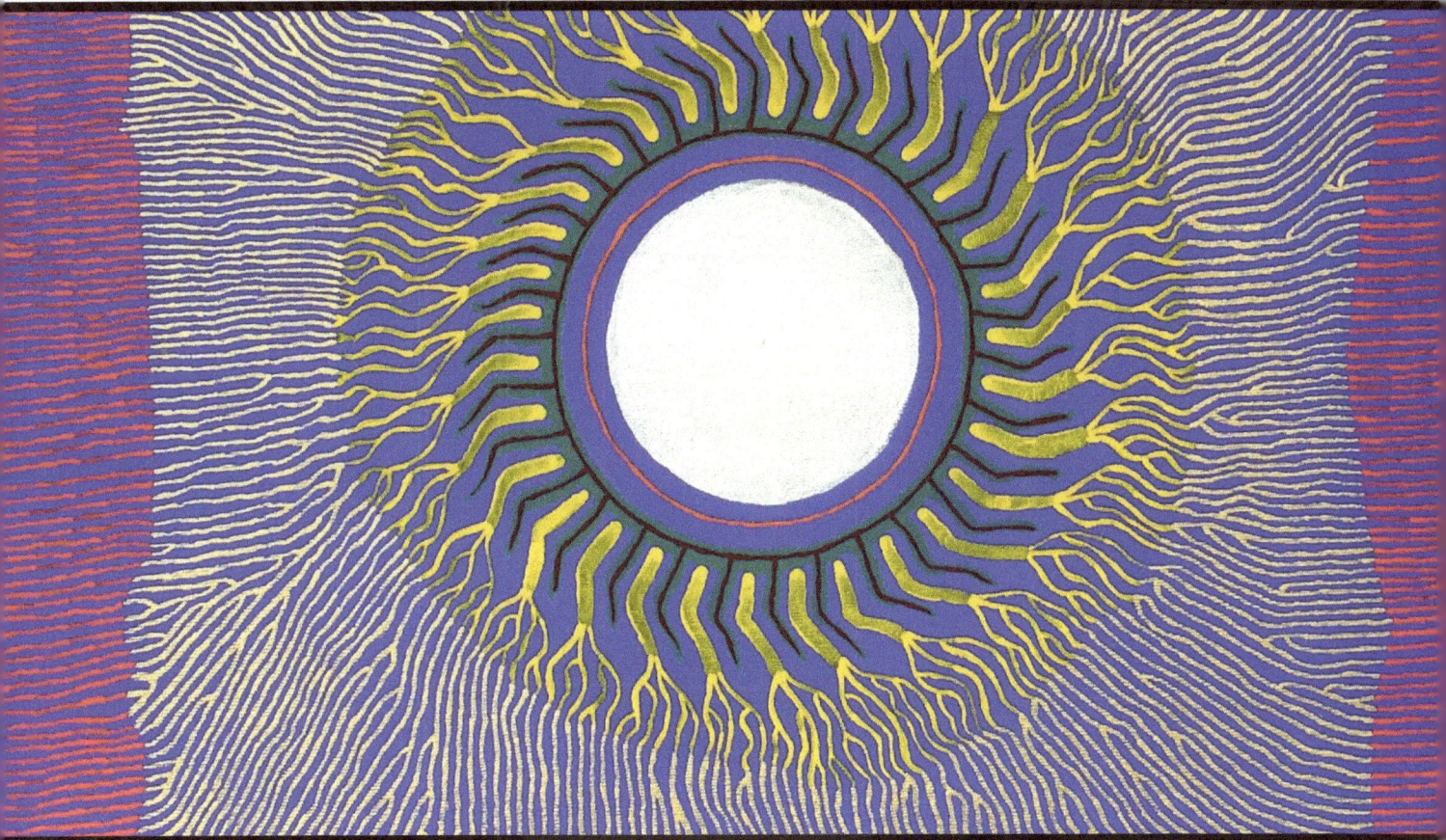

Now this DOES call for outrage

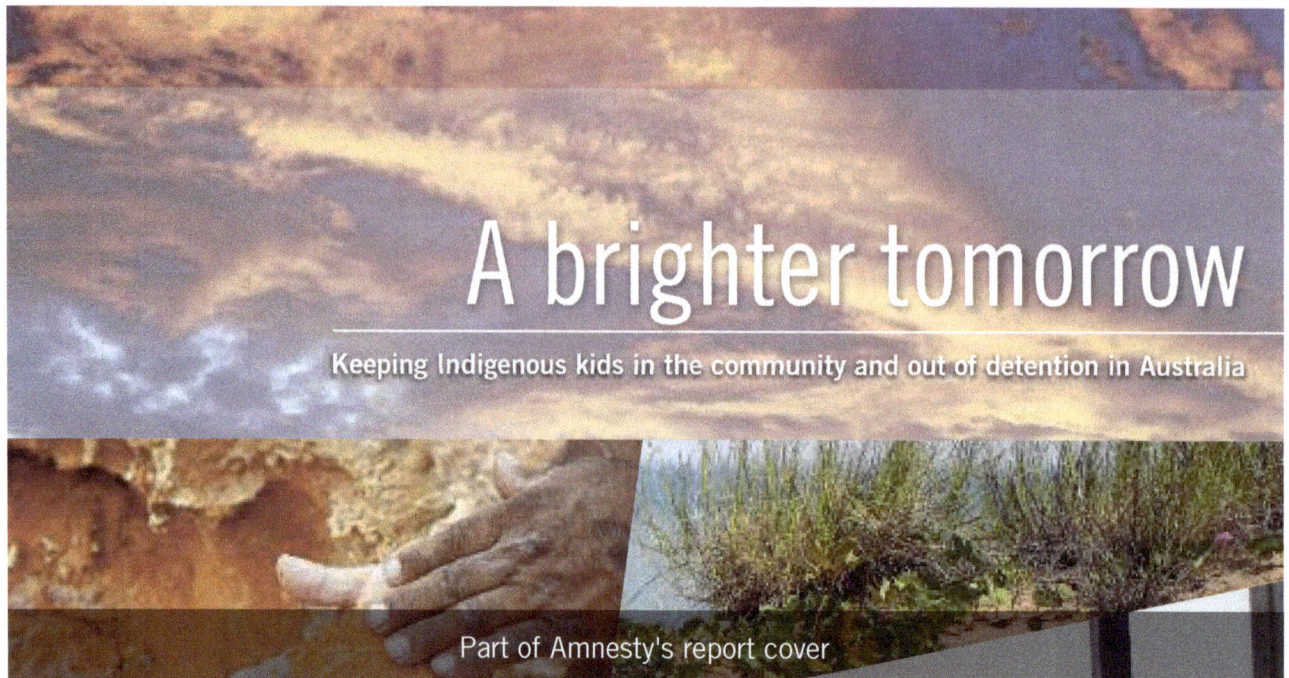

A brighter tomorrow

Keeping Indigenous kids in the community and out of detention in Australia

Part of Amnesty's report cover

| Author: | Darren Parker | Published: | June 04, 2015 |

"Our young people do not belong in prison."

This statement by Aboriginal and Torres Strait Islander Social Justice Commissioner Mick Gooda opens a new report, which makes a strong call for action to end the over-representation of Indigenous youth in the criminal justice system.

The report should inspire widespread outrage, according to researcher Darren Parker, a Ngunawal man and Phd Candidate at the Melbourne Law School. (The report's recommendations are published in full at the bottom of this post).

"Be outraged at the Indigenous youth imprisonment rate!"

Darren Parker writes:

Australia is currently immersed in the 'outrage' of a 'war dance' and an imaginary 'spear' held by an Aboriginal footballer.

Meanwhile, back in reality, an Amnesty International report on the over-representation of Indigenous youth in the criminal justice system was published that is more rightly a source of outrage.

As Aboriginal and Torres Strait Islander Social Justice Commissioner, Mick Gooda, states: "This is a national emergency. This must change, urgently."

The urgency for drastic action to reverse the over-representation of Indigenous young people in juvenile detention centres is immediate. If Australia neglects this, it will face losing another generation of Indigenous peoples to failed government policies, according to the Amnesty International report.

The report, Brighter Tomorrow: Keeping Kids in the Community and out of Detention in Australia, states that rates of Indigenous youth imprisonment are the highest they have been since the Royal Commission into Aboriginal deaths in custody handed down its report in 1991.

This represents 20+ years of failed policies, if not, sadly, even longer. The fact that the imprisonment rates have increased to such levels since the Royal Commission is all the more damning of the current situation in Australia.

The report states that between 2013-14, Aboriginal and Torres Strait Islander children were 26 times more likely to be imprisoned than non-Indigenous children. 26 times! A truly shocking statistic when you consider that Indigenous youth make up approximately 5% of the population of 10-17 year olds, but make up over half (59%) of youth in detention.

Additionally, according to 2012-2013 figures, 1 in every 28 Indigenous boys aged 10-17yrs had spent time in detention, compared to 1 in 544 for non-Indigenous boys.

Indigenous representation among girls in detention was even higher – one in 113 Indigenous girls aged 10-17yrs had spent time in detention, compared to one in 2,439 for non-Indigenous girls. This represents a massive skew in the criminal justice system against Indigenous youth.

Many of the reasons Indigenous youth are incarcerated are preventable. Be outraged at that.

Further, the comparative effects of these rates are all the more alarming when viewed within the continuum of funding uncertainty, shortfalls and government cuts to specialised Indigenous legal services. This means that many Indigenous young people do not always get the legal assistance they require or deserve.

Furthermore, numerous government inquiries have shown that the Aboriginal and Torres Strait Islander Legal Services (ATSILS) and Family Violence Prevention Legal Services (FVPLS) who provide specialised, culturally sensitive services for Indigenous people, including young people, are significantly underfunded.

In the foreword of the report, the Social Justice Commissioner tacitly recognises that even where there is underfunding, it is money being poorly directed. Additionally, current approaches to Indigenous youth encountering the criminal justice system are severely lacking.

He says: "We need an approach that starts to address the underlying causes of crime and starts to divert resources away from imprisonment and into local communities. This is a justice reinvestment approach that suggests that both early intervention and community responses are necessary to achieving long-term change."

'Justice reinvestment' and 'long-term' approaches are certainly at the core of the report's 16 recommendations. All of which are practical and straightforward in implementation, even in recognising the Commonwealth/State jurisdictional sphere. The implementation of the report's recommendations would radically alter the current Indigenous youth criminal justice trajectory away from human rights catastrophe.

Additionally, the implementation of some recommendations may even make Australia look like it takes international law seriously, such as raising the age of criminal responsibility from 10 years of age to the international standard of 12 years of age. Implementing this recommendation would mean that Australia was actually upholding its obligation under an international treaty it ratified.

Critically, the importance of the recommendation should not be lost. As most recent data indicates (Table S76b), Indigenous children make up more than 60% of all children under 12 years of age detained in Australia. That is, more than one in two 10-11 year olds in detention are Indigenous! Be outraged at that.

Be outraged that Western Australia, Queensland and the Northern Territory have, respectively, the highest rate of over-representation of Indigenous youth in detention; the fastest growing rate of Indigenous youth detention; and the highest proportion of youth in detention who are Indigenous. That two of them were named again by the UN Committee on the Rights of the Child for substantial failures in complying with minimum international standards is perhaps more enraging.

Rather than moving in ways that work toward justice reinvestment programs as outlined in the report, both the Western Australian and Queensland governments have recently implemented laws that are more punitive in nature.

In Queensland, the law allows the courts to treat 17-year-olds like adults under the Criminal Code. Last year the Newman government enacted another law requiring that kids who turn 17 in detention with more than six months left on their sentence be transferred to an adult prison.

In Western Australia, a recent decision to toughen "three-strike" mandatory sentencing laws to allow all three strikes to be awarded concurrently could see children jailed for three months on their first court appearance.

The report also recommends including justice targets within the national 'Closing the Gap' strategy. It recommends that a dual target to close the gap between Indigenous and non-Indigenous Australians, in incarceration rates and rates of experienced violence. Perhaps be outraged that there have never been any justice targets implemented at the COAG level or in the Closing the Gap strategy.

Further, the report recommends recognising foetal alcohol spectrum disorders (FASD) as a disability before the courts, and making a national commitment to a justice reinvestment approach to find community-based solutions to youth crime. Additionally, the report recommends that urgently finalising a diagnostic tool for FASD is critical in this regard. Maybe be outraged that there isn't even an official diagnostic tool for a medical condition that is connected with high rates of involvement in the justice system.

Or perchance, be outraged that the report recommends that Australia and its states/territories standardise and integrate all data collection. Because even now, nearly 25 years after the Royal Commission into Aboriginal Deaths in Custody, pathetically Australia still cannot standardise or integrate its own data collection!

It is abhorrent that there are approximately 450 Indigenous children in detention across Australia every night. Even more abhorrent is that we do very little to combat this when indeed we could. Be outraged at that!

Follow on Twitter: @darren__parker. Ngunawal, Phd Candidate at the Melbourne Law School. Recovering Academic.

Recommendations for the Australian Government

1

Legislate in order to override state and territory-based laws that do not conform with the Convention on the Rights of the Child, including by the introduction of legislation to the effect that:

- Notwithstanding any state or territory law which provides otherwise, in sentencing or considering a bail application for any person up to and including the age of 17, the court must observe the principle that detention is a measure of last resort.

- Any state or territory law that requires the imposition of a mandatory minimum sentence on a child or young person up to and including the age of 17 is invalid.

- Any state or territory law treats a person up to and including age 17 as an adult for the purpose of criminal prosecution is invalid.

- Any state or territory laws that treats a person below the age of 12 as criminally responsible is invalid, and the doctrine of doli incapax continues to apply to 12, 13 and 14-year-olds.

2

Immediately withdraw the reservation to Article 37(c) of the Convention on the Rights of the Child.

3

Ratify the Optional Protocol to the Convention Against Torture (OPCAT) without delay, and create an independent National Preventative Mechanism (NPM) under the guidance of the Subcommittee on the Prevention of Torture (SPT). Allow both the NPM and SPT access to all places where people are deprived of liberty, including youth detention facilities.

4

Take immediate steps to become a party to the Third Optional Protocol to the Convention on the Rights of the Child on a communications procedure.

5

Ensure that ongoing funding is made available to so that the managing and coordinating role played by the NATSILS can continue.

Ensure sufficient ongoing funding is available to continue the work undertaken by the Family Violence Prevention Legal Service (FVPLS).

6

Work with the state and territory governments to quantify the level of unmet legal need currently experienced by Indigenous young people and their families; and

Take immediate steps to make up the shortfall in funding to ensure that all young people facing criminal proceedings are granted full access to legal assistance.

7

Commence work with all state and territory governments, through COAG, to identify and address gaps in the collection of standard and disaggregated data related to youth contact with the justice system. This should include taking immediate steps to integrate information on arrest and police diversion into the Juvenile Justice National Minimum Data Set (JJ NMDS) and better link JJ NMDS data with child protection and adult corrections data.

8

Work with the Western Australian and Northern Territory governments to ensure that they provide JJ NMDS data in the required standard format.

Source: Brighter Tomorrow: Keeping Kids in the Community and out of Detention in Australia

9

Begin a process, through COAG, to develop justice targets to reduce Indigenous youth detention rates and create safer communities (through reduced rates of experienced violence). Such targets should be developed in consultation with Indigenous Peoples and their organisations that represent offenders and victims.

Relevant sub-indicators under the target might include the following (disaggregated by age, gender, remoteness and disability status):

- The rate at which Indigenous young people are cautioned or otherwise diverted by police compared to non-Indigenous young people.

- The rate at which Indigenous young people are held in un-sentenced detention compared to non-Indigenous young people.

- The rate at which Indigenous young people are referred to court conferencing by police and courts compared to non-Indigenous young people.

- The rate at which Indigenous young people are diverted by the courts into programs compared to non-Indigenous young people.

- The rate at which Indigenous young people are given non-custodial orders compared to non-Indigenous young people.

- The rate at which Indigenous young people receive custodial sentences compared to non-Indigenous young people.

- The rate at which Indigenous young people reoffend compared with non-Indigenous young people.

- The rate at which Indigenous young people are victims of crime compared with non-Indigenous young people.

- The number of Indigenous-led and designed programs as diversionary options available to the courts and community-based alternatives to detention.

10

Take a leading role, through COAG, to identify the data required to implement a Justice Reinvestment approach, including by tasking a technical body with assisting states and territories and coordinate a national approach to the data collection.

11

Work with state and territory governments to ensure that the adoption of a justice reinvestment approach occurs in close consultation with Indigenous communities and their representatives.

12

Recognise Fetal Alcohol Spectrum Disorders (FASD) as a disability under the National Disability Insurance Scheme and on the Department of Social Services' List of Recognised Disabilities.

13

Provide sufficient resources to Indigenous community-designed and led initiatives to address the effects of FASD to ensure that it is treated as a disability rather than becoming a criminal justice issue.

14

Urgently finalise an official diagnostic tool for FASD.

15

Work with state and territory governments to identify areas of unmet need for bail accommodation. Fund Indigenous community controlled bail accommodation and support services to ensure that Indigenous young people are not held in detention on remand solely due to a lack of other options. Particular focus should be given to young girls and boys in out-of-home care, and those with mental health issues and cognitive impairments, including those with FASD.

16

Work with the state and territory governments to develop youth bail legislation requiring that pre-trial detention should occur only as a last resort where there is a risk of flight or where release would interfere with the administration of justice. Under the uniform youth bail legislation, pre-trial detention should occur only after a case-by-case assessment of necessity and proportionality.

Source: Brighter Tomorrow: Keeping Kids in the Community and out of Detention in Australia

More support needed for Aboriginal youth in contact with juvenile justice in SA

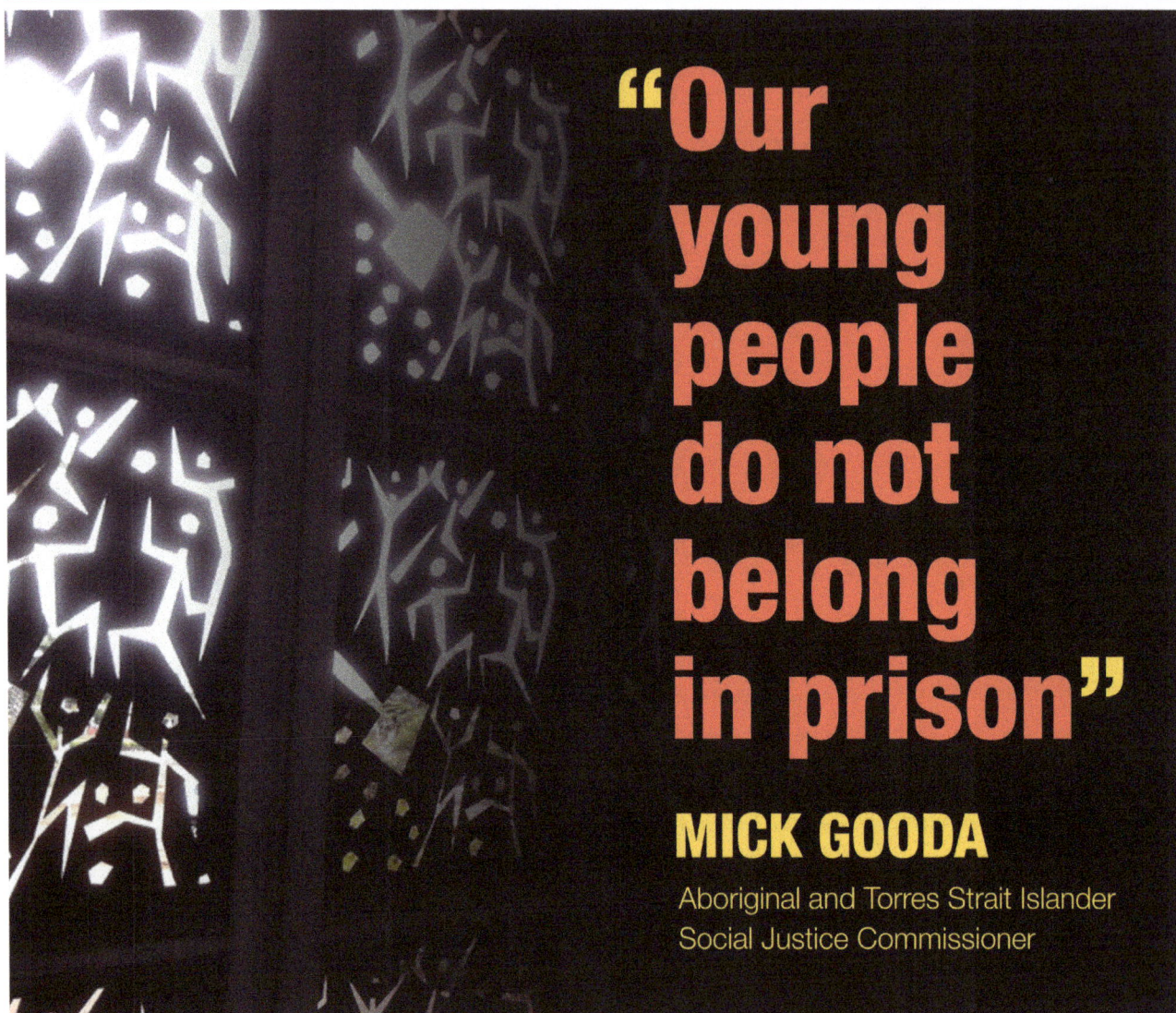

"Our young people do not belong in prison"

MICK GOODA

Aboriginal and Torres Strait Islander Social Justice Commissioner

Author:	Summer May Finlay	Published:	April 04, 2016

Young Aboriginal people who are in contact with the juvenile justice system in South Australia would benefit from greater access to diversionary programs and to Aboriginal mentors or support workers, reports Summer May Finlay.

Summer May Finlay writes:

We know our young people are incarcerated at significantly higher rates than other Australians, and South Australia is no exception, where Aboriginal young people aged between 10-17 years old are only 4 percent of people in that age bracket in Australia but are 46 percent of young people in detention. They also make up 34 percent of young people under community-based supervision.

These statistics made South Australia's rate of contact of Aboriginal young people with the juvenile justice system the second highest in the country.

For Dale Agius, a Kaurna, Narungga, Nadjeri, Ngakaraku man, one of the issues is the lack of appropriate diversionary programs.

It is well known that if a young person experiences incarceration at an early age, they are less likely to complete school or become employed if they had never been in contact with the criminal justice system. This is why diversionary programs are so important.

We also need to make sure that if young people to come in contact with the justice system, they have a voice all the way through and that there are adequate support programs on release, according to Mr Agius.

Mr Agius has worked in the justice sector in a variety of roles for 15 years, including Community Correction, Aboriginal Liaison, Aboriginal Case Management as well as being the Aboriginal Programs Officer working in therapeutic programs for high risk Violent and Sexual offenders in Correctional Services Psych Services Unit (Rehabilitation Programs Branch). He has also worked for the Department of Premier and Cabinet and State Government.

More recently, Mr Agius was the Executive Officer to the South Australian Commissioner for Aboriginal Engagement where he advised and supported the Commissioner on relevant policy topics including justice. Currently he is the Ministerial Advisor Liaison Officer to Kyam Maher MLC, the South Australian Minister for Aboriginal Affairs and Reconciliation. In this position he forms the link between the Division of Aboriginal Affairs and Reconciliation, the community and the Ministerial staff. He is also a current member of the Youth Parole Board, which in South Australia is called Youth Review Board.

Need for Aboriginal involvement

There is clearly no quick or easy solution to addressing these issues, which is why it's important Aboriginal people are involved in all aspects across the justice system, including policing, incarceration, incarceration management and engagement, exit transition planning and ongoing support post detention.

Aboriginal engagement at all levels of the justice system ensures our kids are getting an opportunity to be involved in their rehabilitative process and are adequately supported, says Mr Agius.

He believes "part of my role [on the Youth Review Board] is to engage other youth parole Board members who may not be as aware of some of the challenges faced by Aboriginal young people, and to present the systemic barriers and challenges faced with access to services."

"It's important to have an Aboriginal voice at that level," he says.

"Without an Aboriginal person on the Board, they don't always hear the voice of the young Aboriginal person. And it can be difficult to take their views into account and include them in the process."

When a young person comes before the Board, they are represented by a case manager or case coordinator, who works with the young person while in detention and helps them with an Exit Plan. Exit Plans are a structured pathway plan for what the young person is going to be doing when on conditional

release. The Exit Plan is then presented to the Board by the case manager or coordinator.

Youth voices matter

However, this system is not perfect, says Mr Agius. He believes that sometimes young people will agree to questions during the development of the Exit Plan because they believe the case manager or coordinator know best.

But Mr Agius believes in the youth having a say, "they know the areas they are being released to, and what challenges lie ahead.

"It's reasonable to say that the youth should be engaged in the development of their Exit Plan," he says.

"It demonstrates that they are thinking of ways to stop behaviours and attitudes which lead to coming into the justice system."

Some Aboriginal young people have an Aboriginal mentor or Aboriginal support worker, and he has noticed that these young people seem to have a stronger connection with their mentors and support people when they are Aboriginal.

Mr Agius says:

" *I would like to see more Aboriginal mentors, and more Aboriginal support people come and present to the youth Board. (This ensures) there is continuous connection between the youth and the Aboriginal mentor, from detention to reintegration back into the community. The worker can present options to the Board who may not be up to speed on which services are available.*

I feel that this would lead to more participation by our young people in their Exit Plans. This participation would bring a clearer focus on where they are headed post release and lead to better outcomes.

It is a privilege to have Aboriginal mentors or support workers attend a youth review Board hearing. They clearly present a progressive pathway for completing vocation or education opportunities to the benefit of our young people.

It's a shame not all young Aboriginal people coming before the Board have the option of an Aboriginal mentor or support worker. We just need more.

Diversionary strategies needed

Mr Agius says we also need "more diversionary strategies that are responsive to the needs of our youth. We have one really good program called the "The Journey Home, and The Journey to Respect program".

The program works with young Aboriginal people who have had issues with offending attitudes. The program presents the young person with a realistic model, which empowers them to identify their heritage, connection to country, place, while taking responsibility for their behaviour. This leads to the young person engaging in the process and developing solutions and alternatives.

While the program is great, not all young Aboriginal people who have been in detention have access to it. Mr Agius says "to really reduce the rate of young people coming in contact with the justice system, we need to make sure all our young people have access to programs like these."

Beyond programs like this, young Aboriginal people need other support programs, which aren't always available in their areas such as outreach alcohol and other drug services, employment, education and training services and accommodation.

More services needed in regional and remote areas

In regional and remote areas, services can be limited or non-existent. Mr Agius says "the availability of services can limit our youth opportunities post release".

He would like to see all Aboriginal young people have the support of the services they need in their own communities.

"There is actually nothing in operation that is a coordinated exit strategy in addressing young Aboriginal offenders' needs," he says.

At times, immediate release back into the community is not an option for these young people and some may need to remain in metropolitan areas. If immediate release back into their community is not an option due to the lack of services, there needs to be a coordinated service release response which could assist in eventually returning youth back to their communities after fulfilling service treatment goals in the city.

Mr Agius acknowledges that there is a lot to do to reduce the number of young Aboriginal people coming in contact with the justice system.

As an individual, he is doing what he can to get the best outcomes for our kids. He is undertaking a Bachelor of Arts and majoring in Social Science in Human Services and Psychological Science so he can increase his understanding of what is needed.

"I am studying because of my passion for justice and interest in psychology," he says.

"My interests extend to justice more broadly though I am finding that there is a higher demand for these services in the Aboriginal space."

One day he hopes this is not the case.

Call for overhaul of Queensland youth detention

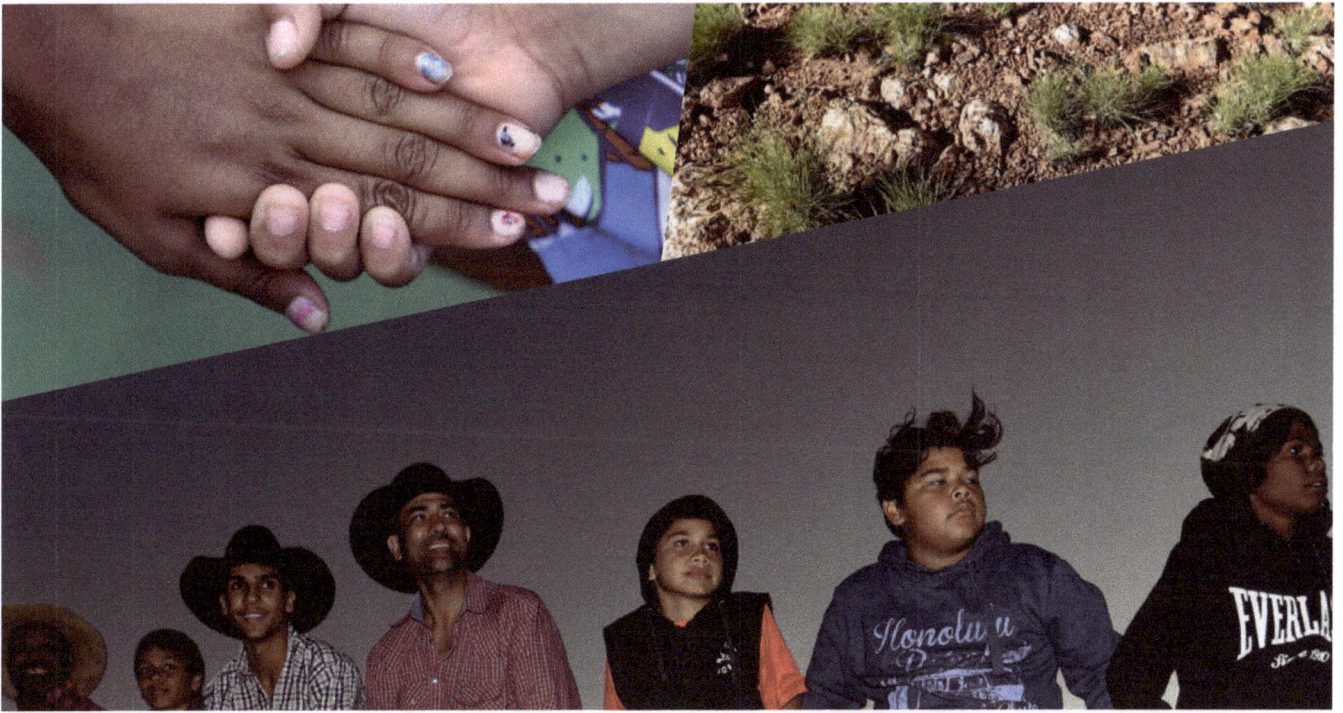

| Author: | Amy Coopes | Published: | August 31, 2016 |

Amy Coopes writes:

Indigenous children in Queensland are 22 times more likely to be locked up than their counterparts and account for a staggering 65 percent of those in youth detention on any given day despite comprising just 8 percent of the state's 10 to 17-year-olds, according to a damning new Amnesty study.

Published in the wake of incriminating new footage showing a 17-year-old Aboriginal teenager **forcibly restrained and fitted with a spit hood** by seven officers inside the Brisbane Corrections Centre and the NT's Don Dale scandal, Amnesty's **Heads Held High** report makes for sobering reading.

According to the report, Queensland leads Australia in locking up 10 and 11-year-olds and holding children on remand, with 83 percent of juvenile offenders held without bail and two-thirds of these Indigenous children.

Queensland is the only state in Australia to hold 17-year-olds in adult prisons.

Claire Mallinson, director of Amnesty International Australia, said these practices flew in the face of international law, which states children should be released from pre-trial detention as soon as possible and only detained as a last resort.

"Decades of harsh policies have seen too many kids, especially Indigenous kids, trapped in the criminal justice system," said Mallinson.

While reforms were underway in Queensland, the report documented troubling new findings including use of dogs,

mechanical restraints and invasive search procedures and self-harm.

Importantly, it highlighted that significant cultural barriers were at play and presented a critical reform opportunity that remained overlooked. Just two of 16 organisations contracted to work with youth justice were Indigenous-led groups.

"Queensland is fortunate to have many trailblazing Indigenous leaders. Their work connects kids to culture, keeps them out of children's prisons and in their communities," said Mallinson.

" All sides of politics should harness Indigenous innovation and expertise to create a stronger and safer Queensland for everyone. This is an opportunity to break with the past that has failed so many kids.

Among barriers highlighted by the report:

- lack of access to culturally-appropriate legal advice
- refusal of bail on grounds, including children's home environment
- lack of culturally appropriate diversionary options for Indigenous juvenile offenders

" *Aboriginal and Torres Strait Islander children are more likely to end up behind bars because they are more likely to be disadvantaged, removed from their families, absent from school, experiencing violence, racism and trauma, abusing substances, and to have a disability or mental illness, among other contributing factors.*

Twenty-five years ago, the Royal Commission into Aboriginal Deaths in Custody (RCIADIC) found that these social and health issues can be determinants of contact with the justice system, and need to be addressed in order to end the over-representation of Indigenous people in custody.

It recommended an Indigenous-led, evidence-based justice reinvestment trial to address these underlying causes of offending, as well as greater funding and support for Indigenous-driven solutions.

The report also called for the age of criminal responsibility to be raised to 12 (currently 10 in all Australian jurisdictions), for all 17-year-olds to cease being held as adults and immediately transitioned into juvenile detention, and the enactment of an enforceable Human Rights Bill protecting the rights of children and Indigenous people.

In addition, it recommended appointment of an independent Inspector of Custodial Services and federal ratification of the Optional Protocol to the Convention Against Torture.

These calls will be echoed tonight in a new documentary, Prison Songs, which goes behind the barbed wire of Darwin's Berrimah jail to share the stories of Aboriginal and Torres Strait Islander inmates.

"*Prison Songs* reveals the truth about incarceration in this country and the urgent need for action: we need to look to Aboriginal and Torres Strait Islander peoples for the solutions." said Shane Duffy, co-chair of Change the Record.

"Better investment is needed in early intervention, prevention and diversion strategies – smarter solutions that increase safety, address the causes of crime, and build safer communities.

"Culture also has an important part to play to break the cycle of incarceration; helping to light a path to a better life, away from the criminal justice system."

Australia's first musical documentary, with lyrics by Keating: The Musical's Casey Bennetto and Shellie Morris, Prison Songs screened on NITV.

'It was a lightbulb in my head. Hang on, I'm black'

Justice system tensions have been squarely in the spotlight again this week, with riots outside the Kalgoorlie courthouse following the death of 14-year-old Elijah Doughty, who was killed by a motorist over the weekend.

Racist commentary over the incident on social media had "absolutely inflamed the situation" according to acting police Commander Darryl Gaunt, but he denied Doughty's death had been a race crime.

"There is nothing to suggest at all that it's a racist issue. It's the death of a child who happens to be Aboriginal," said Gaunt.

Social media begged to differ.

" *#Kalgoorlie 'riot' was reaction to young boy being mowed down / stabbed to death. Stop demonising black people for continued suffering.*

— Dr Anita Heiss (@AnitaHeiss) August 30, 2016

Chris Graham over at New Matilda has put the incident into broader historical context and is worth a read, as is this piece.

Separately, Brisbane Indigenous Media Association worker Leon Petrou, a Gumbaynggirr man, has spoken out about his brutalisation at the hands of Queensland police in 2013 in a panel discussion.

" *I had to kneel down because the pain was so intense (from the Taser). And when I knelt down the officers came belting into me. Punched my tooth into my top lip there and he put his hand in my mouth and ripped my jaw open. He was poking me in my eyes, full on with his thumb and fingers.*

It was a lightbulb in my head. Hang on, I'm black. They don't like blackfellas. That's how the mentality of this nation goes.

Petrou was acquitted of all charges in 2015.

All this, while Cory Bernardi spearheads a backbench push for the Racial Discrimination Act to be watered down.

For children's sake: raise the age of criminal responsibility

Author:	Madeleine Calleja	Published:	March 26, 2016

States and territories have been urged to lift the low age of criminal responsibility, to stop the remand of children as young as ten.

The recommendation comes from Jesuit Social Services, which has released a discussion paper calling for a wide range of reforms to the youth justice system, in the way it responds to offending in children aged 10 – 15 years.

Madeleine Calleja, Policy Research and Advocacy Officer, Jesuit Social Services, writes below that there is widespread support among legal, social and human rights groups for such reforms.

Meanwhile, beneath her post are details of a recent systematic review from the Campbell Collaboration concluding that custodial sentences, such as prison, are no better than non-custodial sentences in reducing re-offending.

"Despite this evidence, almost all societies across the world continue to use custodial sentences as the main crime control strategy," it says.

Thinking Outside

Alternatives to remand for children
Research Report

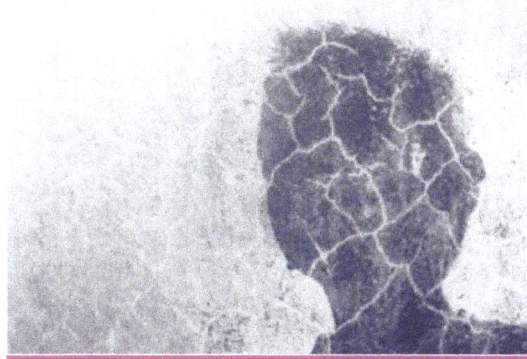

Image from the cover of the Jesuit Social Services report, Thinking Outside: Alternatives to Remand for Children

Madeleine Calleja writes:

Imagine going back to your 10-year-old self. You're standing outside a cinema, watching people stream in to see a new film that you're dying to watch.

You wish you had a few dollars to buy a ticket but you spent the little pocket money you receive on a few lollies at school this week. Perhaps it wouldn't be so bad if you snuck into the cinema, right?

A similar harmless scenario saw a terrified Aboriginal boy arrested and brought before the courts in the Northern Territory, as reported by Julian Cleary from Amnesty International.

This punitive and damaging response is a result of Australia's low minimum age of criminal responsibility – 10 years – which sees vulnerable children enter the youth justice system at far too young an age.

Recognising the unique vulnerability and risk of ongoing offending for children at this young age, Jesuit Social Services released a discussion paper, "Too much too young: Raise the age of criminal responsibility to 12", calling for a wide range of reforms to the youth justice system, in the way it responds to offending in children aged 10 – 15 years.

We recommend that the criminal age of responsibility be raised from 10 to 12 years and a graduated response for 12 – 15 years is ensured to reflect the varying stages of development during these middle years. This was supported by over 30 legal, social and human rights groups.

We are also calling for specialist Koori Children's Courts in each jurisdiction, recognising the unique vulnerability of Aboriginal children. Statistics show that compared with their non-Indigenous peers, Aboriginal children aged 10 – 14 years are:

* 6–10 times more likely to be proceeded against by police

* 23 times more likely to be under community-based supervision

* 25 times more likely to be in detention

Children who enter the youth justice system at a young age are often society's most vulnerable. Evidence shows that children who offend at a young age are more likely to: be involved with child protection; have come from disadvantaged areas; be developmentally vulnerable; have experienced child abuse, neglect, mental illness and homelessness; and be disengaged from school.

For Aboriginal children, there is the added impact of intergenerational trauma, grief and loss. The negative impact of colonisation has seen generations of Aboriginal people experience racism, dispossession, early deaths of family and community members, the forced removal of children, as well as other discriminatory policies.

The over-representation of Aboriginal people in the justice system also means that young children grow up familiar with life in prison, knowing relatives and community members who have spent time there. For some Aboriginal young people, being incarcerated can seem part of life's trajectory.

Experts in children's brain development agree that children under 12 lack the capacities for full criminal responsibility, capacities that don't fully mature until around 15 years. During the middle years the pre-frontal cortex undergoes a significant amount of development. This part of the brain is responsible for impulse control, planning and decision-making, making children susceptible to peer pressure and sensation and reward-seeking behaviour.

Out of step

Many people are unaware that Australia's minimum age of criminal responsibility is much lower than international standards, with 68% of countries having an age of 12 or higher.

UN experts on children's rights advocate for an absolute minimum age of 12 years, but ideally higher, to ensure the child is emotionally, intellectually and mentally mature enough to be held criminally responsible.

According to Andrew Jackomos, Victorian Commissioner for Aboriginal Children and Young People, "our Koori kids come into contact with the justice system younger and return more quickly. We must raise the age of criminal responsibility and reinvest our prison dollars into innovative community-led solutions that build the resilience of our Aboriginal children and their families and keep them connected to kin, culture and each other".

The earlier children come into contact with the justice system, the more likely they are to have longer criminal careers.

All states and territories should raise the age of criminal responsibility to 12 and provide a more effective, graduated response to anti-social behaviour for 12 – 15 year olds including specialist Koori Children's Courts and a legislated framework for diversion.

Madeleine Calleja is Policy Research and Advocacy Officer, Jesuit Social Services. Jesuit Social Services has a long history of working with young people in the justice system, including those from Aboriginal and Torres Strait Islander background. For more information, visit www.jss.org.au

Further reading and listening

- Custodial sentences, such as prison, are no better than non-custodial sentences in reducing re-offending, according to this summary of a recent systematic review by the Campbell Collaboration.
  Fourteen high-quality studies comparing custodial and non-custodial sentences are included in the analysis. The studies span the period from 1961 to 2013 and are mostly from the USA, Europe and Australia.

  In terms of rehabilitation, short confinement is not better or worse than "alternative" solutions. The review says other non-custodial approaches to offender rehabilitation also need to be evaluated, such as those provided through employment or other social networks.

- Washington Post Wonkblog: Poor white kids are less likely to go to prison than rich black kids. This article reports on US research suggesting that racial discrimination is a bigger factor than social and economic disadvantage when it comes to over-incarceration. "Race trumps class, at least when it comes to incarceration," said one of the researchers involved.

- Listen to Summer May Finlay and Amy McQuire talking about #JustJustice and related issues on the Brisbane-based 98.9FM, part of the National Indigenous Radio Service

"Think outside the bars"

Author:	Debbie Kilroy	Published:	November 21, 2016

Vulnerable children are bearing the brunt of governments' failure to address the underlying issues contributing to over-incarceration, according to Sisters Inside CEO and human rights advocate Debbie Kilroy.

Debbie Kilroy writes:

Governments must start to think "outside the bars" and address the underlying issues that contribute to the over-incarceration of Aboriginal and Torres Strait Islander people.

It's time for all governments to do more to address poverty, homelessness, education, violence against women, mental health and drug addictions.

Our prisons are full of the poor, the sick, the disabled, the young, the vulnerable and ever increasingly women.

Criminalisation and imprisonment cannot continue to be the default for those social issues in our country.

Building more prisons does not reduce crime. Nor does locking up children and young people contribute to a safer society. Vulnerable children are bearing the brunt of governments' failure to address these wider health and social issues.

Queensland leads Australia in locking up 10 and 11 year-old children, and must raise the age of criminal responsibility for children to twelve years, the global average.

No child should be imprisoned, no matter how old they are. All children should be protected. Indigenous children are most impacted by this policy.

Queensland also has the highest rates of children on remand in Australia. Between 2011 and 2015, the rate of unsentenced young people in detention in Queensland increased.

Of the 168 young people in prison in Queensland in the June quarter of 2015, 141 (84 per cent) were unsentenced. Of those who were unsentenced, 61 per cent were Aboriginal and Torres Strait Islander children.

The Queensland Government has promised to remove 17 year olds from adult prisons, and we welcome this announcement. However, we are concerned that it will not have an immediate impact. Seventeen-year-olds will continue to be deemed as adults in criminal matters until the legislation is passed and then for another 12-month period. On any given night in Queensland, 40 to 50 young people aged 17 are sharing accommodation with adult prisoners

There's an old saying that a justice department that spends most of its money on prisons is like a health department that spends most of its money on cemeteries

The trauma of incarceration impacts on children for the rest of their lives. It comes as no surprise then that, where 17-year-olds are treated as adults, there is evidence that they are more likely to be criminalised and imprisoned again.

Some of these children imprisoned on remand were ultimately acquitted, yet the damage of their imprisonment stayed long after release.

For many years, various inquiries (most notably the Royal Commission into Aboriginal Deaths in Custody) have recognised the link between social disadvantage and criminalisation.

Repeated studies have found that Aboriginal and Torres Strait Islander children are more likely to end up behind bars because they are more likely to be disadvantaged, removed from their families, absent from school, experiencing violence, racism and trauma, addicted to substances, and to have a disability or mental illness.

These are all social issues that can be addressed in the community if we all really valued our children.

It is critical we end the over-representation of Aboriginal and Torres Strait Islander children in the prison system, stop locking up children on remand, and stop using imprisonment in preference to alternative decarceration strategies.

In 2014-2015, the Queensland government wasted $89.2 million on imprisoning children, the second highest expenditure on youth imprisonment in Australia. It cost an average of $1,445 per child per day to keep them in prison.

There's an old saying that a justice department that spends most of its money on prisons is like a health department that spends most of its money on cemeteries.

Our children, our Indigenous children, are all precious resources and deserve an equal opportunity to grow up in loving and supportive families, with access to health and education resources.

There is deep concern, particularly in the absence of the protections of a Human Rights Act in Queensland, that 17-year-old children are being imprisoned in adult prisons. We are equally concerned about violations of human rights, systemic violence against children prisoners and practices which meet the international definition of torture, being routinely imposed on children in both adult and youth prisons throughout Queensland.

Sisters Inside is horrified by the rates of imprisonment of children in Queensland and the evident human rights abuses they routinely experience in both youth and adult prisons.

The failure of youth prisons to respond effectively to the needs of children has most notably been detailed recently through media coverage of the alleged mistreatment of children at both the Don Dale Youth Detention Centre, the Cleveland Youth Detention Centre and in the last few days in Victorian youth prisons – including the use of tear gas, restraints, spit hoods, beatings and extreme isolation to punish children.

In its recent report, Amnesty International described a systemic culture of secrecy and mistreatment of children, mainly Aboriginal and Torres Strait Islander children, in Queensland youth prisons.

The report identifies an alarming number of human rights abuses uncovered through a Freedom of Information request (including use of dogs to scare young Aboriginal girls, isolation for 22 hours a day, handcuffs during family visits, invasive search practices and extremely high rates of self-harm).

The report recommends that the Queensland Government develop an enforceable Human Rights Bill, in consultation with Indigenous and community sector organisations that incorporates, among others, international law and standards on the rights of children and Indigenous Peoples. (Recommendation 15)

Young people are being increasingly criminalised in Queensland, compared with other Australian states. In the four 4 years to 2015, there were decreases in the youth prison population in all states and territories except Queensland and the Northern Territory, where the number of young people in prisons on an average night increased. In Queensland, the number in youth prisoners increased from 130 in the June quarter 2011 to 168 in the June quarter 2015.

Revelations about the mistreatment of a 17-year-old Aboriginal boy in an adult prison highlight what Sisters Inside and some other NGOs have been stating for many years. We have long had detailed, consistent anecdotal evidence of the violations of human rights routinely directed against child prisoners in both youth and adult prisons.

This incident was extreme and degrading. It was punishment unlawfully administered and reflects the lack of skill among prison officers in dealing with young people. We have multiple examples of mistreatment akin to torture of young people in adult prisons. The very existence of a

boys' yard suggests that the prison system recognises the inappropriateness of keeping children in adult prisons.

The fact that this child, who had no previous experience of (youth or adult) imprisonment, did not have access to the boys' yard (reportedly, due to overcrowding) only further highlights the critical urgency of moving these children out of the adult prison system. Seventeen-year-old girls do not have a girls' yard as they are placed directly into the mainstream prison population.

The incarceration of 17-year-old children in adult prisons represents a failure of both the moral and legal obligations of the Queensland Government, and we call on them to act now.

Debbie Kilroy is the Chief Executive Officer of Sisters Inside, which she established to fight for the human rights of incarcerated women and to address gaps in services available to them and their children.

Sisters Inside is an independent community organisation that advocates for the human rights of women, girls and their children in youth and adult prisons. More information here: http://www.sistersinside.com.au/

Please help to avoid a disaster for kids in the Northern Territory

Author:	Julian Cleary	Published:	June 21, 2016

Changes to the NT Bail Act would result in many more children, particularly Indigenous children, being locked up.

In the open letter published below, Julian Cleary from Amnesty urges NT independent MLA Larisa Lee to use her influential vote to "avoid a disaster for kids".

He also describes this latest development as part of a broader picture of punitive systems in the NT that penalise children, rather than investing in their futures.

Open letter to Independent MLA Larisa Lee, regarding changes to NT Bail Act

21 June 2016

Dear Ms Lee,

I am writing this letter to you in the hope you can help to avoid a disaster for kids in the Northern Territory.

The NT government is planning to pass laws within the next few days that will normalise locking up children who haven't even been to trial.

What has happened to the idea that people are innocent until proven guilty?

Your vote will be extremely powerful. You will probably have the deciding vote – and with that you can make sure kids as young as 10 aren't automatically separated from their families and held in jail while they wait for their day in court.

The government is saying publicly that this is about cracking down on serious property offenders.

But a presumption in favour of pre-trial imprisonment also applies where a child has twice previously been convicted of things like attempted stealing or attempting to remove an object from a public place.

The Don Dale Youth Detention Centre is an old adult prison. The former Corrections Commissioner Ken Middlebrook described it as only fit for a bulldozer.

But instead of decommissioning the prison, it was filled with a growing number of children the NT government is choosing to lock up rather than support and rehabilitate.

This is a youth detention system where allegations of staff mistreatment and abuse of children have been rife and where

> *By sending more unsentenced kids to Don Dale, the government will be stubbornly and wastefully continuing down a failing and discredited path that will not help anyone*

staff training has been characterised as seriously inadequate in a review done by the former head of Long Bay prison (NSW).

Darwin barrister John Lawrence QC recently said: "The stories I'm getting you wouldn't believe in a modern-day society, the way they're treating these kids".

As you're probably aware, 95 per cent of the children who are locked up in the Northern Territory are Indigenous.

I recently heard it summed up like this: "Don Dale – you come out worse!" This was a line from one of the young Indigenous stars of a brilliant show about Katherine that is now touring the country.

By sending more unsentenced kids to Don Dale, the government will be stubbornly and wastefully continuing down a failing and discredited path that will not help anyone. Not the community that wants to see property crime reduced. And certainly not these children or their families and communities.

Victims of crime and those who are – legitimately – concerned about community safety are far better served by investing in services to support young people and their families, and programs to address the reasons why they are offending.

In other words, we need resources to go into better education and employment opportunities; family violence prevention; drug and alcohol services; and proper housing. We need to support Indigenous people and organisations to develop local solutions to the local issues they are best placed to understand.

Yet, the NT government is choosing not to fund youth services and programs to work with children and young people to give them every chance of success. As the NT News recently observed, this government allocated $1.2 million towards youth justice programs in 2016/17, down from the $2 million spent in 2015/16.

A three million dollar funding cut in 2012 forced the closure of a youth drop-in centre and the end of night-time activities run by local Aboriginal organisations in Alice Springs. As local, long-time youth worker Blair McFarland puts it "Now we've got kids on the street – go figure!"

While they cut services that give kids a safe, supportive space, a sense of purpose and hope for the future, the NT government is investing heavily in ensuring these children sink further into the quicksand that is the justice system.

Instead of investing in helping to pull them out of this quicksand, the government is planning to build a bigger sandpit.

In the recent budget, they allocated an extra $2.5 million to "meet demand" at the Don Dale Youth Detention Centre and $4.5 million in operational funding for the Territory's prisons to cater for "increased prisoner numbers."

When it comes to children and young people, the government is choosing to spend more and more on cramming them into prison. We know this sets kids up to fail and makes them more likely to offend in the future.

As an independent voice in the Legislative Assembly I ask that you stand up against this dangerous and counterproductive path.

It is time for us all to get smarter about preventing offending while ensuring children are not consigned to a life in prison by installments.

We should be giving every child every chance to fulfill their limitless potential.

Please don't support the changes to the Bail Act.

Yours sincerely,

Julian Cleary

Indigenous Rights Campaigner for Amnesty

Western Australia: wake up to yourself

| Author: | Summer May Finlay | Published: | August 05, 2015 |

Comments by the Chief Justice of Western Australia and **associated media reports** reveal a simplistic, unhelpful view of the complex factors contributing to the over-incarceration of Aboriginal people, according to public health practitioner Summer May Finlay.

Finlay suggests that, rather than perpetuating negative stereotypes of Aboriginal people, the WA Government and justice systems need to take stock of their own contributions to over-incarceration.

Summer May Finlay writes:

Comments **made** in Perth by the Chief Justice of Western Australia, Wayne Martin, at the Senate committee inquiry into Aboriginal and Torres Strait Islander experiences of law enforcement and justice systems, hurt Aboriginal people.

He stated that Aboriginal children intentionally commit crimes so they are incarcerated so they can have a safe place to sleep and get a good meal. He also said that Child Protection Officers were fearful of removing children because of the Stolen Generations. These comment have been used as headlines by some media outlets.

The comments effectively absolve Western Australia and the Chief Justice himself of any responsibility for the issues facing Aboriginal people in that State.

Without understanding the context of Aboriginal affairs in Western Australia, his comment implies that the responsibility for these children lies solely with parents. The comments continue to perpetuate the myth that all Aboriginal parents are neglectful at best and abusive at worst.

There is no doubt that parents have responsibility for their children but what also needs to be recognised – although this rarely happens – is the impact that past and current policies have on Aboriginal people.

Western Australia is a State that has the highest Aboriginal adult and juvenile incarceration rates. Aboriginal adults are **70% more likely** and Aboriginal children are **58 times more likely** to be incarcerated in Western Australia than in other states. This is the State that continued to remove children until the mid 1970s for no other reason then they were Aboriginal (**estimated up to 30%** between the early 1900s and 1970s).

It has been found that Aboriginal people are **74% more likely** to be reconvicted at any given time than those who receive a non-custodial penalty, yet Western Australia is less likely to divert Aboriginal juveniles than their **non-Aboriginal counterparts**.

There is evidence that out of home care has detrimental effects on Aboriginal children, due to lost connection to family, culture and country

In **2009**, a 12-year-old Aboriginal boy was charged with receiving stolen goods; a $.70 Freddo Frog. This is a State which in 2014 **tried to introduce laws** allowing the Minister to permit access to Aboriginal sites if he deems it appropriate regardless of what Traditional Owners wanted.

Western Australia **in 2014** reduced its education budget, cutting 110 Aboriginal and Islander Education Officer positions. This is a State which this year, despite the ongoing health disparity between Aboriginal people and other Australians, has halved its **Aboriginal health budget**.

This is a State which wanted to close Aboriginal communities because they are not considered financially viable, regardless of the connection people have to country. Western Australia has time and time again shown its lack of concern for the wellbeing of Aboriginal people – and then lays the blame for their own disadvantage at their feet.

Youth incarceration needs to be framed as a social issue that requires involvement from parents and the state for a successful solution. Diversionary programs, such as Justice Reinvestment, which is being **trialled in New South Wales** and considered in **South Australia**, need to be introduced and utilised. This would give young Aboriginal people options.

The Chief Justice also suggested that Child Protection officers were reluctant to remove Aboriginal children for fear of another Stolen Generation, implying more children need to be removed.

It is well documented that Aboriginal people are more likely to experience high levels of stress, racism, financial difficulties and higher rates of chronic disease. Where is the recognition that support is needed for Aboriginal parents who are finding life challenging? Or that early support and working with people will assist them to give their children a better start in life?

There is evidence that out of home care has detrimental effects on Aboriginal children, due to lost connection to family, culture and country. Research has **also shown** that children removed from their families were almost twice as likely to come in contact with the justice system.

Shouldn't we be considering early support programs for struggling families in an attempt to break the cycle of poverty and incarceration? With an estimated 30 per cent of children removed from their families in Western Australia, is it any wonder some people are struggling as parents?

Through its justice system, child protection laws, heritage act, budget cuts and proposed closures of Aboriginal communities, Western Australia has continued to marginalise and discriminate against Aboriginal people.

Rather than working with Aboriginal people on solutions to the issues they face, it seems the State would rather blame them. The State ignores the complex set of factors that are at play when a young person comes in contact with the court system. These factors vary from young person to young person.

Over-simplifying the issues does nothing to assist young people and their families. Western Australia needs to consider the role it plays in the continuing high levels of incarceration of Aboriginal young people.

The very fact that the comment was made and then seized on by the media continues to promote stereotypes of Aboriginal people, without considering the broader social issues at play. It continues to demonstrate Australia has a long way to go in developing healthy race relations.

People in position of power and the media who rely on stereotyping in their description of Aboriginal people do so much harm.

Rather than stereotyping, what we need is a mature debate about the issues and roles and responsibilities – not just of Aboriginal people, but also of our state and federal governments.

We need an approach to reducing incarceration which is holistic and considers all the factors including education, health, housing, country, Culture and early support programs.

I suggest that the Western Australian Government and the Chief Justice need to take stock of their own failings.

Maybe then real gains might be made to reduce incarceration rates of young people and we can see #JustJustice.

9. Health leadership

"Australia cannot claim to be a great nation until we address the underlying causes of the high rates of incarceration of Aboriginal and Torres Strait Islander peoples

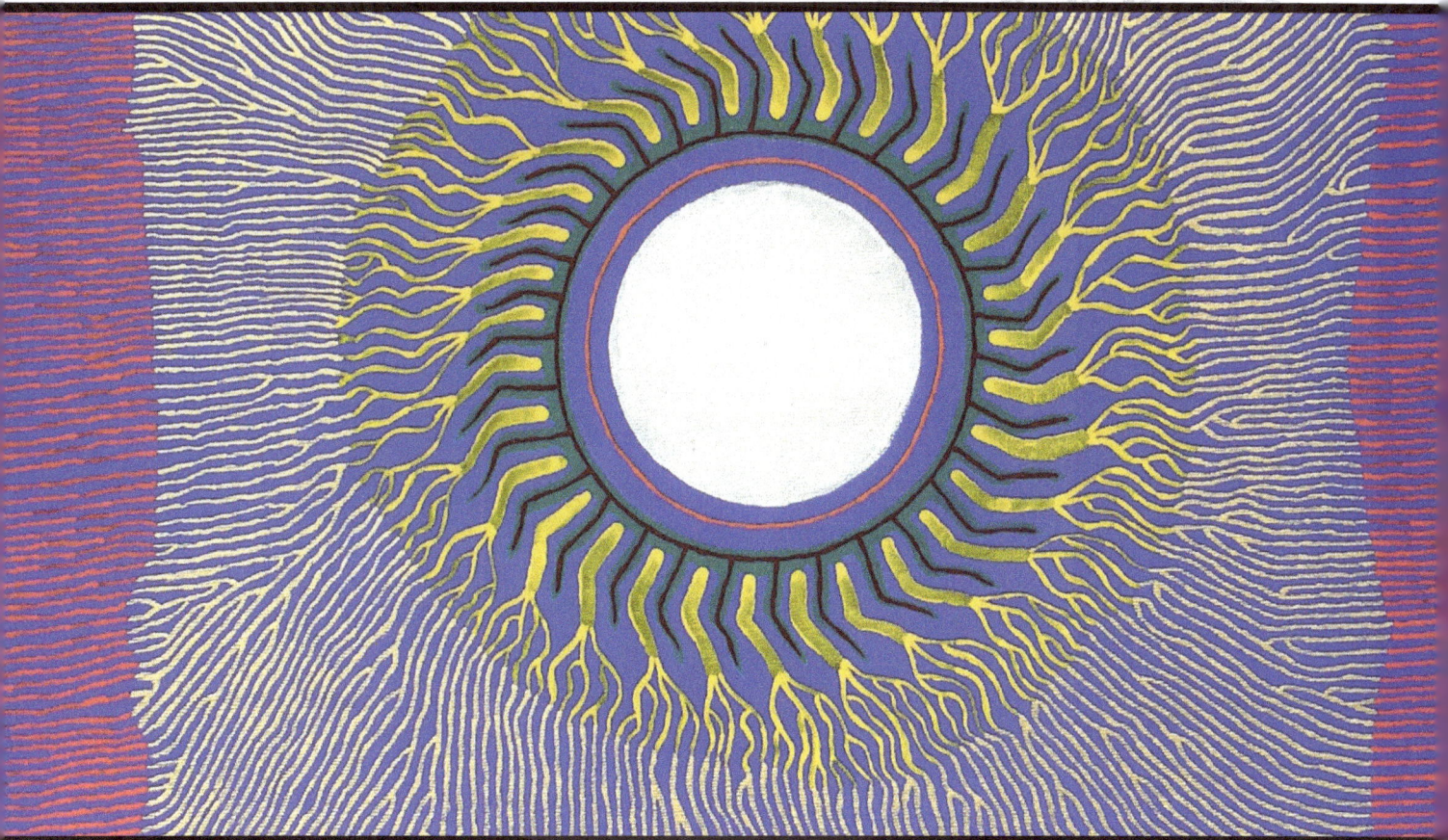

Health professionals urged to step up and advocate for therapeutic justice systems

| Author: | Wayne Applebee, Paul Collis and Holly Northam | Published: | September 13, 2016 |

Cultural interventions, mentoring programs and increased funding for Aboriginal and Torres Strait Islander legal and health services are some of the ways forward for tackling the over-incarceration of Aboriginal and Torres Strait Islander people.

These solutions were identified during recent #JustJustice broadcasts (watch the full clips below) with Dr Paul Collis, a Barkindji man, an author and academic at the University of Canberra, and Mr Wayne Applebee, an Elder and PhD researcher at the University.

The first interview was conducted before ABC TV's Four Corners program aired graphic footage of young people being abused at the Don Dale detention centre in the NT. A second interview – which also included a nursing and midwifery academic from the University of Canberra, Dr Holly Northam – was conducted after these revelations.

The interviews include a rousing call for the health sector and wider Australian institutions and organisations to stand up and advocate for an end to punitive law and order policies, and for action on the underlying determinants of incarceration.

In particular, alcohol and drug problems should be addressed as health concerns rather than as criminal justice issues.

Dr Collis and Mr Applebee have longstanding experience in justice issues, being involved in a circle sentencing court in the ACT, as well as developing an intervention program called Circuit Breaker. This aimed to provide mentoring to help develop prisoners' cultural connections and life skills, for example in self-care and managing budgets, in order to help break the cycle of incarceration (more information is available here – the program is not currently funded).

In the second interview, Dr Northam also critiques the use of spit-hoods on young people in detention, and calls for those who create and uphold systems that victimise young people to be held accountable. "We have a responsibility as a society for changing what's happening," she says.

Interview One

Dr Paul Collis describes the importance of cultural solutions; of finding ways for adults and children who are in prisons or detention to be supported in cultural programs and connections. Art therapy, including the telling of life stories, can help. More use should be made of artist cooperatives, which can provide income and a space for people to work, connect and participate. There should be more funding for men's and women's groups.

In gaols, people do not learn how to practise responsibility; it is taken away from them. Prisoners and released prisoners should have greater access to mentoring and cultural programs and on-country camps, as with Mt Theo program (see page 23 of this document for more information).

To keep governments accountable and ensure money is spent on prevention rather than prisons, non-Indigenous Australia has to engage more deeply with these concerns, and the wider media also needs to get more informed.

Mr Wayne Applebee discusses the importance of supporting people who have been institutionalised in the justice system to develop life skills for independent living, whether it's learning how to cook, or to use computers.

He calls for implementation of the recommendations of the Royal Commission into Aboriginal Deaths in Custody, and for proper funding of Aboriginal legal services which are currently massively under-funded. The situation is now so

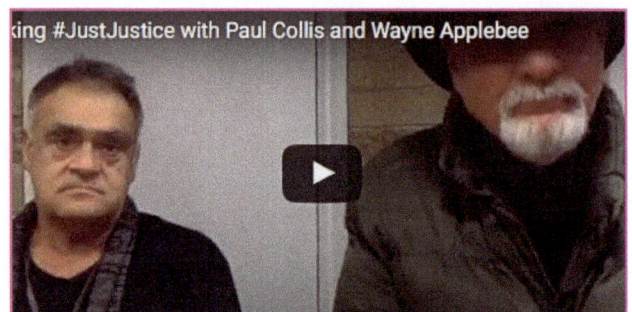

king #JustJustice with Paul Collis and Wayne Applebee

dire in many places that people virtually have to plead guilty to receive legal assistance.

Summary of Interview Two

Mr Wayne Applebee describes how the revelations of brutality towards young people in the Don Dale detention centre in the NT resonated with his own experiences in the Mount Penang Training School for Boys in NSW in the 1960s. He warns that violence begets violence, and says history shows that some of the young people detained in such violent institutions in the past went on to commit acts of violence themselves, after being brutalised in the system. He calls for those who inflict violence upon young people to be held accountable. He also recommends the implementation of Justice Reinvestment in the ACT, and says justice systems should be therapeutic, seeking to help rebuild peoples' lives and opportunities, rather than brutalising.

Dr Paul Collis, who has taught prisoners in a number of jails, says that jail is a very traumatic experience, particularly for young people. "You either survive or you don't," he says. He calls for far greater effort and investment in stopping recidivism and helping people to adapt to life outside institutions. "They learn to survive in the system but not to survive life, they don't learn decision-making, normality," he says. He is optimistic that the national outrage about the treatment of young people in the Don Dale facility suggests there has been a sea change in community attitudes since the Royal Commission into Aboriginal Deaths in Custody's recommendations 25 years ago. "The whole country has said, no we're not that kind of person... we want that stopped," he says. "We didn't have that when we had the Royal Commission into Black deaths."

Dr Holly Northam calls for a far greater focus on the health and wellbeing of young people caught up in juvenile justice systems, and says these systems should be underpinned by principles of restorative justice. She questions the use of spit-hoods in the justice system, given that health care systems manage the risk of patients spitting without having to resort to such devices. She calls for health professionals to step up in demanding changes to punitive systems that are currently victimising victims. "As a society they are our victims; we have to be accountable [that] they are in this situation because we have created the environment that has put them there," she says. "As a healthcare worker, I think we have to start taking responsibility. We can't blame the victims. We have to be accountable as a society for our children." Australia should learn from best practice in other countries and stop throwing money at ineffective, harmful systems of incarceration, she says.

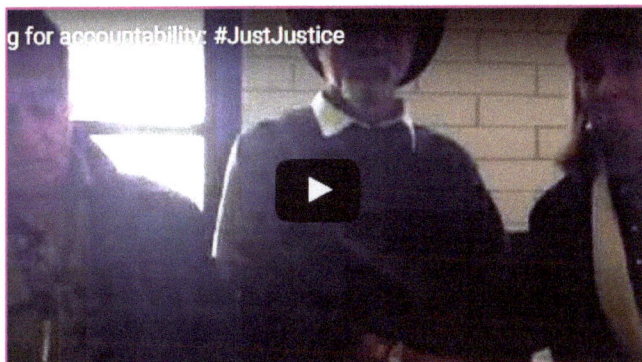

Public health leader calls for accountability in justice policies and politics

Author:	Michael Moore	Published:	April 12, 2016

Tackling the over-incarceration of Aboriginal and Torres Strait Islander people requires some significant behaviour changes from powerful interests, including politicians and policy makers, according to Michael Moore, CEO of the Public Health Association of Australia.

His comments are timely in the week marking the 25th anniversary of the Royal Commission into Aboriginal deaths in custody, when a significant editorial in The Age newspaper has called for State and Federal leaders to act on this "national emergency", and to peel back mandatory sentencing.

Michael Moore writes:

The disproportionate incarceration of Aboriginal and Torres Strait Islander people does not "just happen".

It is the predictable outcome of governments' policies. It is driven by decisions made at the political level, encouraged by a "them and us" attitude in the tabloid media and by the environment in which people grow.

Disproportionality in incarceration is driven, for example, by laws such as "three strikes and you're in" and other mandatory sentencing laws.

> *The disproportionate incarceration of Aboriginal and Torres Strait Islander people does not "just happen"*

These laws fly in the face of our democratic institutions by interfering with the separation of powers. Judges and magistrates lose the ability to take into account the circumstances in which criminal activity has taken place, the seriousness of the issue and the likelihood of re-offending.

Failure to recognise the social determinants of health and failure to respond effectively to the Royal Commission into Aboriginal Deaths in Custody has developed into a situation where even the Chief Justice of Western Australia, Wayne Martin, told a parliamentary committee in August 2015 that "young Aboriginal people consider jail a 'rite of passage'". It is an issue that Nyungar man, Associate Professor Ted Wilkes, has been warning about for some time.

According to the Australian Bureau of Statistics, whilst Aboriginal and Torres Strait Islander peoples make up two per cent of the Australian population, as of last year Aboriginal and Torres Strait Islander people accounted for 27% of the total prisoner population in Australia.

This equates to a rate of 2,235 per 100,000. Compare this to a rate of 146 per 100,000 for the non-Aboriginal and Torres Strait Islander population.

Calling for a better future for young people

Last year Amnesty International released a report calling for a 'Brighter Tomorrow' for young Aboriginal and Torres Strait Islander people. Currently these young people are 26 times more likely than their non- Aboriginal and Torres Strait Islander peers to be detained in a juvenile facility.

Sadly Australia is not alone in this. Canadian Aboriginal people face strikingly similar over-representation within the corrective system. Just over three per cent of the Canadian population is Aboriginal, yet Aboriginal people make up 24% of the prison population (provincial/territorial correctional services).

If things were on the improve, we would probably have been calling for them to improve even more quickly. Sadly, this is not the case. The incarceration rate of Aboriginal and Torres Strait Islander people continues to climb disproportionately.

Since 1989, at the time of the Royal Commission into Aboriginal Deaths in Custody, the imprisonment rate of Aboriginal and Torres Strait Islander people has increased 12 times faster than the rate for other Australians.

Our great shame

Indifference provides a key explanation of why there is a growing Indigenous incarceration rate in Australia and other parts of the world.

On one hand there is lip service – on the other there is appropriate action. We need more of the latter. There are people who commit serious crimes and are appropriately incarcerated. However, in many of the cases of imprisonment of Aboriginal and Torres Strait Islander people, it is for trivial offences.

Creative Spirits identifies many of the reasons for such high rates of imprisonment in Western Australia as unpaid fines, inability to make it to court or not receiving the court mail, unlicensed driving, disorderly conduct and provocation by police.

To our great shame, Australia now indefinitely incarcerates people who have committed no crime. This is an anathema to people who genuinely believe in human rights. Our treatment of refugees is appalling. However, we also have also other laws in place that are questionable in terms of human rights and are certainly questionable in terms of genuine democracy.

Mandatory detention laws cut judges out of the equation and effectively incarcerate people without a fair hearing, without taking the full range of circumstances in to account and fly in the face of the democratic concept of 'separation of powers'. They have a disproportionate impact on the more vulnerable members of our community. In Australia this is first and foremost Aboriginal and Torres Strait Islander people.

Within the last few years States and Territories have been increasingly willing to build on this sort of appallingly prejudicial legislation.

As Rosalea Nobile and Terry Hutchinson **write**, "in 2014 Queensland's conservative Liberal National Party government made a number of amendments to the Youth Justice Act 1992 (Qld) ('YJA'). Of critical importance is the new breach of bail offence (s 59A) and the reverse onus provision (s 59B). The effect of these changes was compounded by the removal of the sentencing principle of 'detention as a last resort'". The authors point to these laws cumulatively increasing the likelihood of young people becoming entrenched in the criminal justice system.

Law and order campaigns are regularly considered good politics. They rarely result in good policy. They have contributed to longer sentences, to mandatory sentencing, less ability to appeal and less tolerance with very little evidence of efficacy – particularly amongst the most vulnerable in our community.

Australia cannot claim to be a great nation until we address the underlying causes of the high rates of incarceration of Aboriginal and Torres Strait Islander peoples.

Michael Moore is CEO of the Public Health Association of Australia (PHAA), and President of the World Federation of Public Health Associations.

> *Mandatory detention laws cut judges out of the equation and effectively incarcerate people without a fair hearing, without taking the full range of circumstances in to account and fly in the face of the democratic concept of 'separation of powers'*

Calling for improved services in custodial and forensic systems

| Author: | Dayna Veraguth | Published: | February 03, 2016 |

The quality of care provided to Aboriginal and Torres Strait Islander people in custodial and forensic systems needs improving, according to Dayna Veraguth, a Diversional Therapist with extensive work experience in juvenile justice and hospital settings.

Below, she explains the rationale for a new resource that aims to help increase awareness of culturally safe and effective, evidence-based wellbeing programs in these settings.

You can download the resource at this website: *Challenge Yourself to Reduce Aboriginal incarceration*.

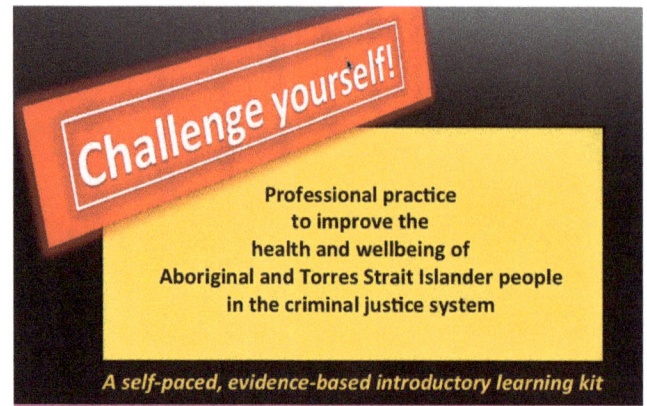

A resource to improve professional practice

Dayna Veraguth writes:

Health professionals working in custodial and forensic systems have a responsibility to improve the care they provide to Aboriginal and Torres Strait Islander people.

This will require a significant shift for many health professionals working within these systems, to ensure their practice is culturally safe and that their clients have access to effective, evidence-based programs.

It is also important that these staff become more familiar with Aboriginal and Torres Strait Islander concepts of healing and social and emotional wellbeing, so that these holistic approaches can be integrated within frontline services.

In particular, it is important to incorporate more cultural and spiritual elements into the daily lives of Aboriginal and Torres Strait Islander people in these settings.

As well, these settings also need to make conscious efforts to increase the employment and presence of Indigenous health workers.

In NSW, the Justice Health and Forensic Mental Health Network (JHFMHN) annual report, 'Year in Review 2013/14' makes clear that there is a desire at an organisational level for practice to reflect current policy and guiding frameworks.

The JHFMHN annual report outlines the strong partnerships that exist, and highlights the various services that are linked to Aboriginal Community Controlled Organisations, both upon a person being detained or admitted and upon release.

However, in my experience, Aboriginal and Torres Strait Islander people admitted to high secure acute wards have limited access to "high quality and culturally appropriate mental health services and supports", although the importance of this is recognised in the Council of Australian Governments (COAG) Roadmap for National Mental Health Reform.

Ensuring there are cultural connections for people who are held in such wards, often for long periods of time, even years, is important for improving their health and wellbeing.

Frontline clinicians can help drive change in program delivery, through being empowered themselves, through improving their attitudes and everyday practices with individual patients, the programs they deliver or the programs and issues for which they stand as advocates.

It is well known that there is a workforce shortage of Aboriginal and Torres Strait Islander health workers, while research shows that many non-Indigenous health workers feel overwhelmingly challenged when working with Aboriginal and Torres Strait Islander patients and their families (clustered into the following common themes, 'don't know how', 'too scared', 'too hard', and learning to practise regardless).

It is thus crucial that efforts are made to improve the competence of non-Indigenous health workers in these settings.

Challenge Yourself

I have developed a resource to help increase awareness of culturally safe and effective, evidence-based wellbeing programs specifically for Aboriginal and Torres Strait Islander people in custodial and forensic systems.

It is a self-paced, evidence-based learning kit, called 'Challenge Yourself' and is available at **this website**.

It is anticipated that this resource will enhance individual health workers' personal practice through self-reflective activities and increased cultural understanding.

It will help non-Aboriginal health workers to reflect on whether their clinical practice may in fact be a hindrance to social and emotional wellbeing through emphasising ill health. Or they may be diverting resources away from service provision and programs that have been proven to be effective for Aboriginal and Torres Strait Islander people.

We need to build up a community of health workers who are leading change collaboratively from the ground up, in line with policy.

Frontline health professionals are in an ideal position to scrutinise existing and proposed programs and enact change by advocating with Aboriginal and Torres Strait Islander people in line with what does work.

While most health professionals want to do the right thing by the patients in their care, as Dr Ernest Hunter highlights, **'good intentions' alone are not enough**.

The literature reflects that there is huge space for improvement in the current attitudes and views of non-Aboriginal health workers towards issues of health equity, including but not limited to eliminating racism and understanding the strength of Indigenous culture and self determination.

Also needed are culturally appropriate rehabilitation programs as well as the need for an increase in connections to culture through the local community and increased links to patient's own communities.

I would also like to acknowledge **'Respecting the Difference'**, an Aboriginal cultural awareness training framework.

This training was to have been completed by all staff by the end of 2015 as part of the 'Good Health Great Jobs – NSW Health Aboriginal Workforce Strategic Framework 2011-2015'.

While it is unlikely that all staff have completed it and the policy is set for review late in 2016, the training is well-designed. It is comprised of a two-hour online course and a one-day face-to-face training and is extremely valuable.

Dayna Veraguth is a Diversional Therapist with extensive work experience in juvenile justice and hospital settings. This is an edited version of a paper she submitted as a UNSW Master of Forensic Mental Health student.

Many thanks to Dr Megan Williams, a Senior Research Fellow with the Muru Marri Collaboration in the Centre for Health Research at Western Sydney University, for facilitating this publication, and to Dayna for sharing the resource with Croakey readers.

Calling for answers to these five questions about critical justice gaps for Indigenous LGBQTI people

| Author: | Dameyon Bonson | Published: | May 19, 2016 |

At the United Nations Permanent Forum on Indigenous Issues in New York this week, human rights and public health advocate Dameyon Bonson has been drawing attention to a lack of data and research into the prevention of suicide for Indigenous LGBQTI people (lesbian, gay, bisexual, transgender, queer and intersex).

Similar concerns were also raised at the inaugural Aboriginal and Torres Strait Islander Suicide Prevention Conference, held recently in Alice Springs, as reported by The Guardian.

In the article below, Bonson highlights critical data gaps surrounding the incarceration of Indigenous LGBTQI people, providing a useful briefing for policy makers and funders.

Dameyon Bonson writes:

As the #JustJustice series is showing, we know many of the solutions to reducing the over-incarceration of Aboriginal and Torres Strait Islander people; the gaps are in creating the political and policy will to make this happen.

In one area, however, the gaps are far more fundamental.

When it comes to Indigenous LGBTQI people, very little is known about our interactions with policing and justice systems. We know even less about how policing and justice systems are responding to our particular needs.

However, the answers to these do need to be informed by a yet to be determined, central cultural capability mandate that takes into account one's gender, sexuality and their identification as an Aboriginal and/or Torres Strait Islander.

The reason for this is two-fold. Historically we know that Aboriginal and/or Torres Strait Islander people receive an unjust experience in the justice system (see both the coronial inquiry into Ms Dhu and the Royal Commission into Aboriginal Deaths in Custody).

When we look abroad, Indigenous LGBTQI people, in this case Native Americans, experience even more prejudice and discrimination than their heterosexual counterparts and LGBQTI people of any other racial/ethnic backgrounds.

The important nature of this is the high risk of suicide and self-harm this places on the inmate, and to the susceptibility to hate crimes; of a phobic nature and racial.

Transgender inmates are particularly vulnerable, suggest recent newspaper reports in Australia and New Zealand. However, it is noted that 'inmates who are known or perceived as gay, especially lesbians and gay men with stereotypically effeminate or butch characteristics, face "a very high risk of sexual abuse."'

Given that the #JustJustice series is providing a briefing paper to politicians, policymakers and others with the power to help reduce the over-incarceration of Aboriginal and Torres Strait Islander people, below are the five questions I'd like to see answered.

1. Reliable data about the incarceration of Aboriginal and/or Torres Strait Islander LGBQTI people.

I believe that nobody should be forced to disclose their sexuality upon incarceration; however, if indeed this is self-identified, this information must only be used to protect the individual. Like other at risk groups in prison, this information would strengthen a request to be placed in a more protective area. This may simply be a tick of a box or a written answer.

2. Reliable data about the crimes experienced or committed by Aboriginal and/or Torres Strait Islander LGBQTI people.

Reliable data about crimes against and committed by Aboriginal and/or Torres Strait Islander LGBQTI people would ensure a far greater picture of the level of criminality affecting this group of people. Questions could be asked about: a) the type of crime committed by an Aboriginal and/or Torres Strait Islander LGBQTI person; or b) a crime has been committed against an Aboriginal and/or Torres Strait Islander LGBQTI person.

3. What types of services are needed for Aboriginal and/or Torres Strait Islander LGBQTI people interacting with police and justice systems?

The first step would see the Custody Notification Service informed of the type of issues and experiences faced by Aboriginal and/or Torres Strait Islander LGBQTI people and their needs around safety. Ideally, this would be Aboriginal and/or Torres Strait Islander LGBQTI; however, a fact sheet is a great start. It could explain what the escalated risks are and the appropriate support. It is my view that a third party organisation could also provide this culturally capable support.

4. What is the impact of policing and justice on the health of Aboriginal and/or Torres Strait Islander LGBQTI people? What is the relationship between contact with policing and justice systems, and suicide for Aboriginal and/or Torres Strait Islander LGBQTI people?

Without the raw data, we can only go on anecdotes and media reports. The highest profile case of a transgendered Indigenous Australian is that of Veronica Baxter. Ms Baxter, despite living her life as a woman, was placed in a men's prison. Her death, after a coronial inquiry, was determined to be due to suicide.

The Gender Centre in NSW does highlight the Management of Transgender Inmates. However, how this management is applied appears to be discretionary. A friend who is a Sistergirl told me of an Aboriginal and/or Torres Strait Islander transwoman, also a Sistergirl, who was recently was murdered in the NT. Her trans* identity was not recorded. This raises questions about whether the murder was a hate crime.

5. How can policing and justice systems be made culturally secure for Aboriginal and/or Torres Strait Islander LGBQTI people?

The information needs to be decided upon, by Aboriginal and/or Torres Strait Islander LGBQTI people, on what is culturally capable within the policing and justice systems. Until then, there is the risk of guesswork and more harm than good being done.

I hope that a national Aboriginal and Torres Strait Islander LGBQTI conference will be held next year. I am working on this, and it is anticipated that such a gathering will provide a framework for the health and wellbeing of Aboriginal and Torres Strait Islander LGBQTI people, including those within the justice system.

Dameyon Bonson is the founder of Black Rainbow Living Well, a self-determining non-profit movement dedicated to creating more than hope for Aboriginal and Torres Strait Islander people who are diverse in gender and sexuality. Amongst other things, Black Rainbow advocates for the human rights of Aboriginal and Torres Strait Islander LGBQTI people in the criminal justice system, and to address gaps in the services available to them. It aims to work alongside Aboriginal and Torres Strait Islander LGBQTI people in prison in determining the best way to fulfil this role. Dameyon lives in Broome, WA.

Forget Vegemite-based policy. Here are some sensible recommendations for reducing alcohol-related harms

Author: The Hon Sharman Stone MP   **Published:** August 10, 2015

Indigenous Affairs Minister Nigel Scullion's foray into Vegemite-based policy has won global headlines for a suggestion that the product should be restricted in some remote communities to stop moonshine production – even Time Australia inhaled.

But the weight of opinion – including from public health experts, police, and scientists – seems to suggest the recommendation should be, uhm, toast…

Public health expert **Dr John Boffa** has raised the potential for the media splash to do harm, by stereotyping

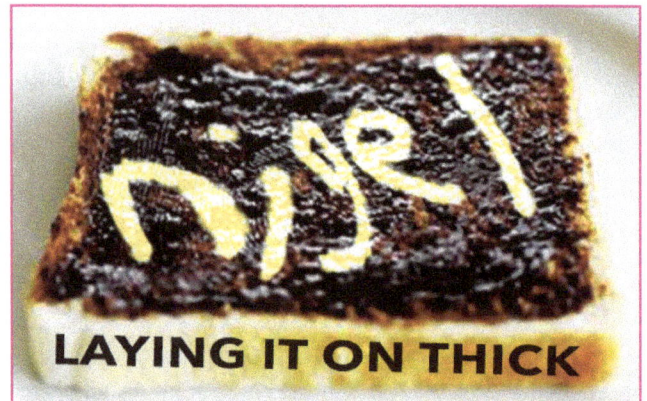

LAYING IT ON THICK

Aboriginal people, encouraging people to experiment with Vegemite, and by undermining effective, community-led strategies to reduce alcohol-related harms. He told radio this morning: "Some stories aren't worth telling."

Strangely enough, there hasn't been anywhere near this level of media attention for a recent House of Representatives Standing Committee on Indigenous Affairs report that made a raft of sensible recommendations for addressing alcohol-related harms.

Croakey thanks **Dr Sharman Stone**, who chaired the Inquiry into the harmful use of alcohol in Aboriginal and Torres Strait Islander communities, "Alcohol, hurting people and harming communities", for permission to cross-post her introduction to the report, as part of the #JustJustice series.

Below her article are the report's recommendations – for anyone interested in actual policy, and particularly in reducing the over-incarceration of Aboriginal and Torres Strait Islander people.

The Hon Dr Sharman Stone MP writes:

The consumption of alcohol at high risk levels is a national issue, however, the focus of this inquiry is the harmful use of alcohol in Aboriginal and Torres Strait Islander communities.

Many reports and studies have recommended stemming the flow of alcohol to address the problems, but usually these works do not analyse why a person drinks at levels which cause them and their loved ones harm. The social and economic determinants of harmful alcohol use such as unemployment, poor housing, racism, trauma, poor education and peer pressure mean that Aboriginal and Torres Strait Islander communities are overly impacted by the harm caused by alcohol consumed at high levels.

A recent Amnesty reports note that it costs $440,000 per year to keep one young person in detention in Australia. This report recommends that justice reinvestment strategies should redirect these resources to overcoming

the deprivation and despair in so many Aboriginal and Torres Strait Islander communities.

This report addresses strategies and treatments found to help in addressing the harmful use of alcohol. Community led solutions are always the key to uptake and success. Unfortunately slow government processes, for example approving community produced alcohol management plans and the short length of project funding, often frustrates community initiatives.

The magnitude of the problem caused by high risk consumption of alcohol is often hidden by the lack of collection of useful data for example at the time of hospital admissions, when children are put into out of home care because of their neglect, when people are incarcerated because of alcohol related crime and when children are born with Fetal Alcohol Syndrome (FAS) or Fetal Alcohol

Spectrum Disorder (FASD) at some of the highest rates in the world.

The committee found examples of the world's best practice at places like Groote Eylandt and Fitzroy Crossing. These communities, led by women's initiatives, have demonstrated courage and determination to tackle alcohol harm to provide a safe environment for their families and community. The committee commends them and hopes that their strategies can be used as examples of a way forward for other communities.

FASD or FAS is creating generations of children whose brain damage will reduce their potential to live lives full of promise and well-being. The rates of FAS and FASD in some Aboriginal and Torres Strait Islander communities in Australia are amongst the highest in the world and yet FAS and FASD are not recognised as a disability for many social security allowances and payments.

The lack of knowledge about, and recognition of FASD and FAS extends beyond the failure to have it officially recognised for social security and NDIS purposes, it also needs to be understood in schools, the criminal justice system and in the health sector.

The committee found that impacts of alcohol on children in communities represents a national tragedy as it is manifested in children growing up with fathers, and increasingly mothers, who are incarcerated, as the children's abuse and neglect leads to the need for out of home care at record levels, missed schooling and too often ultimately become young alcohol addicts or abusers of other illicit substances.

This committee urges adoption of these recommendations as a matter of urgency given the extent of harm and intergenerational afflictions when alcohol is consumed at such high risk levels.

Social and economic determinants of harmful alcohol use

Recommendation 1

That the Commonwealth Government, states and territories, at the late 2015 Council of Australian Governments (COAG) meeting, place harmful impacts of alcohol on the agenda for coordinated action. This should:

- formally recognise the social and economic determinants of harmful uses of alcohol namely poverty, mental health, unemployment, an ongoing sense of grief and loss, alienation, boredom, cultural acceptance of drunkenness, ease of access and cost of alcohol, peer pressure 'to drink' and epigenetics in some Aboriginal and Torres Strait Islander communities and for some individuals

- ensure that within each specific target of Closing the Gap in Indigenous Disadvantage, the impact of alcohol is recognised in all strategies and targets including addressing the social and economic determinants of high risk drinking, and

- develop a framework, methodology and resource allocation for the collection and publication of a national standardised wholesale alcohol sales dataset. The framework and relevant agreements should be in place by December 2015 with comprehensive data available no later than February 2017.

Recommendation 2

That all strategies developed or funded by the Commonwealth or other governments are developed in partnership with the relevant Aboriginal and Torres Strait Islander peoples and/or their organisations.

Health and alcohol-related harm

Recommendation 3

That the Commonwealth develops a public awareness campaign, highlighting the risks of alcohol consumption, focussing on:

- where to find help to reduce harmful drinking

- where to find help to reduce alcohol related violence, and

- providing information on other diseases associated with risky drinking.

The campaign should have sections targeted for populations in the criminal justice system and the education system.

Best practice strategies to minimise alcohol misuse and alcohol-related harm

Recommendation 4

That the committee recommends:

- the introduction of a national minimum floor price on alcohol, and

- prompt consideration be given to the recommendations of the Henry Tax Review on volumetric tax.

Recommendation 5

That the states and territories conduct detailed analysis of any demand increase for liquor licences particularly in areas of high risk drinking, with a view to moving towards a risk-based licencing system similar to that of New South Wales.

Recommendation 6

That the Commonwealth takes steps to ensure a nationally consistent and coordinated approach to alcohol advertising, including:

- Banning alcohol advertising during times and in forms of the media which may influence children

- Banning alcohol sponsorship of sporting teams and sporting events, including but not limited to those in which children participate or may be involved, and

- That the Australian Communication and Media Authority change the Commercial Television Code of Practice to ensure that alcohol is not able to be advertised before

8.30pm and that no exemptions are given for alcohol promotion during sport broadcasting.

Recommendation 7
That governments at all levels:

- prioritise Aboriginal and Torres Strait Islander community driven strategies to reduce the harmful effects of alcohol

- ensure that communities are empowered to develop the strategies that will work for their communities, and

- cooperate and facilitate any work in Aboriginal and Torres Strait Islander communities which aims to change the liquor trading hours in their community.

Community Alcohol Management Plans and other community driven strategies need to be reviewed and processed within a maximum of a six month period, including where any alterations are recommended.

The current backlog of Community Alcohol Management Plans in the Department of Prime Minister and Cabinet need to be cleared by January 2016.

Recommendation 8
That the Northern Territory Government re-introduce the Banned Drinker's Register and set up a comprehensive data collection and evaluation program which monitors criminal justice, hospital and health data.

Best practice alcohol abuse treatments and support

Recommendation 9
That the Commonwealth re-establish the National Indigenous Drug and Alcohol Committee.

Recommendation 10
That the Commonwealth develop a protocol for the recording and sharing of effective, evidence-based practices in Aboriginal and Torres Strait Islander communities, in particular such practices that have relevance to Aboriginal and Torres Strait Islander communities. This protocol should be available by December 2016.

Recommendation 11
That where the Commonwealth funds Aboriginal and Torres Strait Islander alcohol treatment and support programs, these are funded over a longer cycle for at least four years, particularly for well-established and successful programs.

Recommendation 12
That the Commonwealth and key Aboriginal and Torres Strait Islander groups ensure access to training and career pathways for alcohol treatment and support workers. The employment conditions should be fair and equitable.

Recommendation 13
That the Department of the Prime Minster and Cabinet ensure that a full range of evidence-based, best practice treatments are available in order to meet the needs of all Aboriginal and Torres Strait Islander people, regardless of where they live. The treatment services should provide for families, follow-up services, and include detoxification and rehabilitation.

Prevention Strategies

Recommendation 14
That Commonwealth, states and territories, through the COAG process implement justice reinvestment to reduce the number of Aboriginal and Torres Strait Islander people incarcerated as a result of harmful alcohol use.

Recommendation 15
That the Northern Territory Government prioritise the resourcing of voluntary alcohol treatment and rehabilitation programs in place of the Alcohol Mandatory Treatment program.

FAS and FASD

Recommendation 16
That the Commonwealth, as a matter of urgency, increase its efforts to ensure that consistent messages:

- about the risks of consuming any alcohol during pregnancy, and

- about the importance of supporting women to abstain from alcohol when planning pregnancy, when pregnant or breastfeeding to reduce the risk of Fetal Alcohol Syndrome and Fetal Alcohol Spectrum Disorder are provided to the whole community.

Recommendation 17
That the Commonwealth, as a priority, ensure that the National FASD Diagnostic Tool and accompanying resource are released without any further delays.

Recommendation 18
That states' and territories' teacher training, education and in-service systems provide:

- information and education on alcohol and drug exposed children's behaviour, and

- details of the impact on the child's mental health and their achievement at school.

Recommendation 19
That the Commonwealth:

- include FAS and FASD as recognised disabilities for Carer's allowance to allow fast–tracking of the application

- include FAS and FASD as a recognised disabilities in the Better Start for Children with a Disability initiative, and

- include FASD in the operational Guidelines for the National Disability Insurance Agency.

Recommendation 20

That the Commonwealth, in consultation with the FASD Technical Network, include in the appropriate table in the Social Security Tables for the Assessment of Work-related Impairment for Disability Support Pension Determination 2011:

- A person with Fetal Alcohol Spectrum Disorder who does not have an IQ below 80 should be assessed under this Table.

Recommendation 21

That the Commonwealth, in consultation with the FASD Technical Network, and relevant organisations from the criminal justice system system:

- develop a model definition for cognitive impairment, and

- conduct a review of Commonwealth law and policy to identify where eligibility criteria need to change to ensure that people with FAS and FASD and other cognitive impairments can be included.

Determining patterns of supply and demand

Recommendation 22

That the Australian Institute of Health and Welfare review and update the methodology and instrument of the National Drug Household Survey to obtain reliable estimates on Aboriginal and Torres Strait Islander and non-Indigenous illicit drug and alcohol use. These changes should be implemented for the conduct of the 2017 survey.

Recommendation 23

That the Australian Bureau of Statistics conducts a review of the relevant sections of the National Aboriginal and Torres Strait Islander Social Survey and the National Aboriginal and Torres Strait Islander Health Survey to ensure international best practice is adopted in the instrument and conduct of surveys on alcohol consumption.

Dr Sharman Stone is a former Federal MP. She was chair of the House of Representatives Standing Committee on Indigenous Affairs committee at the time this article was published.

AMA joins calls for Closing the Gap justice target, and justice reinvestment approach

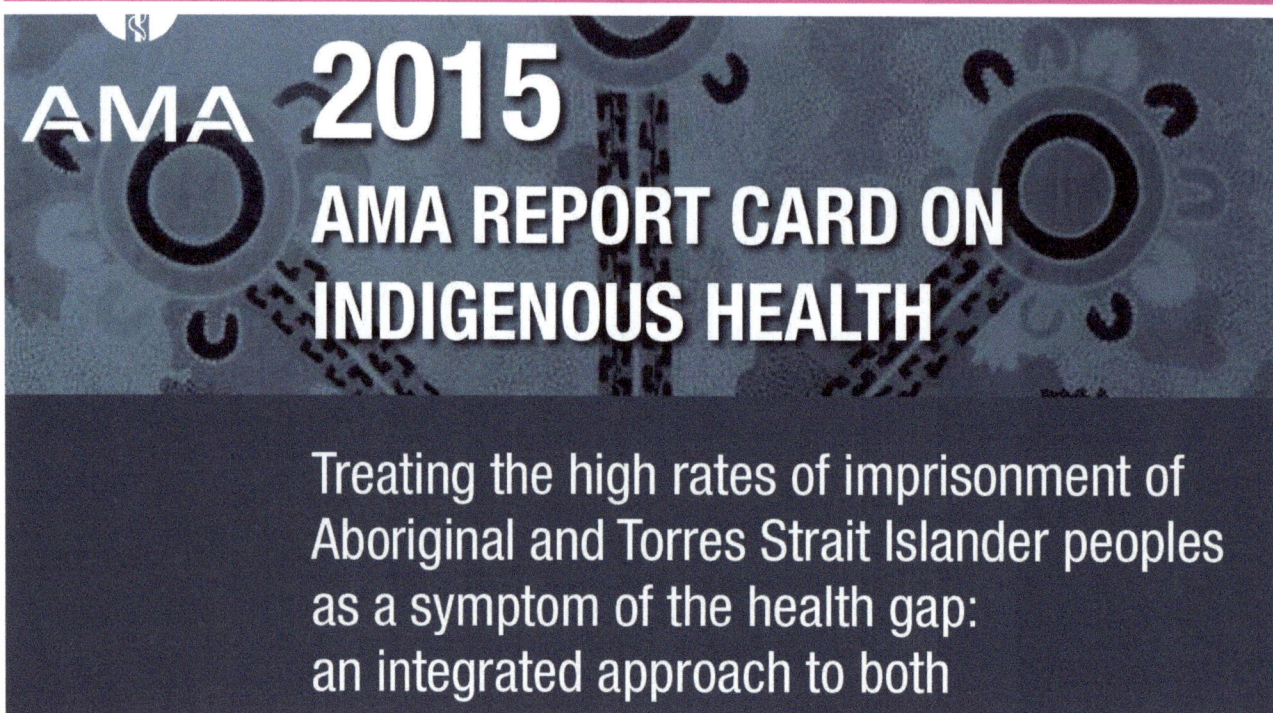

AMA 2015
AMA REPORT CARD ON INDIGENOUS HEALTH

Treating the high rates of imprisonment of Aboriginal and Torres Strait Islander peoples as a symptom of the health gap: an integrated approach to both

| Author: | Marie McInerney | Published: | November 25, 2015 |

Marie McInerney writes:

The **Australian Medical Association** joined growing calls on all Australian governments to commit to setting a target for closing the gap in the rates of Aboriginal and Torres Strait Islander imprisonment.

The call comes in the AMA's **2015 Report Card on Indigenous Health**, which sees a clear link in the poorer health and justice outcomes experienced by Aboriginal and Torres Strait Islander people in Australia, and stresses the need to invest in Aboriginal community controlled health organisations and an Aboriginal and Torres Strait Islander workforce. It says:

"It is not credible to suggest that Australia, one of the world's wealthiest nations, cannot solve a health and justice crisis affecting three per cent of its citizens."

The AMA call follows the recent promise that a **Shorten Labor Government** would support justice targets, justice reinvestment and other measures to "close the justice gap" and address the over-incarceration of Aboriginal and Torres Strait Islander people.

It also comes as a Western Australian **coronial inquiry** is hearing distressing details about the death in custody last year of Ms Dhu, the 22 year old Aboriginal woman held at the South Hedland police station for unpaid fines. See this **tribute** from Labor Senator Sue Lines.

Excerpts from the AMA 2015 Report Card on Indigenous Health

The AMA cites latest estimates that Aboriginal and Torres Strait Islander people will live around 10 years less than non Aboriginal and Torres Strait Islander people, and evidence that the imprisonment rate of Aboriginal and Torres Strait Islander peoples is 13 times greater than non Aboriginal and Torres Strait Islander peers. It says:

" *Among the divides between Aboriginal and Torres Strait Islander peoples and non-Indigenous people in Australia, the health and life expectancy gap and the stark difference in the rates of imprisonment are among the most well-known.*

This Report Card treats the two gaps as connected. While acknowledging the complex drivers of imprisonment in any individual's case, it considers the 'imprisonment gap' as symptomatic of the health gap. In particular, the AMA believes it is possible to isolate particular health issues (mental health conditions, alcohol and other drug use, substance abuse disorders, and cognitive disabilities are the focus of this report card) as among the most significant drivers of the imprisonment of Aboriginal and Torres Strait Islander peoples, and target them as health issues as a part of an integrated approach to also reduce imprisonment rates.

Further, this Report Card examines how the situation is compounded by a health system and prison health system that, despite significant improvements over past decades, remains – in many critical areas – unable to respond appropriately to the needs of Aboriginal and Torres Strait Islander prisoners.

The Report Card says the year 2016 marks two anniversaries that make its findings and recommendations timely:

- the 25th anniversary of the Royal Commission into Aboriginal Deaths in Custody (RCIADIC)

- the 10th anniversary of the 2006 AMA Indigenous Health Report Card, Undue Punishment? Aboriginal and Torres Strait Islander People in Prison: An Unacceptable Reality.

It calls for a national target for 'closing the gap' in the rates of imprisonment of Aboriginal and Torres Strait Islander peoples, arguing the case in the context of the Australian Government's Indigenous Affairs priorities (employment, school attendance and community safety) and controversial Indigenous Advancement Strategy.

" *A prison record, after all, can be a major barrier to employment. Families with members in prison are put under tremendous financial and emotional stress with the major impact being felt by children – potentially affecting school attendance and performance. Further, inherent in reducing imprisonment rates is reducing violent offending by Aboriginal and Torres Strait Islander people, and thereby making communities safer. As noted, acts of violence are*

the most common reason for the imprisonment of Aboriginal and Torres Strait Islander people, at double the rate of their non-Indigenous peers. And fellow Aboriginal and Torres Strait Islander people are all too often the victims.

It notes the growing movement in Australia advocating for justice reinvestment, including by the Just Reinvest NSW campaign and Change the Record and in the call for a trial from the Senate Legal and Constitutional Affairs Committeee in 2013.

" *The AMA supports this call, but would like to see a greater commitment to justice investment principles being used to fund early intervention and diversion efforts, particularly for people with mental health problems, substance use disorders, and cognitive disabilities, in Aboriginal and Torres Strait Islander communities.*

It recommends that governments adopt an integrated approach to reducing imprisonment rates and improving health through much closer integration of Aboriginal Community Controlled Health Organisations (ACCHOs), other services and prison health services across the pre-custodial, custodial and post-custodial cycle, and says key elements of this approach would be:

- a focus on health issues associated with increased risk of contact with the criminal justice system and imprisonment. In particular, mental health conditions, alcohol and drug use, substance abuse disorders and cognitive disabilities;

- service models that incorporate both health care and diversionary practices. These models would be developed by ACCHOs working in partnership with Australian governments and prison health services. Such would define the roles, and integrate the work of, ACCHOs, other services and prison health services to provide the integrated approach;

- preventing criminalisation and recidivism. The former, by detecting individuals with health issues that can put them at risk of imprisonment while in the community and working with them to treat those issues and prevent potential offending; and

- continuity of care. That is, (a) from community to prison – with a particular focus on successfully managing release. And (b) post-release (from prison to community) – with a focus on successful reintegration of a former prisoner into the community and avoiding recidivism. Important elements of continuity of care include access to health records, and individual case management as available.

It says a critical part of this approach is likely to involve:

- expanding the capacity of ACCHOs and other services as required to establish and/or build on existing interdisciplinary mental health and social and emotional wellbeing teams that can work effectively with or coordinate health care for people at risk of imprisonment while in the community and work to divert them from potential contact with the criminal justice system;

- ensuring that these interdisciplinary mental health and social and emotional wellbeing teams are connected to, or include, culturally competent professionals to work effectively with mental health disorders, substance abuse disorders, and cognitive disabilities; and

- supporting prison health services to be able to deliver a culturally safe and competent service including by employing greater numbers of Aboriginal Health Workers and Indigenous health professionals, and working in partnership with ACCHOs or other services.

" *Because Aboriginal and Torres Strait Islander peoples tend to come into contact with the criminal justice system at younger ages than their non-Indigenous peers, a major focus of this integrated approach is on the health, wellbeing, and diversion from the criminal justice system of Aboriginal and Torres Strait Islander children and adolescents. Culturally-based approaches have been identified as effective in working with this cohort in areas like suicide prevention.*

The AMA anticipates that the integrated approach it is recommending would incorporate access to Elders and cultural healers as a core component.

It says the recommendations further develop the AMA's **2012 Position Statement on the Health and Criminal Justice System** that states Aboriginal and Torres Strait Islander peoples should 'have full access in prison to culturally safe primary health care, including management of chronic illness, social and emotional wellbeing, mental health, and drug and alcohol problems', that their culture are 'respected in the design and provision of health and medical care in prisons and juvenile detention facilities'; and that Aboriginal and Torres Strait Islander prisoners have access … 'to community elders and to relevant representatives of their communities to address their cultural beliefs and needs'.

" *It is the AMA's hope that this Report Card will help build momentum for a national integrated approach to reducing both the Aboriginal and Torres Strait Islander health and imprisonment gaps – one that understands both as aspects of each other. Such an approach is aligned with the integrated, whole of life, and holistic approaches that Aboriginal and Torres Strait Islander peoples have long called for as responses to both.*

It is not credible to suggest that Australia, one of the world's wealthiest nations, cannot solve a health and justice crisis affecting three per cent of its citizens.

The high rates of health problems among, and the imprisonment of, Aboriginal and Torres Strait Islander peoples should be a priority social justice and human rights issue in this context.

The AMA Indigenous Health Report Card 2015 is available here.

To tackle hepatitis C, we need to close the justice gap

Author:	Heather McCormack	Published:	December 22, 2015

Health Minister Sussan Ley's **announcement** of PBS listing for new treatments for hepatitis C has been **welcomed** by Hepatitis NSW as "brilliant news".

Given the high rates of hepatitis C among people in prisons, it is significant that the Government has agreed to fund these medicines for prisoners.

However, tackling hepatitis C will also require public health interventions such as the introduction of needle and syringe programs into correctional centres, and concerted efforts to reduce the over-representation of Aboriginal and Torres Strait Islander people in prisons, according to Heather McCormack from Hepatitis NSW.

Heather McCormack writes:

Throughout the #JustJustice series, we've read about the ways over-incarceration affects the health of Aboriginal and Torres Strait Islander people. Reducing over-incarceration is a positive goal in and of itself. Disproportionate incarceration of Aboriginal and Torres Strait Islander people is unjust to the individuals who are victimised by this discrimination and it is unjust to our broader Indigenous communities.

However, over-incarceration also has significant impacts on a range of life indicators, including education, employment and health. The work we do at Hepatitis NSW emphasises a clear nexus between over-incarceration and Indigenous health: the devastating impact of hepatitis C on people who have spent time in prison.

Hepatitis C disproportionately affects Aboriginal and Torres Strait Islander people, who are over-represented both as people who inject drugs and people who have experienced incarceration.

The rates of hepatitis C diagnosis in Aboriginal and Torres Strait Islander communities are alarming.

The rate of new diagnoses of hepatitis C in the Aboriginal community is between two and ten times higher than in the non-Indigenous community, depending on your location (Resnick & Brener, 2010).

They're also on the rise, while the non-Indigenous community experiences a downward trend. Aboriginal and Torres Strait Islander people make up 2.4% of Australia's population, but we're estimated to make up 8.3% of people in Australia who are living with hepatitis C (McNally & Latham, 2009).

Several studies have estimated hepatitis C prevalence for people in custody at between 34% and 47%. For women experiencing incarceration, it's even higher: between 50% and 70%. This is many, many times higher than the rate of hepatitis C in the general community, which is estimated to be around 1%.

The over-representation of Aboriginal and Torres Strait Islander people in prison settings places members of our community at much higher risk of contracting hepatitis C in prison.

The prison environment is almost perfect for hepatitis C transmission: there is high prevalence of the virus in the incarcerated community and high rates of injecting drug use. Both of these factors are a product of laws that criminalise drug use.

Harm reduction programs lacking

Our current system fills prisons with people who inject drugs, but fails to provide either adequate harm reduction programs for people to use drugs safely or sufficient support for incarcerated people to reduce their drug use. The risks of contracting hepatitis C in a prison environment are so great that imprisonment is an independent risk factor for hepatitis C transmission.

The single most important factor in the prevalence and transmission rates of hepatitis C in Australian prisons is the absence of needle and syringe programs (NSP) in correctional centres.

> *The single most important factor in the prevalence and transmission rates of hepatitis C in Australian prisons is the absence of needle and syringe programs (NSP) in correctional centres*

Despite decades of advocacy for prison NSP by communities affected by hepatitis C and the organisations that support those communities, it has not been implemented anywhere in Australia.

The region to come closest (the Australian Capital Territory) has so far failed to deliver on its promises of prison NSP, primarily due to resistance from prison unions. This is despite evidence from overseas confirming prison NSPs to be safe and effective in reducing transmission of blood borne viruses in people in prison.

Introduction of prison NSP would be the most effective measure possible to prevent transmission of hepatitis C in prison environments.

However, reducing the transmission of hepatitis C among people experiencing incarceration – and in the Aboriginal and Torres Strait Islander populations who are over-represented among them – will take more than prison NSP. We also need to expand access to opiate substitution therapy (OST) in prison.

OST is known to have a measurable impact on hepatitis C transmission rates, but it is obviously most effective if people entering prison have immediate access to it.

While NSW has policies in place to support access to OST for people in custody, we are also aware of some people reporting being denied, or having delayed access to, OST. These delays and restrictions may not have been experienced if they were not in custody. In some other jurisdictions, there is limited OST access for prisoners – or it may even be completely absent.

Other vital measures to reduce transmission of hepatitis C in prison environments include better education about the virus and how it is transmitted, including upskilling peer educators among the incarcerated community.

We need to ensure that FINCOL (the hospital grade disinfectant that is provided to prisoners in NSW) is consistently and easily accessible for people in prison. We need to provide safe tattooing and piercing programs to discourage sharing of tattoo guns and piercing needles.

Widespread treatment of hepatitis C with new direct acting antiviral (DAA) therapies will be a game-changer for incidence and prevalence in prison environments. There are current trials of these new treatments in four NSW prisons as part of the SToP-C pilot.

However, even with a rapid scale-up of DAA treatment for people living with hepatitis C in prison environments, the lack of comprehensive harm reduction measures in prisons,

Other vital measures to reduce transmission of hepatitis C in prison environments include better education about the virus and how it is transmitted

including NSPs, to prevent reinfection will still present a challenge.

All of these steps are important to reducing the rates of hepatitis C in prison environments and hence reducing the impact that hepatitis C has on the health gap for Aboriginal and Torres Strait Islander people.

Beyond band-aids

But it's difficult to argue for the resources to implement them in a system that is arguably underfunded and continually at risk of further cuts.

It's also, in a sense, applying band-aids after the cut has been made: the simple way to lower disproportionate rates of hepatitis C transmission in Aboriginal and Torres Strait Islander people affected by the criminal justice system is to reduce incarceration rates.

Rates of imprisonment in NSW have been rising in recent years – in some demographics, such as female prisoners, Aboriginal and Torres Strait Islanders make up almost all of the increase. There is little sign of a reduction in Aboriginal and Torres Strait Islander over-incarceration occurring anytime soon.

While the range of measures outlined above are key to reducing hepatitis C diagnoses in Aboriginal and Torres Strait Islander people, closing the health gap with regards to hepatitis C also requires closing the justice gap.

Reducing the over-representation of Aboriginal and Torres Strait Islander people in the hepatitis C epidemic necessitates reducing the over-representation of Aboriginal and Torres Strait Islander people in our prisons first.

Heather McCormack is Project Officer – Information & Communications at Hepatitis NSW.

The Hepatitis Infoline 1800 803 990

10. Addressing racism

" *Those of us who benefit from white privilege need to do the most to change unfair systems*

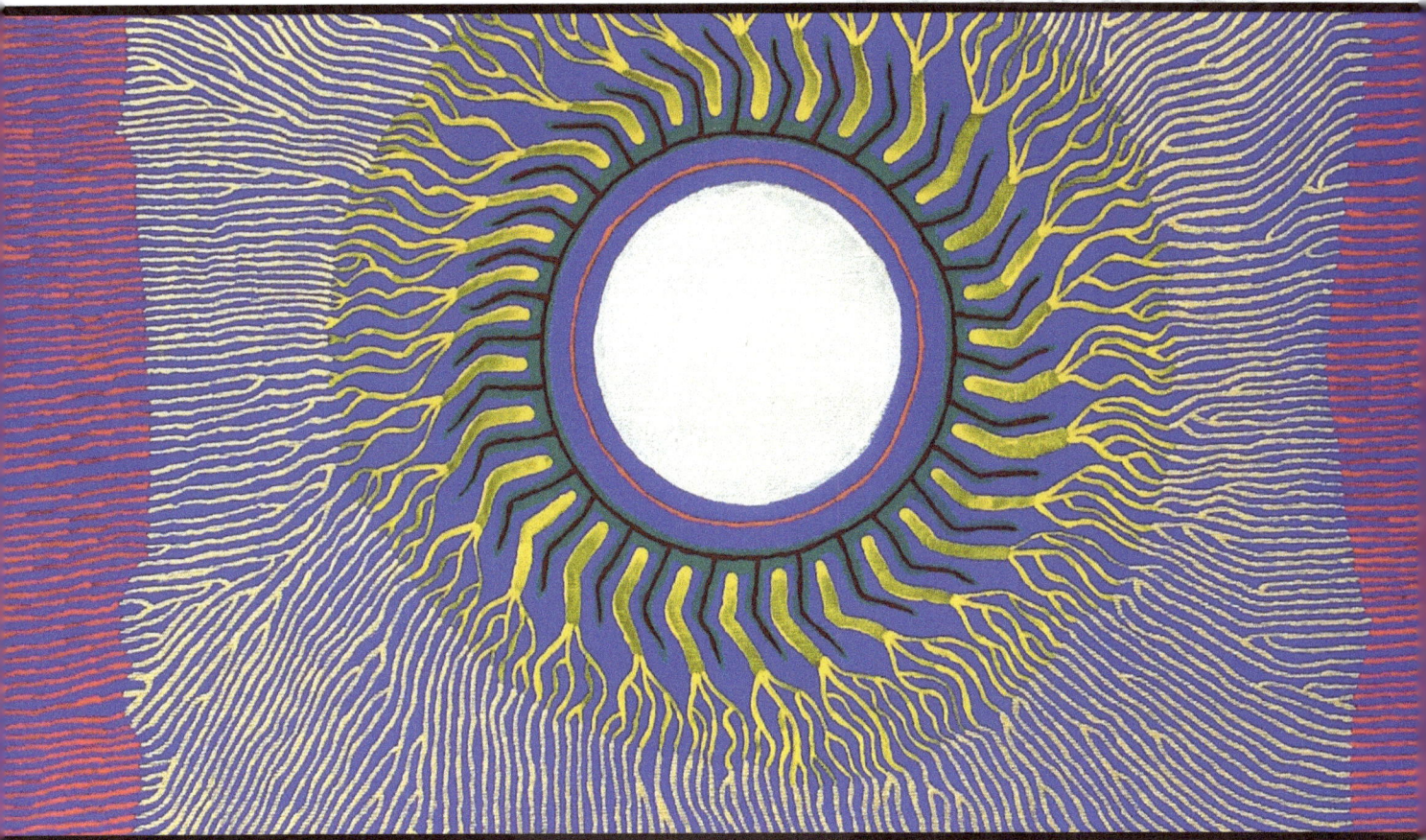

"As a nation, we should be unified in an unwavering commitment to stop Aboriginal deaths in custody"

Author:	Eddie Cubillo	Published:	June 22, 2015

Many of the celebrations of the **800th anniversary of the Magna Carta** as a symbol of liberty and freedom ring very hollow for Aboriginal and Torres Strait Islander people.

However, **one recent conference** examining the Magna Carta legacy did acknowledge the "justice gap", describing the increasing incarceration rate of Aboriginal and Torres Strait Islander peoples as "*one of the most significant social problems anywhere in the developed world*".

The article below is an edited version of a presentation to the **National Access to Justice and Pro Bono conference** by Eddie Cubillo, executive officer of the National Aboriginal & Torres Strait Islander Legal Service (NATSILS).

He gave many examples of how and why the justice system is failing Aboriginal and Torres Strait Islander people. Tragically, just a few days after this speech was delivered, a 40-year-old Aboriginal man **died in custody** in the NT – the second such death there in less than a month.

Meanwhile, the #savetheCNS campaign continues to preserve the **life-saving Custody Notification Service**. How many health professionals are lending their weight to this campaign?

The Magna Carta: what does it mean for Aboriginal and Torres Strait Islander peoples?

Eddie Cubillo writes:

The Magna Carta speaks to us from Medieval England, acknowledging, in writing, that no-one in society is above the law: not the King nor his subjects, not the government nor the governed.

As an affirmation that authority should be subject to law arising from the community itself, Magna Carta is a foundation stone of constitutional and parliamentary government.

However, it is clear that the principles of the Magna Carta are not inclusive of Indigenous Australians.

Below I explore two issues – the Racial Discrimination Act (RDA) and the criminal justice system – and show that equality and fairness before the law remains a problem in this country for Indigenous Australians.

The RDA

The RDA has been suspended on three occasions: to amend the Native Title Act 1993 which removed existing guarantees of rights to Indigenous people; when enacting the Hindmarsh Island Bridge Act 1997; and the Northern Territory National Emergency Response (also referred to as 'the Intervention').

Since the Intervention, discrimination has been felt in a number of ways, perhaps most starkly when Aboriginal people access basic services such as in shops, or otherwise are subject to measures that apply only to them and demonise them as alcoholics or paedophiles.

Consider what our older people would have thought when they saw the convoy of army vehicles rolling in. One comment I heard was that 'this isn't a country at war'. Not surprisingly, people in remote locations did not understand why the military was in their communities. (Many of our elderly people had experienced the bombing of the Top End).

The most humiliating was the signs that were erected outside of our communities. As well, they were subject to the confusion of income management, which in time they found required them to line up, in separate queues in supermarkets, to use a basics card. This brought back old and painful memories of segregation.

The **Kartinyeri case** decided that the Australian Constitution authorises the Commonwealth to pass racially discriminatory legislation.

Suspending the Race Discrimination Act under s51 (xxvi) – to allow the 'Intervention' took the retrograde step of suspending essential anti-discrimination laws in this country and included laws and policies that discriminate against people who are Aboriginal because they are Aboriginal.

This legitimised the views of those who believe that it is OK to treat people differently because of their race.

The ability of the government to act discriminatorily against Aboriginal and Torres Strait Islander under constitutional powers is an affront to the rule of law and the right of all to be treated equally under the law.

Discrimination continues to be felt across a number of other key areas from land rights under native title to criminal justice.

Criminal justice system failings

It is clear that the criminal justice system continues to fail Aboriginal and Torres Strait Islander people, with increasingly dire consequences, as shown by the fact there has been an 88% increase in the number of Aboriginal and Torres Strait Islander people imprisoned between 2004 and 2014.

Discrimination remains a significant issue both in the law and its application. Particular areas of concern include the paperless arrest laws in the NT and mandatory sentencing laws.

Paperless arrests

The Northern Territory's "paperless arrest" laws, introduced late last year, give police the power to lock someone up for four hours for minor offences like making undue noise; swearing in public; or keeping a front yard untidy.

A person locked up under these powers has no effective opportunity to challenge their detention or to ask a court to release them. The police essentially act as both judge and jury

A person locked up under these powers has no effective opportunity to challenge their detention or to ask a court to release them. The police essentially act as both judge and jury.

The Northern Territory's Attorney General said that the new paperless arrest laws make it simpler for police to "catch and release people".

Police have a tough job and every reasonable effort should be made to make their job easier, but efficiency is not the be-all and end-all and it is argued that the law is in conflict with the principle that no person should be deprived of their liberty arbitrarily.

It is clear that the laws are having a disproportionate impact on Aboriginal and Torres Strait Islander people. Of the 700 times that the law was used in the first three months of its operation, more than 75 per cent of those affected have been Aboriginal.

Recently a respected Aboriginal elder passed away whilst in police custody. He had been arrested and detained under a paperless arrest. He died the most inhuman of deaths: without family around, on a cold, concrete floor of a police cell.

As a nation, we should be unified in an unwavering commitment to stop Aboriginal deaths in custody. All governments' laws, policies and practices should support, rather than undermine this end.

This law, which is in flagrant disregard for the rule of law, must be repealed to ensure further tragedies do not occur.

Mandatory sentencing

This eliminates the judiciary's ability to consider appropriate mitigating factors so as to arrive at the most appropriate sentencing outcome; is an arbitrary contravention of the principles of proportionality and necessity; and has a discriminatory effect on Aboriginal and Torres Strait Islander offenders.

According to the Western Australian Department of Justice's Review of the three-strikes laws, over 81% of juveniles sentenced under the laws were Aboriginal.

From 2000 to 2005 approximately 87% of all children sentenced under the mandatory sentencing laws were Aboriginal.

Other issues of concern include:

Overpolicing – For example, police targeting of Aboriginal and Torres Strait Islander people for behaviour in public spaces and/or minor offending; many of Aboriginal and Torres Strait Islander Legal Services (ATSILS) clients occupy public spaces in a more visible way than non-Indigenous people, due to high rates of homelessness and overcrowding.

Bail – An increasingly rigid approach to bail which has had a particularly discriminatory effect on Aboriginal and Torres Strait Islander young people, causing an increase in the number of Aboriginal and Torres Strait Islander young people on remand.

The unnecessary imprisonment of Aboriginal and Torres Strait Islander peoples in regional and remote areas due to a lack of appropriate bail addresses; this is particularly concerning in relation to juveniles.

Fines enforcement – The system of fines enforcement in Western Australia, which is skewed against persons who are disadvantaged and vulnerable.

None of this is to deride the idea of the rule of law and its traditions – it is to say that it has not been applied equally to Aboriginal and Torres Strait Islander people, from the loss of our lands that precedes our current imprisonment rates, to current racially discriminatory laws.

In conclusion

The Magna Carta continues as a symbol of liberty and freedom today. While this affirmation of fundamental freedoms is important, it should also be noted that the Magna Carta and its legacy are problematic.

It can too easily be seen as providing affirmation of this country's past and traditions, while ignoring that the rights and freedoms it contains have certainly not applied equally to all.

The law has been complicit in some of the worst atrocities committed against Aboriginal and Torres Strait Islander people and continuing today. We cannot let the fine spirit and principles of this document be used to ignore this past.

There won't be a single bullet that cures all areas of disadvantage faced by Aboriginal and Torres Strait Islander people, but real constitutional reform would have important symbolic significance to ensure that our foundational document removes the racist elements that still pervade our Aboriginal and Torres Strait Islander people and their communities.

Eddie Cubillo, Executive Officer of the National Aboriginal & Torres Strait Islander Legal Service (NATSILS). On Twitter, follow @Bulgul11

Calling for national action on discriminatory, unfair laws and systems

Author:	Darren Parker	Published:	August 24, 2015

In an earlier article, Darren Parker, a Ngunawal man and PhD candidate at Melbourne Law School, wrote about experiencing racism and violence within his family as a young boy (see page 44).

The article highlighted the importance of the social and cultural determinants of health in any discussion about the over-incarceration of Aboriginal and Torres Strait Islander people.

In the detailed analysis below, he reflects upon his own journey into studying and critiquing the law, and asks: *Is it possible to decolonise Australian law so that Aboriginal and Torres Strait Islander people can attain justice?*

Parker argues that over-representation of Aboriginal and Torres Strait Islander people in the justice system is a national crisis, requiring urgent leadership from all governments that is informed by Aboriginal and Torres Strait Islander peoples' expertise.

Darren Parker writes:

It has always struck me as fascinating how we end up where we do. The factors that play out in our life: those we have no control over, as well as those we do – or at least believe we do. As Douglas Adams stated, "I may not have gone where I intended to go, but I think I ended up where I needed to be."

The two major professions I have pursued in my life (qualified chef and legal academic – and yes, I did it in that order, which seems 'against trend' nowadays) are linked back to my experiences growing up. It is only now, at this point in my life, that I am able to stand back and somewhat appreciate that view.

But if anyone is thinking that this is some type of "well you had to go through what you did to get to where you are...." treatise, you are incorrect. Let me make this absolutely clear, no person should ever experience or be subjected to the horrors of family violence. Ever. I have no idea whether I would have ended up where I am regardless of my family history, because that opportunity was taken from me due to family violence.

However, what I can say is that whilst those horrific experiences were taking place, as mentioned previously, my Mother was a constant touchstone of strength. I don't view her as a victim of family violence, but see her as she is: a powerful Ngunawal woman who commands self-respect, equitable treatment and self-education as cornerstones in her demands for the best of herself and others.

The two professions I have pursued relate to, but are not a direct result of, the circumstances surrounding my experiences in family violence. As a child, helping Mum with the cooking provided me with somewhat of an escape. Later, formal commercial cookery provided something I was desperate for in my early teens and that was, to get away.

On completing my apprenticeship I worked as a chef nationally and internationally, and it exposed me to the delights of foreign foods, peoples and cultures. It was particularly rewarding when meeting and working with other Indigenous people from around the globe because, apart from working in hospitality, we shared many commonalities regarding the 'legal' inequitable treatment of Indigenous people in our respective home nations. Our solidarity crystallised in many of these exchanges.

Over the years and through meetings and discussions like this, my legal curiosity was tweaked more and more.

I recall, however, the first time my interest in the law found its voice. It was during another violent assault by my father against all of us in the family. When the police were called during this particular rampage, they took so long to arrive that there was enough time for my father to methodically assault each of us again.

I remember the attending officers casually walking towards the front door. When I voiced my disgust at their lack of urgency, I was pushed aside and told, "nobody is dead" – I was eight at the time. Then to watch the officers approach my father as if he was an old friend, and hear them being apologetic that they were even attending. Even more galling was watching them walk him out to the paddy wagon *uncuffed* and explaining to him how would be "out" in a matter of hours.

The police didn't ever appear to be concerned by my father's return home after a few hours in the cells, more often without even being charged and usually even more enraged.

Out of experiences like this, I developed a deep revulsion of the police. They never appeared to be in a rush to arrive, nor interested, whenever they were called to our place.

We were known as "blacks" and it was "just a domestic", both expressions I heard the attending police say on more than one occasion – an example of indirect institutional racism, as I was to understand later. But, it wasn't just the actors within the legal system that were demonstrably lacking, it was the system itself, as Mum and I were to discover soon enough.

When I was ten years old and my Mother divorced him, I started learning – experiencing – just how slanted the legal system was. As part of the divorce, the court imposed 'alternate weekends' on me to be spent with him (recognising that the Family Law Act 1975 (Cth) has changed regarding *best interests of the child* since then). I loathed the court and the legal system for forcing me into that situation, of being in his 'care' on alternate weekends. Wretchedly, it was my Mother who had to deal with the repercussions of those visits.

As a child, it didn't occur to me that the legal system's set against a strong, decent hard-working Aboriginal mother as opposed to a white male violent-drunkard with a criminal history was an example of structural sexism. It would be quite some time before ss **60B(3)**; **60CC(6)**; and **61F** of the Family Law Act 1975 (Cth) would be amended to incorporate legal regards for Aboriginal and Torres Strait Islander children. At the time, my mother lived in a state of hyper-vigilance. I won't speak more on this because that is my Mother's story to tell if she wishes.

Experiences like these, among others, prompted me after 15 years as a chef to go back to school and study law. Yet, as I have told many people and students throughout the years, being born an Indigenous person in Australia makes you a legal and political person regardless – so my interest in these areas has always been there.

However, before you think otherwise, I did not study law to wrestle in the heartache that is family law. Neither was it my desire to evangelise or prosecute within the criminal law. It was never my intention to study law for the pure sake of practising it – though I did for a time. No, I wanted to research it – I wanted to teach it.

Moreover, I wanted to research and teach in public law, that is, the person vis-à-vis the State. The reason for my choice was straightforward; studying and also knowing about an unjust system did not allow me to be ad hoc or piecemeal in my approach to law. I wanted to examine, critique and evaluate the law's supra-structure, particularly how the legal system itself, in many direct and indirect ways, is set against Aboriginal and Torres Strait Islander peoples in Australia.

It is for these reasons I have chosen this course of study. Public law provides me with an enormous scope to peer into various areas of the law and reveal its deficiencies, as well as its myopia with regard to Aboriginal and Torres Strait Islander peoples. Public law also goes to the heart of the jurisprudence undergirding the Australian legal system and allows for the exploration, examination and critique of its Eurocentric legal philosophies and practices.

Racist foundation document

The formative political and legal document of Australia – the **Australian Constitution** – is a document more predicated upon a marriage of the former colonies for trade and commerce purposes and for purposes of racial exclusion than it is as 'a people's constitution'. The Constitution was drafted at two conventions held in the 1890s, and neither convention included any women, nor any Indigenous representatives or ethnic communities. Each convention was solely stocked with white land-owning males.

Without going into a drawn-out legal exegesis on the Constitution, its **racist origins are well known**. Suffice to say that the **preamble** sets out the history preceding enactment, and that enactment of the Constitution was supported by 'the people' of the colonies.

The Constitution is silent on Indigenous peoples prior occupation. Whereas the operative provisions within the Constitution – at that time: ss 25; 51(xxvi); 127 – were based upon Aboriginal and Torres Strait Islander peoples' exclusion and discrimination, as they were not considered citizens, thus not a part of 'the people', constitutionally. This was the legal foundation upon which Aboriginal people were part of the Commonwealth of Australia on 1 January 1901.

Given that discrimination and exclusion were the foundations for Aboriginal and Torres Strait Islander peoples in the nation's founding document, it is unsurprising that laws flowing from it are still tainted with much of its origins, as Australian law acts as an agent for colonisation.

This is despite the **best intentions** of the **1967 referendum**. Laws in this country still discriminate against Aboriginal and Torres Strait Islander peoples. Therefore, the question must be asked: *Is it possible to decolonise Australian law so that Aboriginal and Torres Strait Islander people can attain justice?*

Without wrestling with the metaphysics of 'what is justice?' the following addresses the more immediate realities with regard to Aboriginal and Torres Strait Islander people's contemporary treatment in the Australian legal system.

Further, if it is possible to decolonise laws in Australia, what structures and processes are required to achieve such ends?

Unequivocally, discriminatory laws in Australia must be removed from current statutes and decolonising law needs to be understood as legislatively incorporating: listening and responding to Indigenous voices and knowledge; implementing culturally safe systems; and allowing for the retention of community control justice programs. In the sphere of Indigenous incarceration rates and over-representation in the justice system, it is **about changing the record**.

Importantly, discriminatory laws must not be understood as simply being laws encapsulating overt racism such as segregated missions, hospitals, swimming pools, cinemas or exclusion from town halls and other public buildings – all of which, and more, occurred in Australia.

Discriminatory laws take on more multifarious forms than those laws that are obviously racially directed. That is, the Australian legal system discriminates both directly and indirectly against Aboriginal and Torres Strait Islander peoples, as outlined further below.

Overt discrimination

Firstly, lets view some directly discriminatory laws. Below are some screen shots of both the Northern Territory Emergency Response, as well as the Stronger Futures legislative packages that encapsulate the Northern Territory intervention. Both legislative packages, implemented by two different federal governments, were in response to the Little Children are Sacred report.

What is patently noticeable is that despite the rhetoric around 'child protection', the legislation actually is directed towards something else (as the images published at Croakey show, a search for mention of 'child' in the legislation finds zero mentions, whereas a search on 'land' finds 900 mentions). Of note is that both federal governments were able to implement these laws due to the power granted from s51(xxvi) as a result of the 1967 referendum.

Also see Croakey for screenshots showing 10 mentions of 'child' were found in the legislation, and 494 of 'land').

Note: The implementation as a 'special measure' and the suspension of the Racial Discrimination Act.

(Searches of the legislation found 84 mentions of 'child' and 50 of 'land').

Now, the 'Stronger Futures legislative package (with one mention of child), as can be seen at Croakey.

Note: The intended purpose or 'object' of the 'Stronger Futures' package.

The legislative effects of both of these packages are very telling. Moreover, it is easily viewed how each package is expressly directed towards Indigenous people. How both packages have been legally implemented has been in no small part due to the amended scope of the power contained within s51(xxvi). Particularly, whether the power allows for the federal government to implement laws that are detrimental to Indigenous people in Australia.

That is, due to the 1967 referendum removing the exclusion of Aboriginal people from s51(xxvi) and thus granting federal governments the power to legislate regarding Indigenous people. It was a matter of legal interpretation as to whether the power covered the implementation of laws that could be understood as detrimental.

The High Court ruled in the Hindmarsh Island Bridge case, though the court was split 2:2:2 on the scope of the 'race

power' (2 justices did not address the scope of the power) that the power granted under the 'race power' were plenary. Meaning, that government could implement laws either beneficial or detrimental under the power of s51(xxvi).

The legislative effect of the ruling has been that a federal government is able to implement racially discriminatory laws under s51(xxvi) through clear and unambiguous legislation – such as the packages above and the direct references to suspension of the Racial Discrimination Act. Of note, it was also stated by the High Court in the Hindmarsh Island Bridge case, that a law implemented under s51(xxvi) by its nature is discriminatory.

However, if a constitutional amendment were to be implemented to continue to make laws regarding Indigenous people, as suggested by the insertion of s51A, such an amendment, if implemented, may provide that laws passed under such an amendment provide protection against discrimination based upon race. However, it may not provide protection for Indigenous people against laws passed under other parts of the Constitution such as the 'Territories Power in s122.

This means that without a general ban against racial discrimination, as suggested through the insertion of s116A, then discriminatory laws – such as the ones above – may still be passed through other parts of the Constitution, like s122.

Nonetheless, whilst ameliorating directly discriminatory laws can largely be addressed in the manner suggest above, such implementation does not touch upon indirectly discriminatory laws.

Indirect discrimination

I now move onto examples of indirect discrimination in law against Aboriginal and Torres Strait Islander peoples. Again, I use a Northern Territory example initially, before then moving onto the States.

The recent enactment of legislation in the Northern Territory that allows for the paperless arrest of people committing minor offences and the mandatory alcohol treatment scheme have already had a disproportionate effect upon Indigenous people in the Territory.

Wretchedly, it has already resulted in a death in custody and a death in care. Two people that are now gone from this earth due to indirect discriminatory laws and a lack of care that can only be classed as institutionalised violence.

Both of these laws allow for people to be detained without a court process and without legal representation and as can be seen, with devastating results. It is possible that both have breach guaranteed common law rights.

The paperless arrest laws are being challenged in the High Court on the grounds that they lack judicial oversight and places too much power in the hands of police. The NT Coroner has recently called for the paperless arrest laws to be repealed,

warning that they will result in more Aboriginal deaths in custody.

Notwithstanding the laws' constitutional validity, or otherwise, these laws can be repealed today without prolonged judicial deliberation. Both of these laws can be expunged from the statute books through the use of s122 of the Constitution.

As mentioned above, s122 of the Constitution provides the Commonwealth with the power to override territory laws at any time. As the federal parliament did in 1997 when it passed the **Euthanasia Laws Act 1997 (Cth)** which made euthanasia illegal in the territory after a territory law allowed terminally ill patients to decide when to die. So, it is a matter of the political will that is lacking in not repealing both of these indirectly discriminatory territory laws.

This situation is made all the more perverse by the well-known **Royal Commission into Aboriginal Deaths in Custody** ('RCIADC') and its **339 recommendations**. A number of these expressly relate to the need for the decriminalisation of public-intoxication and most importantly, for arrest to be "the sanction of last resort in dealing with offenders".

It is abhorrent that both the imprisonment rates and Aboriginal and Torres Strait Islander deaths in custody have continued to rise, particularly, as the recommendations have remained largely unimplemented.

Now to move onto the States where s122 has no effect. What is there to reduce the ever-growing Indigenous incarceration and over-representation of Indigenous people in the justice system?

Setting aside proposed constitutional amendments for the time, what is required is the implementation of justice targets at an integrated national level, as well as the introduction of statutory justice reinvestment.

It is beyond doubt that State levels of **incarceration** of Aboriginal and Torres Strait Islander people have increased at alarming rates since the findings from the RCIADC were handed down.

Equally beyond doubt is that the Federal and State governments are well aware of these repugnant statistics. Moreover, the need for justice targets aimed at ending the unacceptably high imprisonment rates of Indigenous Australians has also been discussed for **years now**.

Yet, there is still no inclusion of justice reforms as a distinct building block in the Council of Australian Governments ('COAG') framework for the **National Indigenous Reform Agreement** ('Closing the Gap').

This must be rectified immediately, otherwise the statistics will continue on their **detestable upward trajectory**. It has even been acknowledged that a coordinated **whole-of-government approach** is required to ameliorate the deleterious effects Aboriginal and Torres Strait Islander people suffer when in contact with the justice system.

A national crisis: action needed

The over-representation of Aboriginal and Torres Strait Islander people in the justice system is a national crisis, requiring urgent leadership from all governments. And that leadership must be informed through Aboriginal and Torres Strait Islander people's legal and cultural competencies.

Furthermore, with positive initial trials recently being conducted into Indigenous youth justice reinvestment in **NSW** and **South Australia**, it is time for COAG to implement national justice targets and justice reinvestment plans.

Doing so will undoubtedly reduce the current over-representation of Aboriginal and Torres Strait Islander people in the justice system.

It will also allow for justice policies and practices to be informed by principles of self-determination and by the involvement and empowerment of Aboriginal and Torres Strait Islander people at all levels of the system.

"Why aren't I in prison?" … Some questions about white privilege

Author:	Tim Senior	Published:	August 19, 2015

Public health concerns like white privilege and racism were on the agenda at the **Leaders in Indigenous Medical Education Network** conference in Townsville (see more details in **this previous post**).

These are also critical issues to address in efforts to reduce the over-incarceration of Aboriginal and Torres Strait Islander people.

In his contribution to the #JustJustice project, GP Dr Tim Senior investigates white privilege and how it contributes to unfair systems.

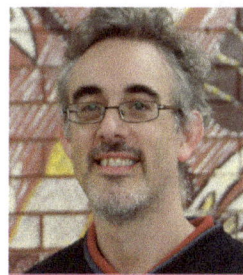

Dr Tim Senior

White privilege: a barrier to #JustJustice

Dr Tim Senior writes:

Why aren't I in prison? To be sure, I haven't committed a crime (unless you count stealing a comb from a newsagents when I was two, which my mum made me take back).

I have been fined for speeding once – and driving offences are **just the sort of thing that can end up with people being put in jail**. Perhaps I should think of that as a narrow escape?

The fact that I *don't* consider this a narrow escape says something about the answer as to why I am not in jail.

Sit down, though. The answer to my question might make you uncomfortable.

The principle reason that I am not in jail, is that I am white. There. I said it.

Why have I come to this conclusion?

Look at the imprisonment rates for Indigenous and non-Indigenous Australians.

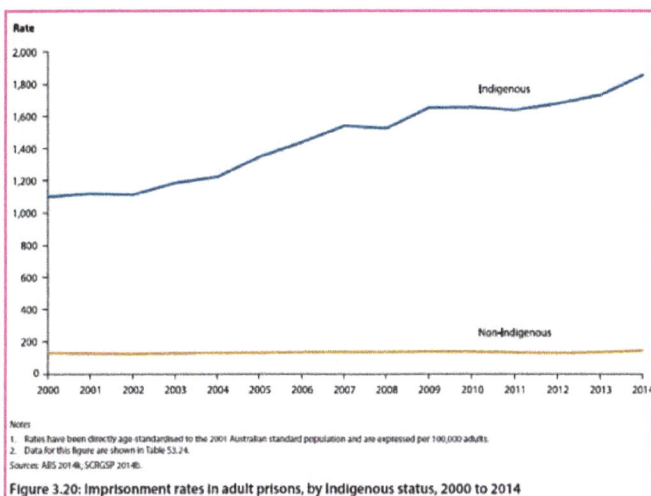

Notes
1. Rates have been directly age-standardised to the 2001 Australian standard population and are expressed per 100,000 adults.
2. Data for this figure are shown in Table 53.24.
Sources: ABS 2014b, SCRGSP 2014b.

Figure 3.20: Imprisonment rates in adult prisons, by Indigenous status, 2000 to 2014

Any explanation is going to have to account for that low, and pretty much flat, rate of non-Indigenous incarceration, and that high and climbing higher rate of Indigenous incarceration.

In the dark recesses of racist Facebook, you might see suggestions that Aboriginal people are just inherently more criminal. This is not only wrong, and explains nothing, it is also a deliberate way of saying "…and I don't want to know."

The reason for the differences in incarceration rates could be that Aboriginal and Torres Strait Islander people are **committing more (or more serious) crimes**, that the police are **more likely to charge Aboriginal and Torres Strait Islander** people for **relatively minor crimes**, or that courts are **more likely to sentence Aboriginal and Torres Strait Islander people to imprisonment**.

There's truth in each of these statistics, but let's ask again: "Why?"

There's a theme that unites all of these reasons, in the society that produces these effects. Naming it provokes deep reactions, but once it is named and explained, it's possible to see its work everywhere.

What is going on here is **white privilege**.

They don't teach this in medical school – **I'll leave you to consider why!** So these ideas are relatively new to me and, as I learn about the unearned privileges I receive, I may be prone to misunderstandings and understatement. That's because, as much as I try, it's hard for me to see the world without my privilege.

Let's think back to that time I was caught speeding. Though I was upset at the time, I never **feared for my safety** from the police officer, and assumed I'd be treated fairly. I never thought I'd be **imprisoned for a minor traffic offence**. I wasn't asked to open the boot, or have the car searched – there was no reason to – but sometimes there is no reason to, and it still happens.

What if the police officer had looked in my car? What would she have found?

Well, echoing a **well known description of white privilege** by Peggy McIntosh (who lists what's in the "invisible knapsack" of white privilege), the police officer would have found a general assumption that the police can be trusted. Also present would be a usually correct assumption that the police officer would be of a similar background to me – why else do the police need specific Aboriginal liaison officers?

Wrapped up in a parcel on the back seat was my belief that if I was unhappy about how I was treated, I'd be able to see a superior police officer, whose background was also similar to mine. Tucked away in a plastic bag was my knowledge that I'd be able to get a lawyer and be seen by a judge who would also be a bit like me.

Aside from this, I'd know that hidden away with the spare tyre, there weren't media stories about people like me that drew on my appearance or race to make me seem scarier or more violent than I am.

And tucked in the glovebox is my CV, which, because it has an English-sounding name at the head, **is more likely to land me a job interview.***

I can go on. The car is full-to-overflowing of my white privilege. Behind the seat is knowing that politicians making the laws mostly have my racial background. I can glance in my rear-view mirror to see that my cultural background is shared by most journalists choosing what is news and how those news stories will be framed. I can also recognise myself in those teachers at school and at uni who were encouraging me and helping to set my course.

It's not just this one interaction with the police where my white privilege might be exposed, either. If the police officer wanted to search my home – more likely to be **rented from someone else if I were Aboriginal** – they'd find white people like me **in my television dramas**, more comfortable about **sitting next to me, or allowing me to shop without suspicion**.

Everywhere I look, in fact, is the message "Yes, you fit in here. You belong." It's nice and comforting. For me, and for other white people like me, life is like **playing the computer game on the easiest setting**.

To say this in public though, can lead to abuse and anger – so called **white fragility**, a state in which even a minimum amount of racial stress becomes intolerable, triggering defensive reactions among white people, such as anger, fear, and guilt.

I'm not saying that white people have it easy, or have no problems, or never go to jail. I'm not saying all white people are racist (though some honesty like this from **Daniel Reeders** would go a very long way to improving the situation).

We are (thankfully) not all Bolt wannabees. It's much more subtle, complex and interesting than that. The structures that we have built society on, and colonised Australia with, have resulted in a whole heap of unspoken advantages to people like me, at the expense of people like my Aboriginal patients.

It's why they relax in the community controlled service I work in – because it says, unlike so much of mainstream Australia's institutions and systems, "Yes, you fit in here. You belong."

There is a common enough understanding that racsim is A Bad Thing, so even those who boo Adam Goodes don't like being called racist. We now need to see and acknowledge the racist structures that we all live in, that exist in out health systems, in our legal systems and across our whole society.

Those imprisonment rates, those health statistics we see are symptoms of those societal structures. That is why we see similar figures right across the world.

Those statistics are the result of white peoples' privilege and how white systems disadvantage and exclude others. It's repeated for **Maori people in New Zealand**, for the **Aboriginal people of Canada**, and for **black people in the US**, which should tell us we're not dealing with an Aboriginal and Torres Strait Islander problem here.

We are seeing the application of a dominant culture to exclude others.

We have to acknowledge this – which means those of us who benefit from white privilege need to do the most to change unfair systems – and perhaps risk losing some of our advantages in the process.

Those advantages can be hard to see. To help bring them to the surface, watch this video that tests your awareness.

Once you start seeing white privilege, like the surprise in this video, you notice it every time you look.

*Yes, one of the authors of that study is now in the Shadow Cabinet!

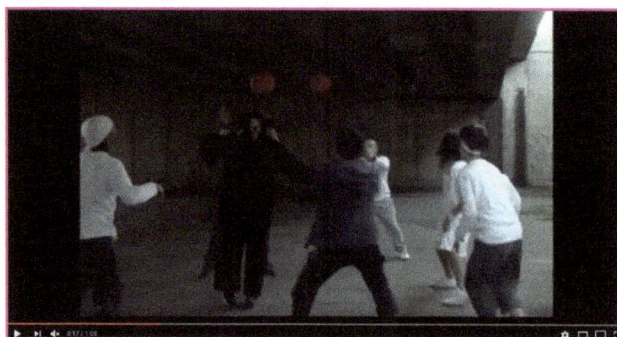

Dr Tim Senior is a GP who works in Aboriginal health, a contributing columnist to Croakey, and author of #WonkyHealth – the e-book. Follow him on Twitter: @timsenior

NT Coroner calls for repeal of "paperless arrest" laws

Author:	Mark Skulley	Published:	August 14, 2015

The findings of an inquest in the Northern Territory into the death of a senior Walpiri man are important reading for those working in the health and justice sectors, highlighting the need for law reform.

Mark Skulley writes:

The Northern Territory Coroner has denounced the so-called "paperless arrest" laws, and called for them to be repealed before more Aboriginal people die in police custody when charged for minor offences.

The landmark finding by the Coroner, Greg Cavanagh, will put pressure on the NT Government to revisit the laws, which have also been challenged in the High Court.

Mr Cavanagh said the laws, introduced last year, were "manifestly unfair", and were irreconcilable with the recommendations of the Royal Commission into Aboriginal Deaths in Custody, which urged that arrest and detention be used as a last resort.

He called for an independent review of responses to alcohol misuse in the Territory, as part of his findings in an inquest into the death of a 59-year old man, Mr Langdon, in the Darwin Watch House on May 21 this year.

The Coroner said it was culturally appropriate to refer to Mr Langdon, a senior Walpiri man who was born in Yuendumu, as Kumanjayi.

"Kumanjayi had the right to die as a free man and in the circumstances he should have done," the Coroner said. "In my view, unless the paperless arrest laws are struck from the Statute books, more and more disadvantaged Aboriginal people are at risk of dying in custody, and unnecessarily so. That is why I recommend their repeal."

Kumanjayi was arrested by police under the "paperless arrest scheme" after he was seen drinking from a plastic bottle in Spillet Park. But he was not causing any disruption before or during his arrest and was at all times polite and cooperative.

The maximum penalty for such a minor liquor offence was a spot fine of $74 with the "victim's levy" of $40, and Kumanjayi was issued with an "on-the-spot fine" for that amount.

> *Mr Cavanagh said the laws, introduced last year, were "manifestly unfair", and were irreconcilable with the recommendations of the Royal Commission into Aboriginal Deaths in Custody*

Although the offence carried no prison term, Kumanjayi was handcuffed, placed in an iron cage in the back of a police van, presented at the watch house with his arms still handcuffed behind his back, searched, deprived of his property, and detained for some hours in a cell.

The Coroner said Kumanjayi, who had chronic health problems, was placed in the cells at 6.44pm. He went to sleep and a later cell check found he had died at 9.07pm.

Mr Cavanagh found shortcomings in the health check process for Kumanjayi, but was confident they did not contribute to his death.

"While the care and supervision of Kumanjayi was adequate in the circumstances, it is clear that there are enormous pressures on Police and Nurses as a result of the paperless arrest scheme and the police initiative known as Operation Ascari II, which encourages the arrest of public drinkers, almost all of whom are Indigenous," the Coroner said.

"That increase in the numbers of Indigenous people in custody is likely to lead to a proportionate increase in the numbers of Aboriginal people dying in custody. This has led me to the recommendation that the law should be repealed."

The Coroner said he was impressed by the "professional and courteous way" that Kumanjayi was handled by police, which was captured on CCTV footage. He also noted "significant improvements" in watch house operations and cooperation with custody nurses who worked "busy shifts".

He agreed with the submission by lawyers for Kumanjayi's family that he was an "old man minding his own business, enjoying the company of family and friends in an early evening of the dry season."

"He had been drinking, but had done nothing to bring himself to the attention of police, beyond being with other Aboriginal people in a park in the Darwin CBD. The only possible reason for his arrest was that he had committed the infringement offence of drinking in a public place."

Mr Cavanagh found police acted lawfully in arresting Kumanjayi and that the arresting officer was a "sincere and conscientious officer", who was trying to achieve the goals of the paperless arrest scheme and Operation Ascari II.

But the "implicit message" from the government and senior police command was that Aboriginal people drinking in designated public areas should be taken off the streets for up to four hours or longer if they needed more time to sober up.

"Kumanjayi Langdon, a sick middle aged Aboriginal man, was treated like a criminal and incarcerated like a criminal; he died in a police cell which was built to house criminals. He died in his sleep with strangers in this cold and concrete cell," the Coroner said.

"He died of natural causes and was always likely to die suddenly due to chronic and serious heart disease but he was entitled to die in peace, in the comfort of family and friends. In my view he was entitled to die as a free man."

The Coroner noted that Kumanjayi was survived by his wife, children and an extended family.

- Read the Coroner's findings here.

Mark Skulley is a freelance journalist. He donated to the #JustJustice crowdfunding campaign, and volunteered his time to contribute articles.

Reconciliation in Australia: where do we stand and how does that help/hinder Closing the Gap?

RACE RELATIONS

All Australians understand and value Aboriginal and Torres Strait Islander and non-Indigenous cultures, rights and experiences, which results in stronger relationships based on trust and respect and that are free of racism.

EQUALITY AND EQUITY

Aboriginal and Torres Strait Islander peoples participate equally in a range of life opportunities and the unique rights of Aboriginal and Torres Strait Islander peoples are recognised and upheld.

UNITY

An Australian society that values and recognises Aboriginal and Torres Strait Islander cultures and heritage as a proud part of a shared national identity.

INSTITUTIONAL INTEGRITY

The active support of reconciliation by the nation's political, business and community structures.

HISTORICAL ACCEPTANCE

All Australians understand and accept the wrongs of the past and the impact of these wrongs. Australia makes amends for the wrongs of the past and ensures these wrongs are never repeated.

Author: Marie McInerney

Published: February 09, 2016

Marie McInerney writes:

My 11 year old son brought home a school work sheet last week for his project on 'Australia as a nation'. It had four pictures on it that he had to decorate: Parliament House in Canberra, a map of Australia, the Australian flag, and an image of the Anzacs.

Nothing about the First Peoples of this nation.

He quietly added an Aboriginal flag in the corner but the message of that sheet goes to the heart of a landmark report released today by Reconciliation Australia on the **State of Reconciliation in Australia**: *Our history, our story, our future.*

One of its findings is that Australians' knowledge of Aboriginal and Torres Strait Islander histories and cultures is limited (only 30 per cent are knowledgeable) but most Australians (83 per cent) believe it is important to know more and strongly support Aboriginal and Torres Strait Islander histories being a compulsory part of the school curriculum.

The report looks at what has been achieved under the five dimensions of reconciliation shown in the image above – race relations, equality and equity, institutional integrity, unity, and historical acceptance – and makes detailed recommendations on how we can progress reconciliation into the next generation. But, with the finding that one in three Aboriginal and Torres Strait Islander people had experienced verbal racial abuse in the six months before the survey, it warns:

" While much goodwill and support for reconciliation is growing across the Australian community, racism, denial of rights, and a lack of willingness to come to terms with our history continue to overshadow the nation's progress towards reconciliation.

The report provides important context for the release tomorrow of the latest Closing the Gap update to Parliament, particularly after the 2015 update was described by then PM Tony Abbott as "profoundly disappointing" with **most of the targets not on track to be met**. Reconcilation Australia says that many reviews have suggested that unsatisfactory progress is not due to the level of spending, but the way funding has been allcoated and delivered:

This criticism was the catalyst for reforms under the Indigenous Advancement Strategy (IAS) in 2014. However, rather than the ambitious IAS reforms resolving many of the issues they were meant to address, early indications are that they were too much, too soon, and have left a trail of anxiety and uncertainty for many service providers

And don't miss the powerful intro to the Reconcilation report from Aboriginal leader Patrick Dodson who warned that Closing the Gap targets are 'doomed to fail' without more input from Indigenous groups and services and questioned Prime Minister Malcolm Turnbull's commitment to Indigenous affairs.

Croakey readers may also like to revisit this 2013 post from Tim Senior on the difference between the work of the Close the Gap and the Closing the Gap campaigns, and why it matters.

This week also saw the release of a welcome evaluation of the Northern Territory Intervention by the Castan Centre for Human Rights Law, which found it had failed to deliver substantial reform on areas covered by Close the Gap goals and violated human rights obligations.

Figure 9: Aboriginal and Torres Strait Islander experience of racial prejudice in the six months prior to the survey

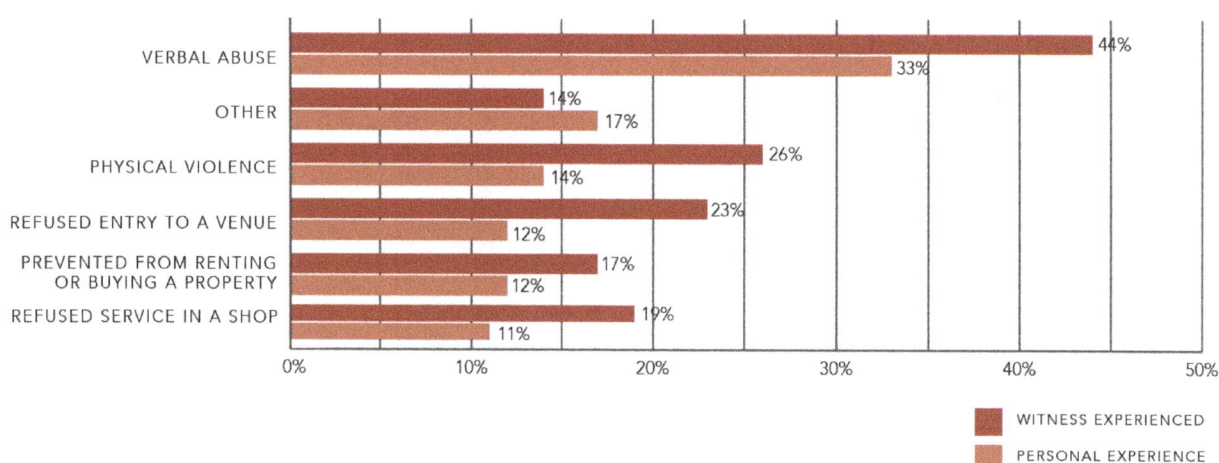

	WITNESS EXPERIENCED	PERSONAL EXPERIENCE
VERBAL ABUSE	44%	33%
OTHER	14%	17%
PHYSICAL VIOLENCE	26%	14%
REFUSED ENTRY TO A VENUE	23%	12%
PREVENTED FROM RENTING OR BUYING A PROPERTY	17%	12%
REFUSED SERVICE IN A SHOP	19%	11%

Source: ARB 2014, Question 12: "In the past six months, have you personally experienced any of the following forms of prejudice on the basis of your race?", and Question 13: "In the past six months, have you seen someone else experience any of the following forms of prejudice on the basis of their race?"

DIMENSION	AREAS FOR ACTION
Race relations	• Overcome racism
Equality and equity	• Renew focus on closing the gap • Recognise and respect the cultures and collective rights of First Australians
Institutional integrity	• Capitalise on the RAP program • Improve the governance of government
Unity	• Achieve a process to recognise Aboriginal and Torres Strait Islander peoples and unite all Australians
Historical acceptance	• Acknowledge our past through truth, justice and healing

Health groups join chorus of concern about excessive force by Queensland police towards Aboriginal woman

| Author: | Statement by multiple groups | Published: | January 21, 2016 |

The push for health in all policies should have a big focus on addressing the impact of police practices on the health and wellbeing of Aboriginal and Torres Strait Islander peoples.

It is noteworthy that health groups, including the Menzies School of Health Research, the Secretariat of National Aboriginal and Torres Strait Islander Child Care, and the Victorian Aboriginal Community Controlled Health Organisation are among signatories to the open letter reproduced below. It is also noteworthy that many health organisations have not signed the letter.

It would be interesting to see an analysis of how much health research funding and public health muscle is devoted to this area more broadly.

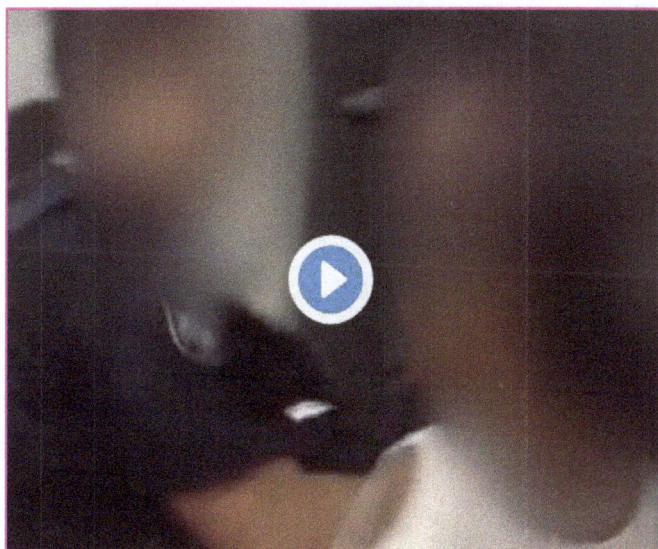

Statement on video depicting excessive force by police towards Aboriginal woman

We the undersigned organisations are deeply concerned by the treatment of an Aboriginal woman by the Queensland Police Service in video footage which emerged over the weekend.

The video appears to show a male officer responding with excessive physical force towards an Aboriginal woman, including repeatedly shoving her as she attempted to get closer to her teenage son. There also appears to be conflicting reports as to the basis for the police entering the home and what they were responding to.

Effective policing relies on having the trust of the community. For Aboriginal and Torres Strait Islander communities, well-documented contemporary and historical factors including racism and deaths in custody have contributed to low levels of trust in the police. This negative relationship hinders the ability to build positive relationships between the community and police, and also impedes the ability of Aboriginal and Torres Strait Islander people to access their rights under the law.

Incidents such as this perpetuate mistrust in Aboriginal and Torres Strait Islander communities towards the police. Sadly, too often communities report this kind of police treatment. These incidents may influence the willingness of Aboriginal and Torres Strait Islander victim/survivors to report family violence to the police in the future.

The undersigned organisations are seeking:

- an independent investigation as to why such force was used towards an Aboriginal mother and on what basis the police were in the home;

- an assurance that policies and practices are put in place to ensure police do not use excessive force, particularly force which adds to the unacceptable levels of violence experienced by Aboriginal and Torres Strait Islander women; and

- the development and implementation of strategies which are aimed at building stronger collaborative relationships between police and Aboriginal and Torres Strait Islander communities, organisations and their representative bodies. These strategies should improve police interaction with the community and build the capacity of police to respond to family violence, mental health issues and other complex situations, in a culturally safe way.

This open letter is supported by the following organisations:

Amnesty International

ANTaR

Australian Council of Social Service

First Peoples Disability Network Australia

Human Rights Law Centre

Menzies School of Health Research

National Aboriginal Torres Strait Islander Legal Services

National Association of Community Legal Centres

National Congress of Australia's First Peoples

National Family Violence Prevention Legal Services Forum

Oxfam Australia

Queensland Association of Independent Legal Service Inc

Save the Children

Secretariat of National Aboriginal and Torres Strait Islander Child Care

Sisters Inside

Uniting Church in Australia, Queensland Synod

Victorian Aboriginal Community Controlled Health Organisation

The indignities that led to Ms Dhu's death are the same indignities her family now face

Author:	Amy McQuire	Published:	October 16, 2016

Amy McQuire, a journalist and Darumbul woman from central Queensland, reflects on the shocking death in custody of Ms Dhu and how the pain and indignity heaped upon her in her final days are now being borne by her family as they seek justice and to shine a light on racism in Australia.

McQuire is the former editor of the National Indigenous Times and Tracker magazine. She is currently a senior reporter with New Matilda and hosts a morning program on radio station 98.9fm, owned by the Brisbane Indigenous Media Association. She is on Twitter at @amymcquire.

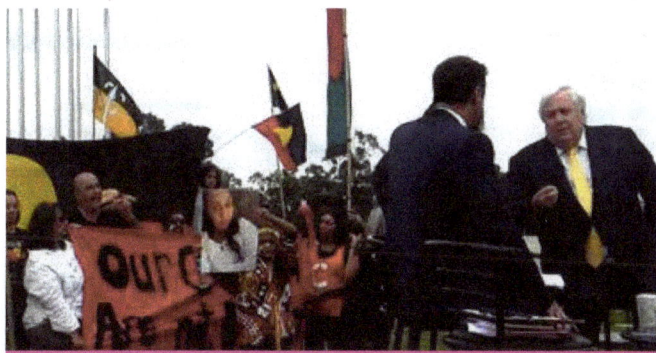

Photo of the Canberra protest supplied by Amy McQuire

With Martin Hodgson, McQuire also premiered This is Curtain – a podcast to "shine a light on the darkest parts of our justice system". You can subscribe here and follow on Twitter at @CurtainPodcast.

Amy McQuire writes:

On the first day of Parliament in 2015, I joined about 100 other people on the lawns of the Aboriginal Tent Embassy in Canberra – a world famous site of black resistance.

Among that 100 were several First Nations grandmothers, whose individual strength had coalesced into a growing movement against the racist child protection system, and a man – Shaun Harris – who had at that point been travelling the country to raise awareness over his niece's death in custody.

Shaun had erected a tent to the side of the embassy, the area furthest from the rose gardens, which had only just started to bloom. At night, he would gather around the fire, talking about his niece with the others camped at the embassy, who had all sacrificed their time and, in some cases, pay packets, in solidarity.

The conversation swung like a pendulum between deaths in custody, policing, child removal and welfare, suspended between sorrow, and anger, and then brief interruptions of laughter.

During the day, I spent time drinking coffee and talking to other grandmothers, hearing their stories of how their grandchildren had been ripped from them. The majority of them could now talk legalese as if they had spent years in law school.

They knew how to rip apart affidavits, most of them full to the brim of inconsistencies, and were in the midst of designing strategies to lobby child protection departments in their own respective states.

They were all here, easily reachable, willing to talk, but they couldn't get anyone to listen. All of the nation's top journalists, the most awarded in the country, were immersed in their press gallery bubble, and no-one, except the Aboriginal media, bothered to walk the short distance to hear them out.

Stories of pain swatted away like flies

But that day, as the first rays hit the parliamentary year, the grandmothers, their supporters – including legends like Aunty Jenny Munro – and Shaun Harris, began their walk past the chalked pavement outside the tent embassy, winding around old Parliament House, and up the grassy expanse that separates it from the new building.

Coincidentally, it was a day of high political drama – when then Prime Minister Tony Abbott avoided a leadership spill but was given six months to get his act together by his caucus.

As usual, the morning television hosts were all lined up on the grass like bobble heads beside each other, using Parliament House as a backdrop.

Channel Ten's Hugh Riminton, Kochie and Sam from Sunrise, and Today's Karl Stefanovic and Lisa Wilkinson were all there, easily accessible, their cameras like a portal into millions of Australian lounge rooms.

Without skipping a beat, the protestors – with their flags and chants – marched straight behind those cameras and began protesting.

But despite the breadth of knowledge making up their rally, and the causes they were fighting for, they were greeted as if they were pesky flies – to be tolerated and ignored, if they couldn't be swatted away.

There was no shock, no surprise from them at how they were treated – just a resignation that this was how things had always been – this was how white Australia and white media treats Aboriginal stories.

But that day, I was struck by one image – and that was a young girl, standing behind Stefanovic and Wilkinson, who were interviewing Clive Palmer.

She was only about 10 or 11. She stood in silence, holding the strength of her ancestors within her tiny body. In her hands was the laminated image of Ms Dhu – Shaun's niece, a Yamitji woman who had died in horrendous pain while being refused medical care in lock-up.

She stood there, separate from the crowd, daring the cameras to pick up the face of an Aboriginal woman who we knew had been let down by a racist justice system.

And it struck me then, that this was the first time Ms Dhu's face had ever been on national commercial television.

It was there that I became keenly aware of the indignities Ms Dhu had faced in life, and the indignities her family continue to face in her death.

Deflecting blame and attention

There is an argument favoured by right wing shock jocks, and certain politicians like WA Premier Colin Barnett — and it goes like this:

"In respect to deaths in custody, avoidable Aboriginal deaths in custody are low and have continued on a downward trend since the 1991 Royal Commission into Aboriginal Deaths in Custody. The rate of avoidable deaths of Aboriginal people in prison in Western Australia is below the Australian average. There has also been a marked decline in the number of Aboriginal prison suicides. These may be the facts, but one death is one death too many."

That was Colin Barnett in WA Parliament last year, responding to the death of Ms Dhu in a South Hedland watchhouse while being repeatedly refused medical attention and health care.

A comment like Barnett's is designed to deflect blame and attention — to act as if this is purely a question of protocol when we know that the vicious cycle continues.

But a breach of procedure doesn't describe the indignities Aboriginal people have to live with every day — and women in particular. They are the continual indignities of being black in this country, and they are the indignities that led to Ms Dhu losing her life in the most disturbing of circumstances.

The reason why we continue to campaign around black deaths in custody is because of this: What happened to Ms Dhu would never happen to a white prisoner. It is not a matter of procedure, it is in itself a symptom of the ongoing colonial project that continually dehumanises Aboriginal people, which leads us to the current day, where Aboriginal life is seen as disposable.

A catalogue of indignities

The indignities that led to Ms Dhu's death — the mocking of her pain, the refusal to believe her over the testimony of the non-Indigenous protectors (the health professionals and police officers), the fact she was criminalised for her poverty despite being a family violence victim — are indignities that are present within the life experiences of our mob, behind and beyond bars. These indignities ensure that even if you aren't confined by physical walls, sometimes the reality of being Aboriginal in this country can feel like a prison in itself.

And you need no further evidence of this than how Ms Dhu's grieving family have been treated following her death. The indignities that led to Ms Dhu's death are the same indignities her family now face.

First of all, they have faced the indignity of not being listened to. Like Ms Dhu, whose pleas of pain fell on deaf ears, her family have had to campaign at their own expense, simply to force anyone to give a damn. They have travelled the length of this country, building contacts, speaking at rallies, simply to break the continual media blackout that engulfs Aboriginal deaths.

They shouldn't have to do this, just like Ms Dhu, who should never have had to plead continually for attention while she was in the death throes of septic shock.

Second — the indignity of being mocked. Like Ms Dhu, who cried out in pain and was believed to have been 'faking' it, Ms Dhu's family have been forced to deal with the daily eruptions of racism while campaigning for their daughter — from the outright casual racism to the more insidious forms. If you go on any online forum, you will see the ignorant comments from people – claiming 'all she had to do is pay the fine like the rest of us do when we get done for speeding. If she did, she wouldn't have had to go to jail.' — somehow attempting to justify the denial of adequate medical care that could have saved her life.

Third, the indignity of exhaustion — like Ms Dhu, her family are exhausted because they continually have to justify their protest, and their grief. No other Australian would be required to explain why their loved one shouldn't have been locked up for no crime, let alone why she shouldn't have died there, with no consequence.

Constantly fighting to take small steps when there is still a mountain ahead, while also dealing with other traumas passed down through generations, is an exhaustion that few other Australians would understand.

Fourth, the indignity of waiting. Like Ms Dhu, who waited and waited for medical attention, only to be let down not once, not twice, but three times when seeking medical attention (she died shortly after making it to the South Hedland Health Campus on her third visit), Ms Dhu's family have been forced to wait for a long drawn out coronial inquiry, which sadly is considered 'sped-up' by Western Australian standards.

For two years they have been grieving, lost in the traumatic experience of 'not knowing'. Ms Dhu's grandmother Aunty Carol Roe repeatedly tried to enquire about her granddaughter's health while she was locked up — and was repeatedly told she was 'fine'. We now know, after nearly two years of waiting, that Ms Dhu was not fine. How much longer will this family have to wait?

And fifth, the indignity of disempowerment. Like Ms Dhu, who lost her liberty and her life simply because she had failed to pay back over $3,000 in fines, Ms Dhu's family have been continually disempowered at every turn — the latest of which has been Coroner Ros Fogliani's refusal to release CCTV footage of Ms Dhu's final hours.

The footage is supposed to be harrowing, and shows Ms Dhu being handcuffed, and thrown in the back of the police van like a carcass — those were her last moments.

Fogliani has the audacity to claim she doesn't want to 're-traumatise' the family — but even presuming to understand their pain and their trauma is disempowering, and harks back to the days of the old protectors on the missions and reserves across this country. The thinking is not that much different — 'we know what is good for you'.

I think there is another indignity here as well — the fact that this CCTV footage is even required in order to wake up a complacent Australia. We shouldn't need to see the footage of the last hours of a dying young woman in order to care. We shouldn't have to be forced to care. But the Don Dale footage on Four Corners has shown us that Australians are blissfully apathetic unless Aboriginal pain is put straight in front of their noses.

Ms Dhu spent three horrendous days in pain, deprived of her freedom, and repeatedly mocked and ignored. And her pain continues as long as her family faces the same indignities.

It is not enough just to have a coronial inquiry that leads nowhere. There needs to be some sort of accountability, an acknowledgement that her pain was just as valid as the pain of a white woman, that her life was just as precious.

Because even in her death, Australia has shown time and time again that it is willing to tolerate the indignities of being black in this country. And unless there is accountability, unless there is some justice — probably in the form of convictions — these indignities will only continue.

Amy McQuire is a journalist and Darumbul woman from central Queensland.

Address systemic racism, homelessness, unemployment, poverty and trauma – for #JustJustice

Author:	Julie Walker	Published:	November 02, 2016

Systemic racism in the justice and wider government systems needs to be addressed in order to tackle the over-incarceration of Aboriginal and Torres Strait Islander people, according to Julie Walker, a Yinhawangka woman from South Hedland in Western Australia.

The criminal justice system is not doing enough to deal with the issues underlying many peoples' interactions with the system, including homelessness, unemployment, poverty and trauma, she says.

Ms Walker, a social worker with long experience in social justice advocacy and initiatives, says the report of the Royal Commission into Aboriginal Deaths in Custody is "Australia's most significant social document", and that many of its recommendations remain relevant today.

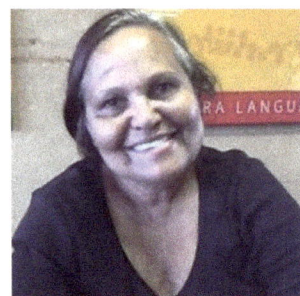

Julie Walker: Calling for an end to top-down decision-making by distant bureaucrats

These include the need for Aboriginal people to have access to culturally appropriate services, including from the education, health, social and justice systems.

The colonial attitudes of the past continued on in policies designed to punish, and bring harm and injury to Aboriginal people, she said, and this was particularly evident in Centrelink policies and practices.

Ms Walker also highlighted the need to stop high rates of removal of children, and to ensure child protection systems catered for children's cultural needs.

"In the Pilbara, 98 percent of the children in DCP [Department for Child Protection] care are Aboriginal; many have English as second or third language," she said.

"When they go into child protection, they go into cultural shock, which is very traumatic…I've seen little ones, two-year-olds, you get a situation where they can't even talk to their carer. It's a really traumatic experience for any child to go through."

Other issues identified by Ms Walker in this interview include:

- The need to understand the historic context of colonisation in order to address contemporary incarceration rates.

"*Aboriginal people were subject to tremendous violence from the onslaught of the first settlers…to understand how Aboriginal people have become criminals in their own country, you need to understand the history of colonisation. In the fight for land and resources, Aboriginal people were sent to prison…*"

- The need for secure funding for community organisations and programs focused on the needs identified by communities. She called for an end to the short-termism of 12-month funding arrangements and to top-down decision-making by bureaucrats far away who don't know the local community.

"*You can't do anything on 12 month funding. They change the goal posts, they change the rules, they change the policies. You get the impression, they really don't want us to do well, they really don't want us to make some changes here. Decision-making doesn't happen on the ground; it's all top-down made by bureaucrats and people who have no understanding, in some cases they don't even know where South Hedland is. They have no idea about the community…but they make the decisions.*"

- The need for Australia to recognise Indigenous sovereignty, and to address the atrocities committed in the past.

Watch the full interview here: https://youtu.be/3bilVSJkNJQ

Is this Justice?

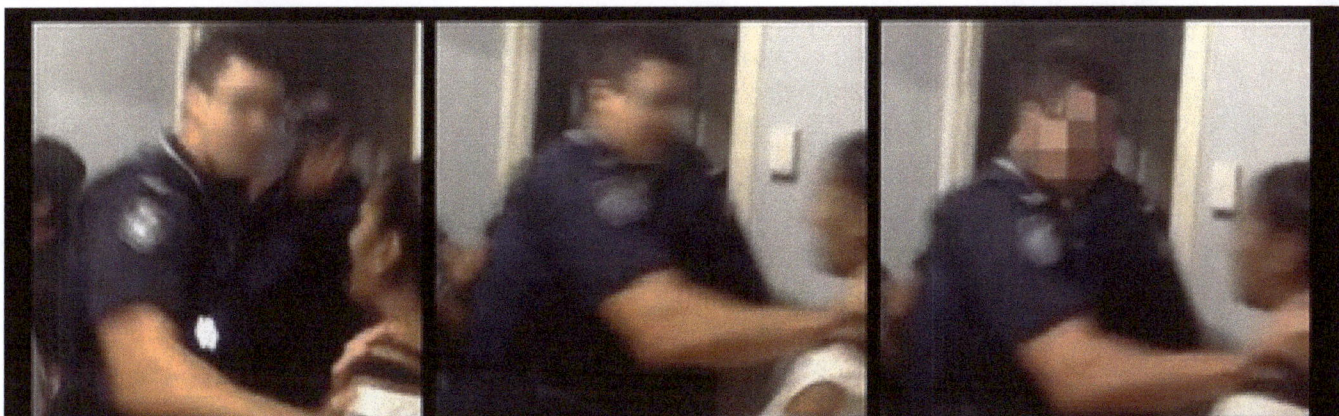

POLICE VIOLENCE IS NOT OKAY
Call on Queensland's Police Minister to launch an independent investigation ▸

Image courtesy of Amnesty

Author:	Kelly Briggs	Published:	January 20, 2016

As Amnesty International **calls for an independent investigation** into police violence against an Aboriginal woman in Queensland, the award-winning Kelly Briggs writes for the #JustJustice series about "the talk" that Aboriginal parents need to have with their children about police.

Kelly Briggs writes:

I am a parent of two Aboriginal boys. When they were 12 or so I sat them down and had the talk with them. Not the birds and the bees talk, the interacting with police talk. I am probably not the only parent of black children to have this talk with their children, and nor will I be the last.

This talk consisted of how to behave, not to let the police antagonise them into anger, to call me immediately if they were taken by the police and above all else, not to talk to them without me present.

If you are reading this, you may be assuming the police would only be speaking to my children if they have done something wrong. This couldn't be further from the truth.

Because of racial profiling (refers to the discriminatory practice by law enforcement officials of targeting individuals for suspicion of crime based on the individual's race, ethnicity, religion or national origin), my children everyday become targets for police.

I am not over reacting; the statistics of Aboriginal imprisonment rates are a major factor in me telling my children to use the utmost caution around the police. Below are the statistics of young people in prison 2013 – 2014.

It is incredibly hard to look at these charts and not infer racial profiling from the results.

As of June 30, there were 9,885 adult prisoners in Australian prisons who identified as Aboriginal and Torres Strait Islander, a 7% increase (620 prisoners) from 30 June 2014 (9,265 prisoners).

Mick Gooda, the Aboriginal and Torres Strait Islander Social Justice Commissioner, who wrote the foreword on Aboriginal justice issues for an Amnesty International Report has said: "We've got cases where a kid in WA got charged with receiving a stolen chocolate frog. Would that happen to a white kid? Probably not."

He goes on to say:

" We have high rates of unresolved intergenerational trauma, which has led to disability, alcohol-related disability, brain injury and mental health issues. It makes a mockery of our justice system if we incarcerate children who have some sort of cognitive impairment, which we increasingly think is the case.

He is right. We need to shift the conversation to why such seemingly mild infractions are treated as criminal, and not for what they are, inter generational trauma being played out on a basic scale. As a country we must begin a conversation about justice reinvestment, where prison is treated as a last resort and not the first.

As it stands, we now have Aboriginals entering prisons with no prior mental health issues or drug addictions but leaving with mental health issues, drug addictions and the stigma of being in prison, no matter how small the offence.

Is it any wonder that Aboriginals do not trust the police after looking at the facts? In 1987 there was an inquiry into Aboriginal deaths in custody. Ninety-nine cases were examined and not one out of those 99 deaths was ruled as the police's fault. 99.

The commission did, however, hand down 330 recommendations, of which not even a handful have been instituted. One of them is the Custody Notification Service, which is only implemented in NSW and Canberra.

It ensures that Aboriginal people have an opportunity to call for legal advice. This service is seriously underfunded and at times relies on assistance from the public.

So before you judge me for instilling distrust in the police, now that you have read my reasons, can you honestly say you would not have the same talk with your children if they were Aboriginal?

Kelly Briggs was the winner of the Social Commentary Blog of the Year award in 2014 by the Australian Writers Centre for her blog. Read her previous Croakey articles here, and follow on Twitter at @TheKooriWoman.

11. Don Dale

"*The treatment of youth imprisoned in the Northern Territory is disgusting and inhumane. The justice system has failed not only the individual but society. Shameful. Sickening*

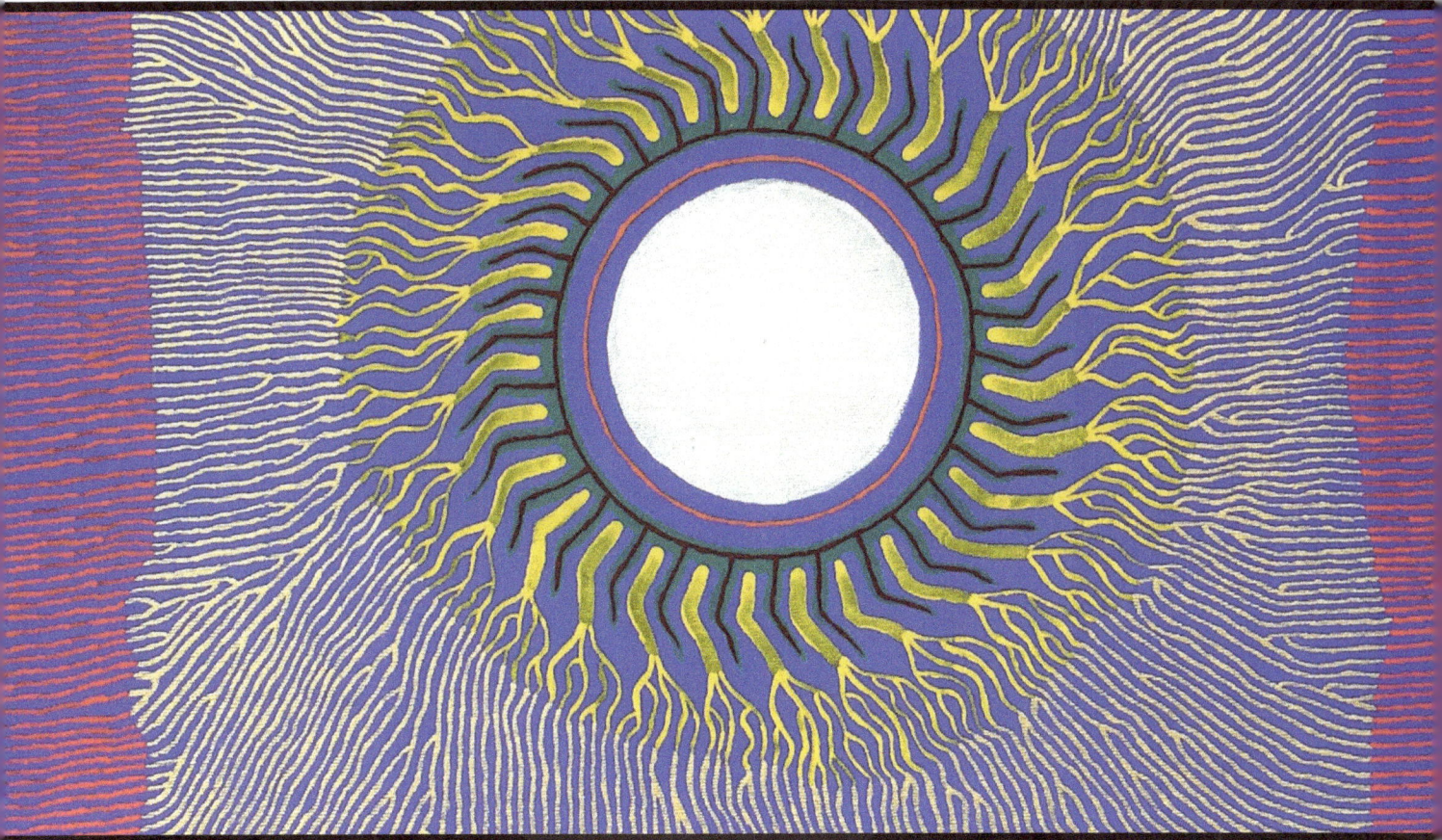

Where's the #JustJustice in NT teenagers being hooded, transferred to adult prison?

Author:	Roxanne Moore	Published:	September 23, 2015

The Human Rights Law Centre has requested a United Nations investigation into the mistreatment of young people at the Northern Territory's Don Dale Detention Centre, after the NT Children's Commissioner report into an alleged 2014 riot by six juvenile detainees detailed "cruel, inhuman and degrading treatment" inside the facility, including prolonged solitary confinement, use of dogs and tear gas, and hooding and cuffing as restraint practices.

In the article below, Amnesty Indigenous rights campaigner Roxanne Moore examines the reports findings and calls on the Northern Territory Government to drastically overhaul the justice system for kids and ensure they are being rehabilitated, not mistreated.

Urgent reform is also needed in the Northern Territory to the 'paperless arrests' laws that allow detention without an arrest warrant. Listen to this report from Radio National's Background Briefing.

Roxanne Moore writes:

A report by the Northern Territory (NT) Children's Commissioner reveals shocking treatment of juveniles at Don Dale Youth Detention Centre.

The report comes after NT Correctional Services staff were found to have used tear gas on kids following an attempted escape on 21 August last year.

Confinement

The recent report shows six Indigenous children were in confinement "for periods of between six and seventeen days" in the lead-up to the tear-gassing incident.

And it gets worse. Some kids were left in confinement for long periods of time without access to water or natural light.

Imagine being locked in a windowless cell, with no fan or air conditioning, or tap water, for three days. It is inhumane and such treatment could constitute torture under both domestic and international law.

One witness told the Commissioner: "The detainees went off and I don't blame them...I would have too. It wouldn't have happened if they didn't keep them in there so long. It is horrible, it stinks...I am surprised it didn't happen sooner."

Riot shields, batons and tear gas

It comes as little surprise that kids tried to break out of the cells. During the commotion, three officers were called in from the adult prison. They were wearing gas masks, and held riot shields and batons – a reaction completely out of proportion.

When one child tried to climb out of a window, audio from camera footage captured an officer using swear words to describe the child. Before realising he was being recorded and laughing it off, the officer was also heard saying he would 'pulverise' the child.

One child later told his caseworker that he thought he was going to die. He and another child hid behind a mattress and said their goodbyes during the gassing.

Kids hooded and fitted with anti-spit masks, sent to the adult detention centre

Following the tear-gassing, the boys – one as young as fourteen – were handcuffed and transferred to an adult prison. To force them into compliance for the transfer, the boys were hooded with anti-spit masks. The youth detention centre did not have the authority to transfer the 14-year-old, but did so anyway. He was transferred back only when they realised it was illegal.

Two children who were not involved in the disturbance were also gassed, transferred and punished.

Why is this particularly concerning for Indigenous youth?

The lack of support given to Indigenous people by our governments has led to a massive over-representation of Indigenous youth in detention. Failure to address the underlying causes of offending, including poverty, intergenerational trauma and substance abuse, compounds the problem.

The NT has one of the highest rates of Indigenous youth in detention. Between July 2013 and June 2014 Indigenous young people averaged 96 per cent of all young people in detention, while making up only around 44 per cent of the population aged between 10 and 17.

Nationally, Aboriginal and Torres Strait Islander young people account for just over 5 per cent of the Australian population aged between 10 and 17, but more than half of those in detention.

What needs to happen now

Our Government needs to drastically overhaul the justice system for kids and ensure they are being rehabilitated, not mistreated.

It is outrageous that Australia refuses to rule out sending kids to adult prisons. Australia must live up to its obligations under the Convention on the Rights of the Child and make sure children are kept separate from adult prisoners.

We also need to advocate for Australia to immediately ratify the Optional Protocol to the Convention Against Torture and set up a National Preventative Mechanism. This will enable us to hold our Government to absolute account for these atrocities.

How you can help

Our Community is Everything campaign, launched in June 2015, focuses on the over-representation of Indigenous kids in detention. Sign up now to support the campaign and let Indigenous kids know you stand with them.

Roxanne Moore is a Noongar woman from the South West of Western Australia. She is an Indigenous Rights Campaigner with Amnesty International Australia, and tweets at @RoxyAmnestyOz. This article was published at Amnesty International Australia and is republished with permission.

Australian and NT Governments urged to stop torture and abuse of children in detention

| Author: | Melissa Sweet | Published: | July 25, 2016 |

Thousands of people have signed a petition calling for a Royal Commission into the torture and abuse of children in Northern Territory youth detention centres following horrific footage and revelations on ABC TV's Four Corners program.

And a Turnbull Government Minister, Ken Wyatt, the Assistant Minister for Health, has called for those responsible to be held accountable.

"I am angry, stunned and ashamed that this is happening in our Country and those responsible must be held accountable," he tweeted.

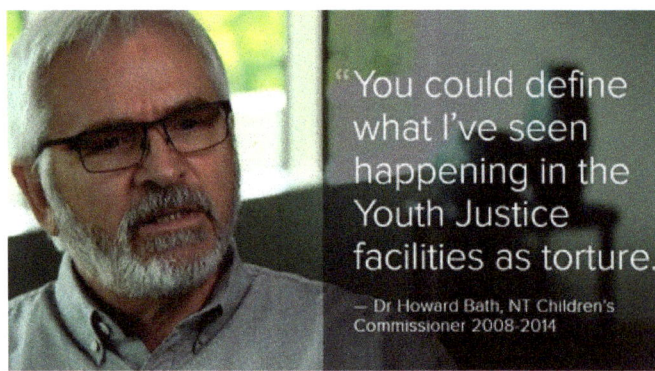

"You could define what I've seen happening in the Youth Justice facilities as torture.
— Dr Howard Bath, NT Children's Commissioner 2008-2014

Dr Howard Bath, former NT Children's Commissioner, on Four Corners

Human Rights Commissioner GillianTriggs called for an independent inquiry into NT juvenile detention in the wake of the "disgraceful" revelations.

(Correction on earlier figures given here. Amnesty figures show: From July 2013 to June 2014 Indigenous young people made up an average of 96 per cent of all young people in detention in the NT (45 out of 47) while comprising around 44 per cent of the population aged between 10 and 17).

Triggs told Q and A that a proper inquiry is needed to determine the facts and "whether people should be charged".

The revelations will put the Prime Minister and Indigenous Affairs Minister Nigel Scullion under renewed pressure to introduce justice targets and to tackle the over-incarceration of Aboriginal and Torres Strait Islander people.

The abuses in the NT are not only down to the Territory Government. The Australian Government's "recalcitrance" in tackling rising rates of incarceration of Aboriginal and Torres Strait Islander people is well documented.

Traumatic footage showed boys being tear-gassed inside their cells, forcibly stripped naked, hooded and strapped to restraining chairs for hours, and isolated in hot, stinking cells for days, without even running water.

Hefty guards were shown holding down the boys, stripping them, assaulting them, and laughing as tear gas was fired into their cells.

A series of legal experts told Four Corners that the treatment amounted to torture, as defined by the United Nations, as well as breaches of the rights of children.

The program also revealed that authorities lied to the public about a so-called riot at the Don Dale detention centre in 2014 (see more details here).

One of the solicitors on the program, Peter O'Brien, has launched an online petition, calling for a Royal Commission to ensure that the perpetrators and responsible institutions are held to account.

Amnesty International has called for the Australian Government to act, to end systemic abuse of children in youth detention.

An Amnesty statement said the abuses shown by Four Corners are a shocking violation of both the UN Convention on the Rights of the Child and the Convention against Torture.

"The Australian Government must immediately launch an investigation into the NT youth detention system, and take action to prevent the abuse of children in youth detention across Australia," the statement said.

It said the issue was a wider problem than the NT, and that Amnesty International is aware of serious allegations about the treatment of children in detention in every state and territory over the past five years.

Amnesty called on the Australian Government to ratify "without delay" the Optional Protocol to the Convention Against Torture, which would ensure independent monitoring of places of detention – including youth detention facilities. The Australian Government has recently claimed ratification of OPCAT is under "active consideration."

Meanwhile, in the run-up to the NT election, a local Making Justice Work coalition has launched this campaign Making Justice Work in the NT_2016 election:

2016 NT ELECTION: SIX ASKS TO MAKE JUSTICE WORK for TERRITORIANS

ask 1 — ABORIGINAL JUSTICE AGREEMENT

Negotiate an Aboriginal Justice Agreement that sets out how the government **and** Aboriginal people will work together to make justice work.

ask 2 — SPECIALIST & THERAPEUTIC COURTS

Commit to establishing and resourcing specialist and therapeutic courts across the Territory's entire justice system.

ask 3 — REHABILITATION & REINTEGRATION

Intensive supervision with community-based services reduced recidivism rates by 18 per cent.

One of the key roles prison must play in our society is rehabilitating people for their return to the community. There needs to be increased funding for rehabilitation, reintegration and employment programs for young people and adults already in the system.

Community-based programs have a greater impact on recidivism than those based in prisons.[i]

i   According to the WSIPP study, the latter reduced recidivism rates by an average of 5–10 per cent, whereas intensive supervision with community-based services reduced recidivism rates by 18 per cent.

ask 4 — REDUCE THE NUMBER OF YOUNG PEOPLE BEING LOCKED UP

The government could employ 3.5 mid-level nurses each year for the same amount it costs to keep one young person in detention.[ii]

The NT locks up young people more often than anywhere else in Australia. Evidence based early childhood programs, like the Nurse Family Partnership Program, have been shown to reduce by more than 75% interactions between young people and the criminal justice system.[iii]

A study by the Australian Institute of Criminology found that young people diverted from the court system were less likely to have further involvement in the criminal justice system.[iv]

ii   See Department of Correctional Services Annual Report 2014-2015.

iii   Tremblay R E, Gervais J, et al. (2008). Early childhood learning prevents youth violence. Montreal, Quebec, Centre of Excellence for Early Childhood Development.

iv   Troy Allard, Anna Stewart, April Chrzanowski, James Ogilvie, Dan Birks and Simon Little, Police Diversion of Young Offenders and Indigenous Over Representation (March 2010) Australian Institute of Criminology.

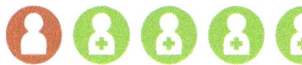

makingjusticework.org.au
@MJW_NT

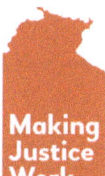

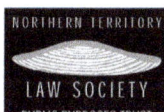

ask 5 — ABOLISH MANDATORY SENTENCING

The government could employ one senior classroom teacher for the same amount it costs to keep one person in prison each year.[v]

Mandatory sentencing does not work to reduce crime or make the community a safer place. Harsher sentences have been shown not to deter offenders.

v   See Department of Correctional Services Annual Report 2014-2015.

ask 6 — COMPREHENSIVE PLAN TO DEAL WITH ALCOHOL

The cost per person of alcohol-related harm in the NT is more than four times the national level.[vi]

Alcohol is a major driving factor behind offending and causes significant harm to our community. The NT needs a comprehensive plan to deal with alcohol – including a review of current laws and policies to identify strengths and shortcomings.

vi   http://www.menzies.edu.au/page/Research/Indigenous_Health/Smoking_alcohol_drugs_and_other_addictive_behaviours/Alcohol/

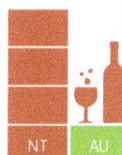

**our rights
our justice
our future**

NORTHERN TERRITORY LAW SOCIETY

Calls for the Royal Commission into NT juvenile justice to have a wide-ranging remit

Author:	Melissa Sweet	Published:	July 26, 2016

Health and justice experts are calling for a wide-ranging examination of Aboriginal and Torres Strait Islander youth justice concerns in the wake of the Prime Minister's announcement of a Royal Commission into abuses in NT systems.

The Prime Minister, Malcolm Turnbull, told ABC radio this morning that he was "shocked and appalled" by the footage aired on ABC TV's Four Corners program last night.

As previously reported at Croakey, thousands of people had signed a petition calling for a Royal Commission into the torture and abuse of children in NT youth detention within hours of the program going to air.

The PM said the Royal Commission would be established as soon as possible, and "the aim will be to have a swift inquiry into the Don Dale Centre with a report as soon as possible". The Commission would also consider "whether there is a culture that spreads across the detention system in the Northern Territory, whether it was specific to that centre". (Read the full transcript of his comments here).

While it is clearly critical that abusive individuals and systems in the NT are held to account, there are suggestions it will be a missed opportunity if the Royal Commission does not examine some of the wider issues, including the need to prevent and reduce incarceration of Indigenous youth in the first place.

Andrew Jackomos, Victoria's Commissioner for Aboriginal Children and Young People, suggested on Twitter this morning that the Royal Commission should look more broadly, into the relationship between First Nations children and justice systems (see his tweets at the bottom of this post).

Senator Patrick Dodson, Labor's shadow assistant minister for Indigenous affairs, called on the Government to take a broader look at the justice system and detention, not just the Don Dale centre.

The Aboriginal and Torres Strait Islander Social Justice Commissioner, Mick Gooda also said the Commission's focus should be wider than the incidents at Don Dale Youth Detention Centre in Darwin.

He said: "It can't be just a royal commission into what happened in Don Dale … I think they've got to look nationally. I think you've got to look at why there are so many of our kids in detention."

As many commentators have noted, the general concerns raised by the Four Corners report are not new or limited to the NT (see this report from Victoria in 2012 about the solitary confinement of children).

The Federal Opposition has issued a statement supporting the Royal Commission, but calling on the Turnbull Government to support the introduction of justice targets through COAG.

Further reaction and comments

Matthew Cooke, Chair of NACCHO, after watching #4corners:

> The treatment of youth imprisoned in the Northern Territory is disgusting and inhumane. The justice system has failed not only the individual but society. Shameful. Sickening.
>
> Government Ministers and Departments should be held to account. How can we expect to have these youth integrated into society after their sentence when they are abused and no doubt scarred for life with mental issues.

Social justice and health advocate, Professor Tom Calma:

> It is deplorable and unacceptable in modern Australia to treat anyone, and especially youth, in a manner shown on Four Corners tonight.
>
> We must treat people with dignity and not in a way that the prison officers trivialised and denigrated the youth at Don Dale.
>
> The system must reform and governments need to invest meaningfully into prevention through Justice Reinvestment initiatives and in in-prison and post release programmes.
>
> If we consider the reasons for the Redress initiative in Queensland we would conclude by suggesting that a redress initiation was needed for Don Dale detainees.

The Royal Commission into Juvenile Detention: a wake up call or a defining moment?

Author:	Ruth Armstrong	Published:	July 27, 2016

Many Australians would have woken yesterday morning after a restless night's sleep, thanks to the disturbing footage of the abuse of teenage boys incarcerated in a Northern Territory Juvenile Detention Centre, aired on Monday night by the ABC's Four Corners program.

The Prime Minister Malcolm Turnbull was up early too: his announcement of "a Royal Commission, in co-operation with the Government of the Northern Territory into the Don Dale Youth Detention Centre" came before breakfast, both in a formal statement and on AM radio. He vowed to "move quickly to finalise Terms of Reference and recommend an eminent person to conduct the inquiry."

As detailed at Croakey, there has been widespread and bipartisan support for the Prime Minister's decision to act on this issue.

The Aboriginal and Torres Strait Islander Social Justice Commissioner, Mick Gooda, captured the collective outrage and mood for urgent remediation, when he told a press conference, "This must be a wake-up call to everyone in Australia. Something has to be done about the way we lock up people in this country, especially our kids."

The distressing scenes depicted in the Four Corners footage have also led to calls for a wider examination of juvenile detention, and the issues which see high rates of incarceration of Aboriginal and Torres Strait Islander youth nationally.

Excerpts from some of the statements emerging from organisations involved in the welfare of young people are posted below. Amidst all the public discussion – and there has been a huge amount of it – there have been several recurring themes, offered here for consideration and further discussion.

What should be the scope and terms of reference of the Royal Commission?

The Prime Minister's initial announcement was that it would be a joint NT/federal Commission into the treatment of children held in the Don Dale Detention Centre, but NT Chief Minister Adam Giles flagged later that, as he and the Federal Attorney General George Brandis worked to negotiate the terms of reference, he would like it to "look at some of the root causes … why children are entering the youth system in the Northern Territory … recognising that there are children who are being neglected, unloved, getting into trouble, causing trouble in the streets, and finding their way into our detention facilities."

The individuals and organisations releasing statements yesterday were in favour of a wide-ranging examination of the NT Juvenile Justice system, with some, including the Change the Record coalition, the National Family Violence Prevention Legal Services and the National Aboriginal Community Controlled Health Organisation (NACCHO) pointing out that the problems were not confined to one Australian Territory, and the Commission should lead to a national examination of both the conditions of juvenile detention and the factors playing into the unacceptably high number of Aboriginal and Torres Strait Islander children and youth in prison.

George Brandis has confirmed his intention that the Royal Commission will be confined to the NT, with "terms of reference sufficiently wide and sufficiently penetrating to get to the bottom of the conduct that was revealed … and the broader question of the extent to which it is systemic conduct in the Northern Territory system…"

Speaking on ABC radio last night, Human Rights Commissioner, Gillian Triggs, proposed a model for a wider inquiry, in which a Royal Commission could respond quickly to the issues at the Don Dale facility and in the Northern Territory, then move to a second phase, "which would be a national inquiry that would get a better sense of just of how diverse the practices are across Australia as a whole".

There is much support for the Royal Commission to encompass a national brief, with the Greens launching a petition today, to extend its remit to all children in prison, including immigration detention. While the Prime Minister reiterated today that it is not his intention to broaden the inquiry, it seems likely that the Commission's reach will continue to be debated in days to come.

What will be needed for the Royal Commission be effective?

The events at Don Dale are a reminder that, 25 years after the Royal Commission into Aboriginal Deaths in Custody, many of the recommendations have not been implemented and young people are still being harmed by the prison system. The Prime Minister has assured us that the Commission will be timely, but its findings will be shaped by the questions it asks.

The Labor party has flagged its interest in helping to shape the Commission, with Senator Patrick Dodson telling ABC AM that he hoped the opposition would be consulted because the matter, "requires bipartisanship in order to give us some confidence that we're not just putting this back in the hands of the political people who are actually running both states, the Commonwealth and the Territory".

Importantly, other organisations, including a coalition of NT Aboriginal organisations and Change the Record and Miwatj Health, have emphasised the need for immediate consultation with Aboriginal and Torres Strait Islander health and community leaders, and the youth justice sector, in developing the terms of reference, and that the Government commit to funding and implementing the Commission's recommendations.

What is the culpability, and what should be the role, of the NT government?

The then NT Minister for Corrections, John Elferink, and NT Chief Minister, Adam Giles, denied specific knowledge of the abuse of children at Don Dale Detention Centre, prior to seeing Monday night's Four Corners footage. Giles has removed Elferink from the portfolio, taking it over himself, but retaining him as Attorney-General and minister for children, families, justice, disability and mental health.

Both men's ignorance is difficult to understand, given that the NT Children's Commissioner had furnished the Government with a report on the problems at Don Dale in August last year, some of the details of which were highlighted in this Croakey #JustJustice article, and which were reported elsewhere in the national and NT media.

Former Chief Justice of the Family Court of Australia, Alastair Nicholson, said yesterday that the NT Government should play no part in the Royal Commission because it was "part of the problem," and will "act as a brake on the freedom of the commission to inquire into what it ought to be inquiring into".

A press release from a coalition of six Northern Territory Aboriginal organisations went further. The group reiterated calls for the NT Government to be excluded from the Commission's process and for local Aboriginal and Torres Strait Islander organisations to be involved in developing the terms of reference, and also called for the federal Parliament to step in to dissolve the NT Government, with spokesperson John Paterson from Aboriginal Medical Services Alliance, Northern Territory saying,

"Any government that enacts policies designed to harm children and enables a culture of brutalisation and cover-ups, surrenders its right to govern."

These sentiments have been echoed by others on social media and on the front cover of today's NT News.

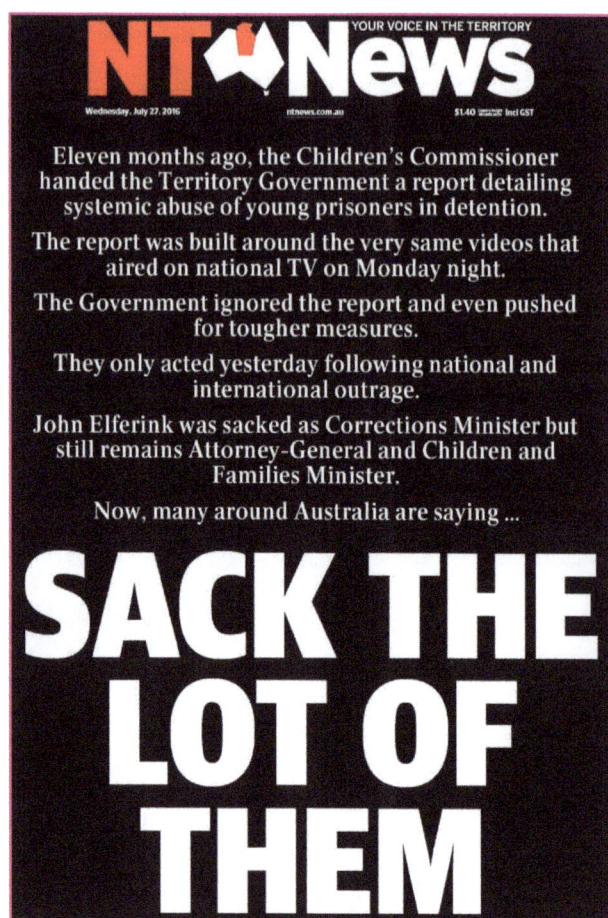

NT News — YOUR VOICE IN THE TERRITORY

Wednesday, July 27, 2016   ntnews.com.au $1.40

Eleven months ago, the Children's Commissioner handed the Territory Government a report detailing systemic abuse of young prisoners in detention.

The report was built around the very same videos that aired on national TV on Monday night.

The Government ignored the report and even pushed for tougher measures.

They only acted yesterday following national and international outrage.

John Elferink was sacked as Corrections Minister but still remains Attorney-General and Children and Families Minister.

Now, many around Australia are saying ...

SACK THE LOT OF THEM

What should happen now, and what else should happen in the longer term?

However quickly it is begun, the Royal Commission will take time to implement change, and it is clear that some things need to happen immediately, especially for the sake of children currently held in juvenile detention.

The Australian Bar Association came up with the following list for a start:

- Immediately commit to building a fit for purpose youth detention facility in the Northern Territory which is to be staffed by appropriately trained personnel.

- Put in place diversion and education programs to prevent youth coming into contact with the justice system in the first place.

- Provide all detainees with access to rehabilitation and education programs to minimise the risk of re-offending and to assist with reintegration back into society.

- Immediately suspend the use of solitary confinement, spit-hoods and mechanical restraints.

The AMA has repeated calls for COAG to introduce a Close the Gap justice target. Others, including the Change the Record Coalition and Amnesty International, have called upon the Australian Government to immediately ratify the Optional Protocol to the Convention Against Torture (OPCAT), which Australia signed in 2009, but has never ratified: Amnesty has collected more than 4000 messages in the past 24 hours, asking the Prime Minister to do so.

The Royal Commission needs to do its work, but what happens in the longer term as a result of our collective "wake-up call" will define us, and make or break us as a nation.

There is a vast wealth of wisdom and knowledge about the solutions to Aboriginal and Torres Strait Islander Youth incarceration, the best of it coming from Aboriginal and Torres Strait Islander peoples and organisations.

As recently as June this year, in the historic, pre-election Redfern Statement (to which the federal government has made no response), Aboriginal and Torres Strait Islander organisations have called for justice targets and funding for a range of strategies to reduce incarceration rates.

Summer May Finlay, who has launched and championed #JustJustice, and is the Public Health Association of Australia Aboriginal and Torres Strait Islander SIG Co-Convener, writes,

> *I am upset, horrified and disgusted. The children in Don Dale and other juvenile justice centres are some of the most vulnerable in Australia.*
>
> *It is outrageous to think that after the report by the NT Children's Commissioner last year that anyone with any responsibility for these children can be blissfully unaware.*
>
> *As a country we have some soul searching to do about our wilful blindness to the treatment of the children who need us the most. We must push for alternatives such as Justice Reinvestment which aims to help kids stay out of detention. We need to hold all governments accountable for ensuring that each and every child in Australia is treated with dignity and respect.*
>
> *We need to make sure that the Royal Commission recommendations aren't put in the too hard basket and implemented because our children are priceless.*
>
> *The Royal Commission Terms of Reference should be national, not just focused on Don Dale.*

The terrible images we saw on Monday night have provided us with a rare moment of clarity, when we can all agree that it is time to end the scourge of young Aboriginal and Torres Strait Islander people being robbed of their liberty, dignity and opportunity by an unfair and heavy handed justice system, and by the circumstances by which they arrive there in the first place.

Calls for reform have been falling on deaf ears for too long.

It is, and should be, a moment of national shame, and of urgency to put things right in the NT and wider juvenile justice system. It is also time to use the knowledge and leadership of the Aboriginal and Torres Strait Islander and other organisations who have been working to expose and solve the problem of over-incarceration of young Aboriginal and Torres Strait Islander people.

The draft terms of reference for the Royal Commission are due to be tabled in the next few days. Now that the Government has been made to take notice we should accept nothing less from them than a commitment to learn what is needed, and do what it takes, to keep kids out of jail.

Statement excerpts, 26/07/2016

NSW Aboriginal Land Council

"Given the shameful over-representation of young Aboriginal people in detention throughout Australia, the Federal Government must consider broadening its investigations to other States and Territories.

Aboriginal families need reassurances that people's basic human rights are being respected in juvenile justice centres in the Northern Territory, New South Wales and other States and Territories.

Unfortunately, Aboriginal people have little faith in the justice system given the inability of governments to tackle increasing imprisonment rates in the 25 years since the Royal Commission into Aboriginal Deaths in Custody.

It's time for governments to work with Aboriginal communities and organisations on alternatives to detention based on education, training, parole support, rehabilitation and community-driven approaches."

NACCHO

"Whilst NACCHO welcomes the swift action of Prime Minister Turnbull, it also hopes that the Royal Commission proceeds with the same immediacy, and delivers answers in a timely fashion."

… This Royal Commission should be the starting point of a wider inquiry that looks at the impacts of detention on mental health, and the devastating suicide rate of the Aboriginal and Torres Strait Island people, particularly young people.

… We need a system that justice system that is best practice and culturally safe for Aboriginal children faced with detention.

Young people should not be risking their lives in detention, and the price they pay for their crimes should not be life long."

AMA

"A Royal Commission will put the spotlight on juvenile justice, and related health issues, and ensure that the inhumane treatment exposed by *Four Corners* never occurs in Australia again.

The AMA Indigenous Health Report Card 2015 – *Treating the high rates of imprisonment of Aboriginal and Torres Strait Islander peoples as a symptom of the health gap: an integrated approach to both* – called on the Australian Government to set a target for closing the gap in the rates of Aboriginal and Torres Strait Islander imprisonment.

"Our Report Card showed clearly that Aboriginal and Torres Strait Islander people are failed by the health and social justice systems in Australia, and the victims are too often young people and teenagers."

Australian Bar Association

" Whilst an independent inquiry into the systemic abuse at the Don Dale centre is necessary, The ABA is calling for immediate action to address the following key issues:

Immediately commit to building a fit for purpose youth detention facility in the Northern Territory which is to be staffed by appropriately trained personnel.

Put in place diversion and education programs to prevent youth coming into contact with the justice system in the first place.

Provide all detainees with access to rehabilitation and education programs to minimise the risk of re-offending and to assist with reintegration back into society.

Immediately suspend the use of solitary confinement, spit-hoods and mechanical restraints."

The Change the Record Coalition

"Prime Minister Turnbull's commitment to establish a Royal Commission to expose the horrific incidences of abuse at Don Dale is a welcome first step. It is vital that those responsible are held to account and that systemic failings are documented and reported back on quickly.

It is also imperative that the terms of reference for the Royal Commission are developed in consultation with the youth justice sector, and that the Federal Government commits to implement all of the recommendations.

The Royal Commission should examine whether these incidences of abuse are more widespread throughout the NT, and the reasons behind the over-representation of Aboriginal and Torres Strait Islander young people in juvenile detention facilities across the country. Nationally, Aboriginal and Torres Strait Islander young people are 24 times more likely to be imprisoned than their non-Indigenous youth.

The CTR Coalition is also calling for the Australian Government to immediately ratify the Optional Protocol to the Convention Against Torture (OPCAT). This would ensure independent monitoring of all places of detention – including youth detention facilities.

We shouldn't be waiting until an inquiry is completed to take steps to prevent to abuse of vulnerable children. OPCAT would provide an important safeguard to protect to the human rights of children, and the Federal Government should act to ratify OPCAT without delay

The Change the Record Campaign has developed a **Blueprint for Change**, which provides a critical roadmap for Government to reduce imprisonment and violence rates."

National Family Violence Prevention Legal Services

"Given the disproportionate representation of Aboriginal and Torres Strait Islander youth within the youth justice system, the establishment of the Royal Commission's Terms of Reference should rely heavily upon engagement with and involvement of Aboriginal and Torres Strait Islander organisations.

The National FVPLS Forum believes the Royal Commission announced today is an initial first step for a broader investigation across all Australian jurisdictions into the treatment of children in juvenile detention and the underlying factors driving engagement with the justice system.

It is imperative a broader inquiry examines the structural disadvantage experienced by Aboriginal and Torres Strait Islander children. Particular consideration should be given to interrelation between family violence, child removal and incarceration. Governments of Australia have to shift from a punitive to a therapeutic approach within the youth justice system."

Australian Council of Social Service (ACOSS)

"ACOSS welcomes the swift action of the Prime Minister in supporting a Royal Commission and urge that he consults with community leaders and stakeholders on the Terms of Reference as a first priority.

In the Northern Territory 96% of those in juvenile detention are Aboriginal or Torres Strait Islander. Nationally, Aboriginal and Torres Strait Islander people make up over 54% of young people in detention.

ACOSS endorses the calls for action by the Northern Territory Council of Social Service for **immediate action that must occur in the Northern Territory**, the call for a Royal Commission, and the call by the Change the Record campaign for Federal leadership to reduce the over-representation of Aboriginal and Torres Strait Islander people in the justice system and end abuse and mistreatment of young people, including by taking immediate steps to:

- Develop terms of reference for the Royal Commission in partnership with Aboriginal and Torres Strait Islander and youth organisations;

- Set targets to reduce the over-representation of Aboriginal and Torres Strait Islander people in the justice system and to reduce violence against Aboriginal and Torres Strait Islander people; and

- Immediately ratify the Optional Protocol for the Convention Against Torture to ensure independent monitoring of all places of detention."

Miwatj Health – Nhulunbuy, East Arnhem Land, NT

" Health institutions have shared with prisons the often deserved mistrust of many Indigenous people who viewed them as another instance of institutionalised racism. To address this, in the 1970s Aboriginal leadership developed the Aboriginal Community Controlled Health Sector. The relevant lessons learned from the past four decades of Aboriginal Community Controlled Health Services are:

- Robust and sustainable Indigenous governance: This can be structured in different ways but needs to be underpinned by accountability to Aboriginal leadership and oversight within culturally appropriate frameworks.

- High levels of Aboriginal employment: The vast majority of the prison population are Indigenous. A significant Indigenous workforce at all levels of the system, from policymakers to frontline staff, is required to reflect the needs of the population it serves.

Aboriginal cultural frameworks embedded in governance and operational structures ensure that Indigenous and non-Indigenous staff share the same values and objectives. This not only will help keep children safe in prison but also will engage in social transformation providing real jobs, with real wages and therefore a reason for kids to stay in school, working upstream to prevent incarceration in the first place.

Yolŋu leadership has demonstrated the effectiveness of this model in East Arnhem Land with improved access to services and better health outcomes within a decade under Miwatj community control. Therefore, we call upon the Australian and Northern Territory Governments to make a real commitment to hold correctional services accountable to Aboriginal communities. Only through ongoing and real commitment to Aboriginal community controlled services more broadly -health, education, legal services- will we advance towards reducing the scourge of Aboriginal incarceration rates."

NT Aboriginal organisations (AMSANT, Danila Dilba, NAAJA, Central Land Council, CAALAS)

A coalition of Northern Territory Aboriginal organisations today called for the federal Parliament to step in to dissolve the NT Government, following the exposure of the NT Government's barbaric abuse of children in detention.

Any government that enacts policies designed to harm children and enables a culture of brutalisation and cover-ups, surrenders its right to govern.

We also urge the Prime Minister to ensure the NT Government plays no role in the development or oversight of the Royal Commission.

It must be entirely independent of the NT Government, and chaired by an appropriate independent expert and must have Aboriginal representation from the NT. Local organisations and those working in this sector must have input into the terms of reference.

The terms of reference must:

- Encompass the entire NT youth justice system, not just issues relating to detention facilities;

- Examine all previous enquiries relating to youth justice in the NT for cover ups and uncover why the recommendations were not implemented.

- Not limit how far into the past the Commission can inquire.

We also call for further immediate interim actions:

- The Commonwealth must appoint an alternative provider of youth detention and child protection/out of home care for the NT. The NT Government cannot continue to deliver these services while our kids remain at risk.

- The youth currently on remand should also be removed from the Darwin and Alice Springs detention facilities immediately and placed in appropriate secure accommodation.

- The office of the NT Children's Commissioner must be appropriately and adequately resourced to perform her statutory duties.

That harm is being done to our children and our community in our name is unacceptable. Those responsible, including ministers, advisers, bureaucrats and corrections employees need to be held to account.

The NT Government has led a concerted and sustained campaign demonising young people and to pass draconian laws inconsistent with recommendations made by successive inquiries, including those of the NT Children's Commissioner.

We are seeking urgent discussions with the Prime Minister to ensure this Royal Commission actually meets the needs of those most affected, and ultimately creates the momentum for reform of the entire youth justice system in the NT."

Dr Ruth Armstrong is an editor at Croakey. With a background in general practice, she worked from 1997-2015 on the editorial team of the Medical Journal of Australia, including as Indigenous Health Editor and Medical Editor and weekly columnist for the MJA's online newsletter, MJA InSight.

More than 100 organisations step up pressure over youth justice Royal Commission

Author:	Open statement from concerned groups	Published:	July 28, 2016

More than 100 organisations (including many health groups) are supporting a call for the Royal Commission into abuses within the NT's youth justice system to take a national approach, independent of the NT Government.

Read their statement below.

"The undersigned organisations strongly welcome Prime Minister Turnbull's Royal Commission into the horrific abuse of children in detention in the Northern Territory, but call for it to be conducted completely independently from the Northern Territory Government and for a broader inquiry into the youth justice system.

The shocking footage revealed in this week's ABC Four Corners episode exposed a broken system, with systemic cruel, inhumane and degrading treatment of children, most of whom were Aboriginal and Torres Strait Islander.

But the issue of over-incarceration of Aboriginal and Torres Strait Islander youth, or mistreatment in detention, is not confined to the Northern Territory.

It is vitally important that a light is now shone on Aboriginal and Torres Strait Islander young peoples' interaction with the youth justice system in each State and Territory jurisdiction.

The Royal Commission should, as a matter of priority, investigate the situation in the Northern Territory, including ensuring those involved in abuse and torture are held to account along with those responsible for the systemic failure.

The terms of reference must be developed in consultation with the Northern Territory Aboriginal organisations and the youth justice sector, and should:

- Encompass the entire Northern Territory youth justice system, not just issues relating to detention facilities;

- Examine all previous enquiries relating to youth justice and investigate why the recommendations were not implemented;

- Not limit how far into the past the Commission can inquire;

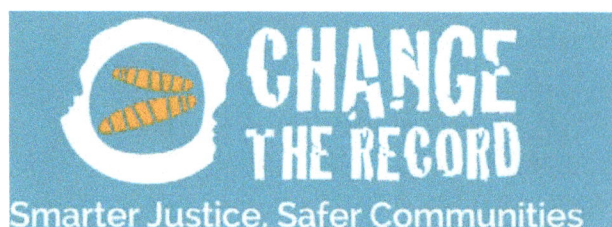

CHANGE THE RECORD
Smarter Justice. Safer Communities

- Ensure the inquiry is completed promptly and that the Government commits to implementing all recommendations;

- Be conducted entirely independently from the Northern Territory Government; and

- Be chaired by an appropriate expert and must have Aboriginal representation from the NT.

As a second step, the Royal Commission must conduct a broader investigation across all Australian State and Territory jurisdictions into the underlying factors driving engagement with the justice system and the treatment of children in juvenile detention.

This could take the form of a separate national inquiry which:

- Examines the drivers of over-representation of Aboriginal and Torres Strait Islander young people in the justice system, including:

  – Social and economic determinants of incarceration including poverty, educational attainment, and health; and

  – Institutional/structural discrimination and racism.

- Considers the interrelation between family violence, child removal, disability, youth suicide and incarceration; and

- Reviews the implementation of the Royal Commission into Aboriginal Deaths in Custody's recommendations.

While it is necessary to shine a comprehensive light on these issues at a national level, government can take steps right now to improve the youth justice system, including:

- Urgent ratification of the Optional Protocol to the Convention Against Torture (OPCAT);

- Raising of minimum age of criminal responsibility to 12;

- Setting meaningful national justice targets through Council of Australian Governments (COAG);

- Developing, through COAG, an intergovernmental approach to tackle imprisonment and violence rates; and

- Investing in effective early intervention, prevention and diversion programs."

Supporting organisations:

1. Aboriginal Alcohol and Drug Services

2. Aboriginal Family Law Services (WA)

3. Aboriginal Family Violence Prevention Legal Service Victoria

4. ACOSS

5. Act for Kids

6. ACTCOSS

7. ACTU

8. Advocacy Law Alliance Inc.

9. African Think Tank Inc

10. Amnesty International Australia

11. Andrew Jackomos, Commissioner for Aboriginal Children and Young People

12. Anglican Social Responsibilities Commission

13. Anglicare SA

14. ANTaR

15. Asylum Seeker Resource Centre

16. Australian College of Midwives

17. Australian Indigenous Doctors' Association

18. Australian Lawyers for Human Rights

19. Australian Physiotherapy Association

20. Australian Youth Action Coalition

21. Autistic Family Collective

22. Barwon Community Legal Service

23. Belconnen Community Service

24. Berry Street

25. Binaal Billa Family Violence Prevention Legal Service

26. Bringing Them Home Committee (WA) Inc.

27. CAAFLU Aboriginal Corporation

28. Castan Centre for Human Rights Law, Monash University

29. Centre for Excellence in Child and Family Welfare

30. Common Grace

31. Community Legal Centres NSW

32. Community Legal Centres Queensland

33. Connecting Home

34. Domestic Violence Victoria

35. Edith Cowan University

36. Elizabeth Evatt Community Legal Centre

37. Families Australia

38. Family Worker Training + Development Programme Inc

39. Federation of Community Legal Centres (Victoria) Inc.

40. First Peoples Disability Network

41. Flemington & Kensington Community Legal Centre Inc. (FKCLC)

42. Healing Foundation

43. Human Rights Law Centre

44. iEmpower

45. Immigration Advice and Rights Centre

46. Indigenous Allied Health Australia Ltd

47. Jumbunna Research Unit, UTS

48. Just Reinvest NSW

49. Justice Reinvestment SA

50. Kingsford Legal Centre

51. Latrobe Valley Bus Lines – Kindred Spirits Foundation

52. Law Council of Australia

53. Life Without Barriers

54. Marrickville Legal Centre

55. MYAN

56. National Aboriginal and Torres Strait Islander Legal Services

57. National Association of Community Legal Centres (NACLC)

58. National Congress of Australia's First Peoples

59. National Ethnic Disability Alliance (NEDA)

60. National FVPLS Forum

61. National Stolen Generations Alliance

62. Northern Rivers Community Legal Centre

63. Northside Community Service

64. NSW Aboriginal Land Council

65. Oxfam Australia

66. People with Disability Australia (PWDA)

67. Plan International Australia

68. Public Health Association of Australia

69. Queensland Aboriginal and Torres Strait Islander Child Protection Peak (QATSICPP)

70. Queensland Advocacy Incorporated

71. Reconciliation WA

72. Refugee Advice and Casework Service

73. SACOSS

74. Save the Children

75. SCALES Community Legal Centre

76. Scarred Tree Ministries of St Johns Anglican Church Glebe

77. Sisters Inside

78. Smart Justice for Young People

79. SNAICC

80. Southern Aboriginal Corporation

81. Sydney Institute of Criminology.

82. Tasmanian Aboriginal Centre

83. The Kimberley Foundation

84. The Youth Junction Inc.

85. Townsville Community Legal Service Inc.

86. UNICEF Australia

87. Uniting

88. Uniting Jaanimili

89. University of South Australia

90. VACCHO

91. VCOSS

92. Victorian Aboriginal Child Care Agency

93. Victorian Aboriginal Children and Young People's Alliance

94. Villamanta Disability Rights Legal Service Inc

95. WA Council of Social Service

96. Winnunga Nimmityjah Aboriginal Health Service

97. Women in Prison Advocacy Network (WIPAN)

98. Women with Disabilities Australia (WWDA)

99. Yarraville Community Centre

100. Yorganop Association Incorporated

101. Youth Advocacy Centre

102. Youth Affairs Council of Victoria

103. Youth Coalition of the ACT

104. Youth Network of Tasmania (YNOT)

105. Youthlaw

106. YouthNow

107. YWCA Canberra

Health and legal groups raise concerns about NT Royal Commission processes

| Author: | Melissa Sweet and statements from various organisations | Published: | July 29, 2016 |

The Government is emphasising its "swift and decisive" action in establishing a Royal Commission into abuse in juvenile justice in the NT – but there are widespread concerns that a lack of proper process will undermine the effectiveness of the Commission.

The Aboriginal Medical Services Alliance NT (AMSANT) is one of three peak NT Aboriginal organisations to have expressed bitter disappointment about the terms of reference and composition of the Royal Commission into the Child Protection and Youth Detention Systems of the Government of the NT.

"Prime Minister Turnbull has comprehensively failed us," AMSANT Chief Executive John Paterson said in a statement issued on behalf of three peak organisations (read full details at the bottom of this post).

"Yet again the Commonwealth Government has refused to consult with Aboriginal people, in spite of Mr Turnbull's commitment, now hollow, to 'do things with Aboriginal people, not to us'.

"We are hurt and furious because, yet again, we have been ignored – this time on the most important matter of the safety of our children."

Other Aboriginal and Torres Strait Islander health leaders – see tweets at the bottom of this post – have also expressed disappointment at the lack of proper consultation and engagement in the processes.

No end of reports and recommendations over the years have stressed the importance of Aboriginal and Torres Strait Islander leadership, whether in addressing over-incarceration or wider health concerns.

When governments fail to enact such advice, they are not only failing to address traumatic situations effectively by utilising the expertise of Aboriginal and Torres Strait Islander people and organisations, but are exacerbating the traumas that many people experience, especially during weeks like this one which revive many personal memories of trauma.

The Australian Lawyers Alliance said the Turnbull Government had missed "a once in a generation opportunity" to deal with the inherent racism of the Australian legal system towards Indigenous people.

The Alliance also queried whether the appointment of former NT Chief Justice Brian Martin was the right choice as Royal Commissioner given the high rates of incarceration of youth and adults, particularly Aboriginal and Torres Strait Islander people, in which the judiciary has played a part.

The Prime Minister announced the Royal Commission will be conducted jointly with the Northern Territory Government and that Martin would investigate:

- failings in the child protection and youth detention systems of the Government of the Northern Territory;

- the effectiveness of any oversight mechanisms and safeguards to ensure the treatment of detainees was appropriate;

- cultural and management issues that may exist within the Northern Territory youth detention system;

- whether the treatment of detainees breached laws or the detainees' human rights; and

- whether more should have been done by the Government of the Northern Territory to take appropriate measures to prevent the reoccurrence of inappropriate treatment.

- The Royal Commission will also make recommendations about legal, cultural, administrative and management reforms to prevent inappropriate treatment of children and young persons in detention, and what improvements can be made to the child protection system.

The announcement followed calls from more than 100 organisations yesterday for the Terms of Reference to examine both specific NT concerns, and to take a wider national focus.

The Government said Royal Commission recommendations and findings were expected to be of use to other jurisdictions when they are considering how their juvenile detention systems can be improved.

Brian Martin has told journalists that racism would be examined as part of his inquiries. Amnesty figures show that from July 2013 to June 2014, Aboriginal and Torres Strait Islander young people made up an average of 96 per cent of all young people in detention in the NT (45 out of 47) while comprising around 44 per cent of the population aged between 10 and 17.

Attorney General George Brandis told ABC radio that the Government had consulted with Aboriginal and Torres Strait Islander Social Justice Commissioner Mick Gooda and Warren Mundine, from its Indigenous Advisory Council. However, the extent of these consultations is not clear.

The Attorney General's comment that the Government didn't hold "some endless public seminar" to consult Indigenous groups on the Royal Commission's scope does not suggest an understanding of the critical importance of ensuring leadership and representation in all processes related to Aboriginal and Torres Strait Islander people.

Gooda later told ABC radio that he had been consulted on the terms of reference of the Royal Commission and had agreed its focus should be on the Northern Territory. He also welcomed that it would examine the underlying causes of over-representation of young Aboriginal people in juvenile justice and consider human rights breaches, which could open up scrutiny on racism.

However he said he wasn't consulted on Martin's selection as Royal Commissioner, and said the government should have at least consulted with Aboriginal Peak Organisations – Northern Territory.

...because at the end of the day, our people have got to have confidence in the process. And at the moment what I'm hearing: there's some lack of confidence in the selection of this person.

This morning Senator Penny Wong suggested the Royal Commission should be extended to include an Indigenous Commissioner.

It's not too late for the Government to respond to concerns, and this suggestion would be a good start.

Also, as many have noted, Governments around the country do not need to wait for the Royal Commission findings to take action to improve the outcomes for Aboriginal and Torres Strait Islander children.

The Lowitja Institute yesterday issued a statement strongly recommending that governments consider Justice Reinvestment so that resources are more effectively spent on services that help young people avoid contact with the criminal justice system in the first place.

"As a society, we must build the pathways to growth, wellbeing and resilience that all children deserve, not allow punishment that destroys," the statement said.

Statement: Royal Commission compromised from the start

Three Northern Territory Aboriginal peak organisations say they are bitterly disappointed that the Prime Minister has ignored their request to be consulted about the terms of reference for the Royal Commission into child protection and youth detention in the Northern Territory, and utterly reject his choice of former NT Chief Justice Brian Martin as the Royal Commissioner.

The organisations are the Northern and Central Land Councils and the Aboriginal Medical Services Alliance NT (AMSANT).

On Tuesday, a wider group (APO NT – Aboriginal Peak Organisations Northern Territory) wrote to Prime Minister Turnbull, seeking an opportunity to comment on the terms of reference and urged him to ensure that the Royal Commission be led by an "independent" expert and include Aboriginal representation from the NT. That wider group included two Aboriginal legal aid agencies, Central Australian Aboriginal Legal Aid Service (CAALAS) and North Australian Aboriginal Justice Agency (NAAJA) which are both unable to comment on today's announcement of the Royal Commission appointment, because they will likely be representing parties before the Commission.

"Prime Minister Turnbull has comprehensively failed us," said AMSANT Chief Executive John Paterson on behalf of the three organisations.

"Yet again the Commonwealth Government has refused to consult with Aboriginal people, in spite of Mr Turnbull's commitment, now hollow, to 'do things with Aboriginal people, not to us'.

"We are hurt and furious because, yet again, we have been ignored – this time on the most important matter of the safety of our children.

"We are also deeply disturbed that NT Chief Minister Adam Giles was party to developing the terms of reference and selecting the Royal Commissioner," Mr Paterson said.

The Aboriginal organisations have challenged the statement by the Prime Minister and his Attorney General that the Royal Commission is independent of government.

"The appointment of Brian Martin does not satisfy any threshold of independence. On the facts and on perception, the appointment is unacceptable," said AMSANT Deputy Chair Olga Havnen.

"Only a few weeks ago Brian Martin delivered to the NT Government a report about the establishment of a regime to investigate corruption, at the instigation of the now disgraced and former NT Corrections Minister, John Elferink. Mr Martin accepted that commission and was paid for it, so how can Mr Turnbull boast his independence from government?

"There are many other eminent former judges around the country who would qualify as truly independent, but the Prime Minister clearly did not canvas that field.

"This appointment is wrong for all manner of reasons, and Aboriginal people in the Territory will not have confidence in the appointment of Brian Martin. As Chief Justice, he sat at the apex of the NT's justice system. He presided over all judicial officers who sentenced young Aboriginal offenders to detention, and he knew them all; he himself sentenced juveniles to detention.

"Worse, although Mr Martin retired as NT Chief Justice in 2010, he was later that same year appointed as an additional judge of the Supreme Court of the Northern Territory and he continues to hold that appointment.

"Finally, we are further upset that the terms of reference are not cast widely enough to include the wider NT youth justice system, rather than a narrow focus on youth detention, and that they do not specify an examination of the huge over-representation of Aboriginal youth in detention.

"Not only does the Northern Territory justice system lock up more juveniles than any other jurisdiction, more than 90 per cent of those detainees are Aboriginal.

"Mr Turnbull has let us down badly," Ms Havnen said.

Statement: Lowitja Institute

The Lowitja Institute welcomes the swift action by the Federal Government in announcing a Royal Commission into Northern Territory juvenile detention in response to the brutal treatment of children detained in the Northern Territory criminal justice system, aired in the ABC Four Corners program on Monday 25 July.

The disturbing revelations show that immediate action must be taken and we welcome the Prime Minister's announcement. We expect that it will result in effective and swift reform of the current youth detention system.

We support the Aboriginal Peak Organisations Northern Territory (APONT) call for the Royal Commission to have independence from the Northern Territory Government, as well as the appointment of Aboriginal Commissioner/s from the Northern Territory. (APO NT's letter to the Prime Minister and media release via AMSANT)

At a more systemic level, however, the program serves to highlight the urgent need to consider alternatives to incarceration for young people, in the Northern Territory and elsewhere in Australia.

As a society, we must build the pathways to growth, wellbeing and resilience that all children deserve, not allow punishment that destroys. We are better than that

Alarming Aboriginal and Torres Strait Islander over-representation in Australian prisons, combined with high rates of recidivism, and an annual government expenditure reaching $3 billion, have led many to claim that incarceration—particularly of young people—is a social policy failure that needs to be redressed. Research commissioned by the Lowitja Institute in 2015 showed that, despite the myth of little sympathy for offenders among the general public—a situation that is often exploited by politicians to perpetuate punitive policies—citizens are open to the idea of alternatives to incarceration, and to the provision of better services and programs that address the social, cultural and economic determinants of crime.

Almost ten years ago in 2007, the Little Children are Sacred Report co-authored by Lowitja Institute Chair, Ms Pat Anderson AO, provided a comprehensive overview of the determinants that impact on Aboriginal individuals, families and communities in the Northern Territory.

Increasingly, the evidence points to the limitations of incarceration as a tool for effective justice, and to the strong link between contact with the criminal justice system and poor health and social outcomes for individuals and families.

As Australia's national institute for Aboriginal and Torres Strait Islander health research, the Lowitja Institute strongly encourages governments to consider adopting Justice Reinvestment. Endorsed by past and current Aboriginal and Torres Strait Islander Social Justice Commissioners, Professor Tom Calma and Mr Mick Gooda, Justice Reinvestment is based on evidence that a large proportion of offenders come from a relatively small number of disadvantaged communities (Social Justice and Native Title Report 2014). Justice Reinvestment impels governments and policymakers to realise the benefits of initiatives that address the health and social determinants of incarceration, rather than continue to implement punitive policies that result in more incarceration, particularly of Aboriginal and Torres Strait Islander Australians.

Imprisonment is expensive: per year, prison beds cost some $100,000 for adults and some $200,000 in youth justice. Rates of incarceration and recidivism, let alone abuses such as illustrated by the Four Corners program demonstrate that these public monies are misdirected. The Lowitja Institute strongly recommends that governments consider Justice Reinvestment so that resources are more effectively spent on services that help young people avoid contact with the criminal justice system in the first place.

As a society, we must build the pathways to growth, wellbeing and resilience that all children deserve, not allow punishment that destroys. We are better than that.

Resources

Download this position statement

APO NT's letter to the Prime Minister and media release via AMSANT

Simpson, P., Guthrie, J., Lovell, M., Walsh, C. & Butler, A. 2014, Views on Alternatives to Imprisonment: A Citizens Jury Approach, The Lowijta Institute, Melbourne

Northern Territory Board of Inquiry into the Protection of Aboriginal Children from Sexual Abuse 2007, Little Children are Sacred: Report of the Northern Territory Board of Inquiry into the Protection of Aboriginal Children from Sexual Abuse, Northern Territory Government, Darwin

Aboriginal and Torres Strait Islander Social Justice Commissioner, Social Justice and Native Title Report 2014, Australian Human Rights Commission, Sydney.

Statement: Australian Lawyers Alliance

The Australian Lawyers Alliance said today that the Turnbull Government had missed a once in a generation opportunity to deal with the inherent racism of the Australian legal system towards Indigenous people.

The Alliance also queried whether the appointment of former Northern Territory (NT) Chief Justice Brian Martin was the right choice at Royal Commissioner given the high rates of incarceration of youth and adults, particularly Indigenous people, in which the judiciary has played a part.

ALA Spokesman Greg Barns said that Mr Turnbull should have heeded widespread community opposition to his view that a Royal Commission into NT youth detention ought to be narrowly focused.

"Youth detention is an outmoded concept and is particularly damaging for Indigenous Australians, as we know. There are thousands of Indigenous young people who are entrenched in the youth detention system across Australia. The revelations of what is happening in the NT should have resulted in a broad Royal Commission. The risk now is that mistreatment and abuse in other parts of Australia will continue, out of sight and out of mind of the narrow Royal Commission in the NT", said Mr Barns.

The ALA also queried the appointment of former NT Chief Justice Brian Martin as Royal Commissioner. "While Mr Martin has had a distinguished career and no doubt has insight into the NT justice system, it would have been preferable to draw upon the expertise and wisdom of a retired judicial officer without this connection to the NT. Detention of young people in the NT has been sanctioned by the courts there, including by Mr Martin and his colleagues. While we have no doubt as to Mr Martin's utmost integrity,

having a former Chief Justice of the NT Supreme Court as the Commissioner opens the inquiry up to perceptions of a conflict of interest.

"It is advisable to also appoint a prominent expert in youth justice matters and Indigenous elders and experts to work with Mr Martin. Youth justice is highly specialised and there are a number of eminent practitioners and judicial officers with that experience. Their input into this Royal Commission is crucial.

"Further, to ensure this commission wins the respect of the Indigenous community and is able to adequately respond to its concerns, engagement of Indigenous elders and experts will be essential," Mr Barns said.

Indigenous groups welcome Gooda, White to lead NT Royal Commission

Author:	Marie McInerney	Published:	August 01, 2016

Indigenous and mainstream justice and rights leaders welcomed the appointment of Aboriginal and Torres Strait Islander Social Justice Commissioner **Mick Gooda** and former Queensland Supreme Court Justice **Margaret White** to lead the Royal Commission into abuse in juvenile justice in the Northern Territory.

The appointments followed the resignation of former Northern Territory Chief Justice **Brian Martin** whose appointment to head the inquiry was widely criticised for lack of consultation with NT Indigenous groups and concern about his past role.

Marie McInerney writes:

National Congress of Australia's First Peoples Co-Chairs **Rod Little** and **Dr Jackie Huggins** said the appointment of Gooda was a "wise choice" that showed the Federal Government was "finally starting to listen to our people". See their full statement.

Huggins said:

It is also great to see that we have a balance of gender and racial expertise. Hopefully this will help ensure some equity in the investigations and the final report.

Little added:

I see this as the first step taken by this government in resetting the relationship with the First Peoples of Australia. Hopefully, they will continue to listen and together we can work through some of the issues and concerns facing my people.

The Change the Record (CTR) Coalition, which campaigns to address over-representation of Aboriginal and Torres Strait Islander people in prisons, also welcomed the Federal Government's "change of heart" on the makeup of the Royal Commission following Martin's resignation.

It said in a statement that the appointment of Gooda "will likely restore the faith lost in the Royal Commission by many Aboriginal and Torres Strait Islander leaders."

CTR Co-Chair Shane Duffy said.

Mr Gooda is a well-respected member of the Aboriginal community and his strong experience in health, law and human rights will enable him to put the Royal Commission back on track.

In a joint statement, Prime Minister Malcolm Turnbull and Attorney General George Brandis said the Federal Government acknowledged the importance of having Indigenous voices on the Commission given the high number of Aboriginal and Torres Strait Islander children incarcerated in the Northern Territory detention system and who are involved in the child protection system. They said:

Over the course of the last week, the Government has been speaking with Indigenous leaders, members of the community and justice advocates.

We have listened, and we have responded.

National Aboriginal and Torres Strait Islander rights advocacy organisation **ANTaR** also welcomed Gooda's appointment, but said it was shocked that the appointment of an Aboriginal Commissioner hadn't been considered at the outset, particularly given Turnbull's earlier vow to do things 'with' Indigenous people not 'to' them. Its statement said:

The process last week flew in the face of that commitment and the government needs to urgently establish good engagement from the start of its term.

'One of Australia's most highly regarded Indigenous leaders'

Gooda is a Gangulu man from Central Queensland who was appointed as Social Justice Commissioner in 2010, and is a current member of the Referendum Council on Constitutional Recognition of Aboriginal and Torres Strait Islander peoples. He was previously chief executive officer of the Cooperative Research Centre for Aboriginal Health and a senior consultant to the Aboriginal Legal Service of Western Australia.

Brandis said Gooda is well known as one of Australia's most highly regarded Indigenous leaders.

He has the respect of both sides of politics, as is evident from the fact he was appointed as the Aboriginal and Torres Strait Island Social Justice Commissioner by a Labor Government and reappointed by the Coalition Government.

With Huggins, Gooda has led the Close the Gap campaign to raise the health and life expectancy of Aboriginal and Torres Strait Islander people to that of the non-Indigenous population by 2030.

He is also a passionate advocate on Indigenous justice issues and vowed to make the over-incarceration of Aboriginal and Torres Strait Islander peoples a priority issue for the remainder of his term as Social Justice Commissioner. He has been a generous supporter of Croakey's #JustJustice campaign, describing Indigenous over-incarceration as a "public health catastrophe".

You can also see his initial response as Social Justice Commissioner to the brutal treatment of children detained in the Northern Territory criminal justice system, aired in the ABC Four Corners program last Monday 25 July, which sparked the Royal Commission.

#JustJustice team member, public health practitioner and Yorta Yorta woman **Summer May Finlay** said Gooda was a "fantastic choice" as Royal Commissioner and a strong advocate in the justice space whose appointment "is a sign the Government has paid attention to Aboriginal people".

Announcing Gooda's Co-Commissioner, Attorney-General **George Brandis** said former Queensland Supreme Court Justice Margaret White was "highly regarded among the judiciary and the legal profession throughout Australia".

According to this ABC profile, White was admitted as a barrister of the Supreme Court of Queensland in 1978, and acted as junior counsel for the Queensland Government in the landmark Mabo case. She was the first woman to be appointed as a Justice of the Supreme Court of Queensland in 1992, serving for more than 20 years.

Brandis told journalists White is long practiced in the conduct of forensic proceedings, including commission proceedings.

Still concerns but groups hail Martin's 'courageous' decision

Change the Record Co-Chair Antoinette Braybrook said the group still had concerns over the involvement of the NT Government in creating the terms of reference for the Royal Commission into the Child Protection and Youth Detention Systems of the Northern Territory, and their involvement going forward.

However, she hoped the Royal Commission created the necessary conditions for positive change and that its recommendations were fully implemented.

This Royal Commission cannot be ignored like the Royal Commission into Aboriginal Deaths in Custody.

We also hope that the Federal Government recognises that the Royal Commission provides an important opportunity for Federal and State/Territory Governments to take action on underlying factors driving the over-imprisonment of Aboriginal and Torres Strait Islander people nationally.

The creation of closing the gap targets on both incarceration and community safety through COAG, and investment in early intervention, prevention and diversion programs designed and implemented by Aboriginal and Torres Strait Islander communities, would lead to the necessary mechanisms to address this national crisis.

As previously reported at Croakey, there were widespread concerns that a lack of proper process, and particularly a lack of proper consultation with Aboriginal and Torres Strait Islander groups, would undermine the effectiveness of the Royal Commission, with bitter disappointment about both its terms of reference and composition.

Opposition Leader **Bill Shorten** called on the weekend for two Indigenous Co-Commissioners to be appointed to join Martin, with Aboriginal Labor Senator **Pat Dodson** saying:

Justice has to be done and has to be seen to be done.

Ahead of the new appointments today, NT Aboriginal peak organisations had welcomed the news that Commissioner Martin was stepping down and thanked him for a "courageous and difficult decision". Spokesperson **John Paterson** said:

We appreciate these past few days must have been a stressful time for him and his family and we commend his action in the face of the controversy that has surrounded the issue.

We welcome his acknowledgement that his decision has been made foremost in the best interests of our children who are the subject of this inquiry.

We wish to make it clear that his stepping down in no way reflects on his standing or capacity and we acknowledge his distinguished legal career.

The peak group, APO NT – Aboriginal Peak Organisations Northern Territory, called on the Federal Government to consult with them on any further appointments, which they said must include strong Aboriginal Co-Commissioners and come from outside of the NT justice system.

Croakey will update this post with their and further responses to the new appointments.

The Australian Human Rights Commission farewelled Gooda today, saying his appointment was fitting, given the wide breadth of the Royal Commission's terms of reference which extend to international law. President Professor **Gillian Triggs** said:

The Commission has no doubt Justice White and Mr Gooda will bring much needed perspective and experience to the Royal Commission.

Mick is a great Indigenous leader who brings a powerful voice to those who need it most.

NT's Don Dale footage: the end result of a 'tough on crime' approach to children

| Author: | Liana Buchanan and Andrew Jackomos | Published: | August 03, 2016 |

Shocking images from the Don Dale detention centre broadcast on the ABC's Four Corners late last month finally sparked a Royal Commission to investigate abuses of children in the Northern Territory juvenile justice system.

Meanwhile, Victoria has seen dramatic media headlines, talk of the need for vigilante-style groups, and demands for tougher responses to "lawless thugs" in the wake of a high profile number of violent break-ins and car-jackings by young people in Melbourne.

It is important that we draw a link between these two sets of stories, say Liana Buchanan, Victoria's Principal Commissioner for Children and Young People, and Andrew Jackomos, Commissioner for Aboriginal Children and Young People, in this article which is published as part of Croakey's #JustJustice series. They warn:

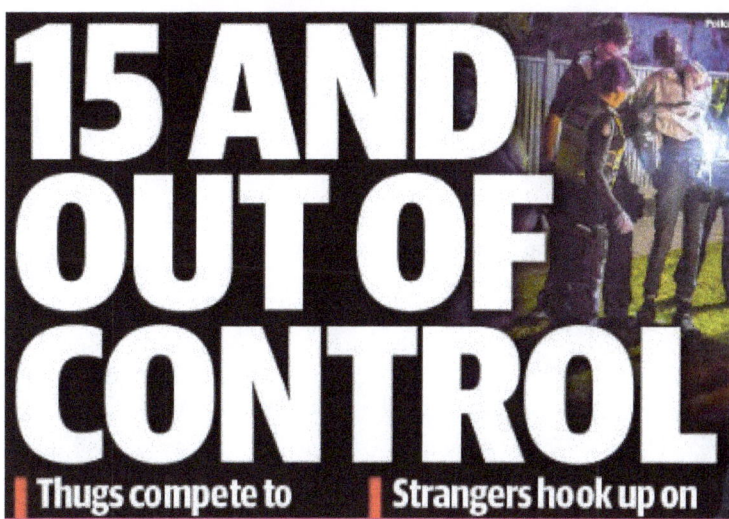

Part of the Herald Sun's front cover - Tuesday, July 19, 2016

"We have to recognise the kind of mistreatment that we watched with distress from the Northern Territory shows us the potential consequence of an overly simplistic, punitive approach to youth crime. It shows us what can happen when we demonise young offenders and ignore what causes them to offend."

Liana Buchanan and Andrew Jackomos write:

The stories about the abuse of children in custody in the Northern Territory are devastating. The footage aired last Monday night showed children being tear-gassed without cause, a child stripped naked and held down by multiple adult men, and the same child left hooded and restrained for hours in the kind of contraptions we associate with Guantanamo Bay. These images have shocked us to the core, and rightly so.

Here in Victoria, we have had several months of media focus on young offenders involved in serious crime. This coverage and the incidents described have resulted in significant community alarm. We have heard reports of neighbourhood groups gathering to keep watch for "young thugs" and sports stores in parts of Melbourne selling out of baseball bats as concerned citizens prepared to take justice into their own hands. Meanwhile news headlines, talkback radio and letters pages have been filled with descriptions of the teenage "monsters" responsible for these crimes and calls for a tougher, harsher approach to young offenders.

We have to connect these two sets of stories. We have to recognise the kind of mistreatment that we watched with distress from the Northern Territory shows us the potential consequence of an overly simplistic, punitive approach to youth crime. It shows us what can happen when we demonise young offenders and ignore what causes them to offend.

A simplistic approach to youth crime focuses on how we feel in response to the crimes committed. This is understandable. Many of the incidents we have heard about in recent months are serious, violent incidents with long-term impact on the victims. That is important and we have to respond to the severity of the incidents and their impact. We also have to focus on what will actually stop this behaviour, rather than being driven exclusively by desire for retribution and punishment.

The evidence shows that locking kids up actually increases the likelihood they'll go on to commit more serious offences, in turn entrenching them in a possible lifetime of crime.

A harsh, punitive approach to the young offenders we detain is also counterproductive. This week we saw evidence of the

Northern Territory's hard line approach to young offenders. The Northern Territory also has the highest youth offending rate in the country. A tough approach doesn't stop kids from offending in the first place and it certainly doesn't stop them reoffending after they leave custody.

This is because a tough approach doesn't address the reasons young people are getting involved in crime in the first place. Two-thirds of children in Victorian youth justice centres are known to child protection, one third have mental health issues and we're 12 times more likely to lock up Koori children than non-Koori children.

The bottom line is many of these children have themselves already been victims of the worst society has to throw at them. When they offend, we need to tackle the causes and support them to turn around, not compound these causes by exposing them to more abuse.

We know nine out of 10 Koori children in out-of-home care are traumatised by family violence. High figures also apply for non-Koori kids. Too many make their way into the criminal justice system. These children need the right services and supports to recover from the trauma they have lived through.

The recent Youth Summit hosted by Victoria's Chief Commissioner of Police identified that we need to invest in youth workers as much as we need to invest in police, that we need to do better at keeping kids engaged in education and we need to strengthen community-based programs to build social inclusion and stop kids feeling their only path to "success" and belonging is through crime.

We need to invest more in diversionary programs. For those kids who do end up in custody, we need to use that opportunity to make sure they do not return.

We have to make sure time in custody is focused on rehabilitation. That principle underpins the approach to youth justice in this state and is enshrined in legislation. Correspondingly Victoria has always had, and still has, one of the lowest youth offending rates in the country.

Thankfully, Victoria's youth custody system does not feature the brutalities we have seen in footage from the Northern Territory. Nonetheless, independent scrutiny of closed environments where children are held is always important.

Independent oversight bodies play a critical role in monitoring youth custody, calling out abuse when they see it, and recommending action to improve the system.

In Victoria, the Commission for Children and Young People provides that scrutiny. Established in 2013 as an independent body with a mandate that includes youth justice, the Commission's capacity to monitor youth justice was strengthened earlier this year when the Victorian Government passed legislation to ensure we have visibility of all serious incidents in youth custody.

As independent Commissioners, we are proud to work in a state that values transparency in the way we treat our most vulnerable.

The bottom line is many of these children have themselves already been victims of the worst society has to throw at them

Using our mandate, we run a program of community visitors who speak to children and young people in youth custody and report on their treatment, conduct ongoing monitoring activities and hold exit interviews with children leaving custody. The Commission has recently initiated a systemic inquiry into the use of isolation, separation and lockdowns in youth justice centres in Victoria and we are also inquiring into an incident of restraint causing injury to a child.

The same transparency is needed for children across Australia. The Prime Minister's quick action on a Royal Commission into the Northern Territory custody issues is to be applauded, but it will not be effective if the recommendations are not acted upon. Our counterpart in the Northern Territory reported publicly on youth justice abuses in September 2015, long before the footage aired on Monday night. In 1991 the Royal Commission into Aboriginal Deaths in Custody handed down recommendations, many of which – 25 years later – have not been funded and implemented. Political will and community concern are vital in driving change.

This week we have seen Australians' reaction to the brutality exposed in the media. This has resulted in the establishment of a royal commission. Community sentiment makes a difference.

We need to continue to express our disgust when we learn of abuse against children and young people and to speak up for those who do not have a voice. We also need to remember that a purely punitive, tough-on-crime response to youth offending can lead to unacceptable and shocking mistreatment of children, as well as being ineffective in making our community safer.

See the Commissioners' website.

Kennett's comments on Don Dale: a personal opinion or beyond conscionable?

Author:	Ruth Armstrong	Published:	August 18, 2016

An Aboriginal and Torres Strait Islander trauma expert has called into question the fitness of former Victorian Premier Jeff Kennett to head one of Australia's most visible mental health awareness and support organisations.

On National Indigenous Radio, Robert Eggington, head of Nyoongah trauma support service at Dumbartung Aboriginal Corporation, called for Kennett's "immediate termination" as Chair of beyondblue, amidst disquiet from Indigenous health advocates about where he and the organisation stand on the mental health needs of children in the juvenile justice system.

Eggington's comments came after Kennett, beyondblue's founding Chair, told attendees at the Country Liberal Party's Northern Territory election campaign launch on Sunday, that the ABC's Four Corners program on the abuse of detainees at Darwin's Don Dale youth detention centre was "unbalanced" and politically motivated.

Former Victoria Premier Jeff Kennett

Kennett also told ABC radio in Darwin that the political response to the Four Corners report – the announcement of a Royal Commission into the NT Child Protection and Youth Detention Systems – was unprofessional.

On Tuesday he reiterated his comments in an opinion article in Melbourne's Herald Sun, and expanded in his concerns about unbalanced reporting and the timing of the program's screening. He concluded the article with the disclaimer, "These comments are my own and not those of beyondblue."

ABC staff involved in the Four Corners report have denied bias, saying the program's screening was not timed for the election, and that the NT Government was given a fair right of reply with then-Corrections Minister John Elferink nominating himself as the sole representative of the Government for the program.

beyondblue responded to enquiries and comments about Mr Kennett's statements on Twitter, with a repeating series of three tweets;

> *As Mr Kennett has made clear publicly, his views on the Don Dale Detention Centre reports & Royal Commission were his own...1/3*
>
> *Mr Kennett's comments were made in a private capacity. 2/3*

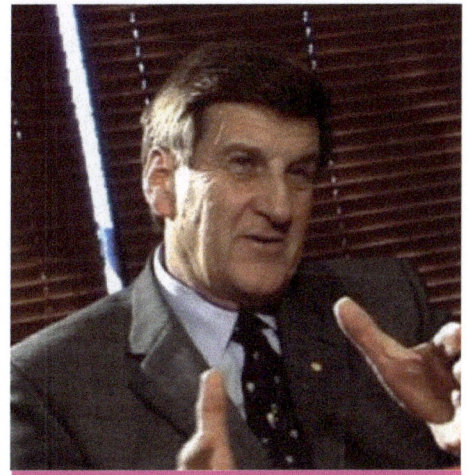

> *beyondblue advocates for protecting the mental health & wellbeing of all Australians on the principle of 'first do no harm' /3*

The organisation has recently been working to raise awareness of the mental health effects of racism on Aboriginal and Torres Strait Islander people with their Invisible Discriminator campaign, but has made no public comment about the allegations of abuse on the NT juvenile justice system or the need for a Royal Commission.

Dr Chelsea Bond, Senior Lecturer in Aboriginal and Torres Strait Islander Studies at the University of Queensland, told Croakey that beyondblue's response to criticisms of its Chair's airing of a personal opinion in a very public forum, and silence on the substantive issues raised by the Don Dale allegations was of concern.

She said:

> *beyondblue's silence about the Don Dale abuse, coupled with the defence of their Chairperson, Mr Kennett who stated that the ABC report was a political issue which attacked prison workers, rather than a mental health issue that harmed Aboriginal children, is deeply disturbing.*
>
> *As an organisation that has insisted that we all #BeTheChange in relation to racial discrimination and mental illness, it was astounding to me, that they would be so indifferent to the mental health needs of Aboriginal*

children in detention. It would appear that much of their advocacy work in relation to the Don Dale abuse has been to advocate for their Chairperson's right to dismiss the reporting of such abhorrent abuse.

That beyondblue has the resources to individually reply to a wide range of Indigenous and non-Indigenous individuals, advocates and health professionals to defend their Chairperson, tells us as much about them as an organisation as it does their Chairperson.

Indeed, Mr Kennett has the right to dismiss the mental health needs of Aboriginal children, but as Chairperson of beyondblue, it is just not right.

A spokesperson for beyondblue told Croakey that there would be no further response to the criticisms of Mr Kennett, beyond the statements already made on Twitter.

12. Time for Action

> *Hearing is the physical act of being able to hear, and listening is the part where you pay attention to what is being said*

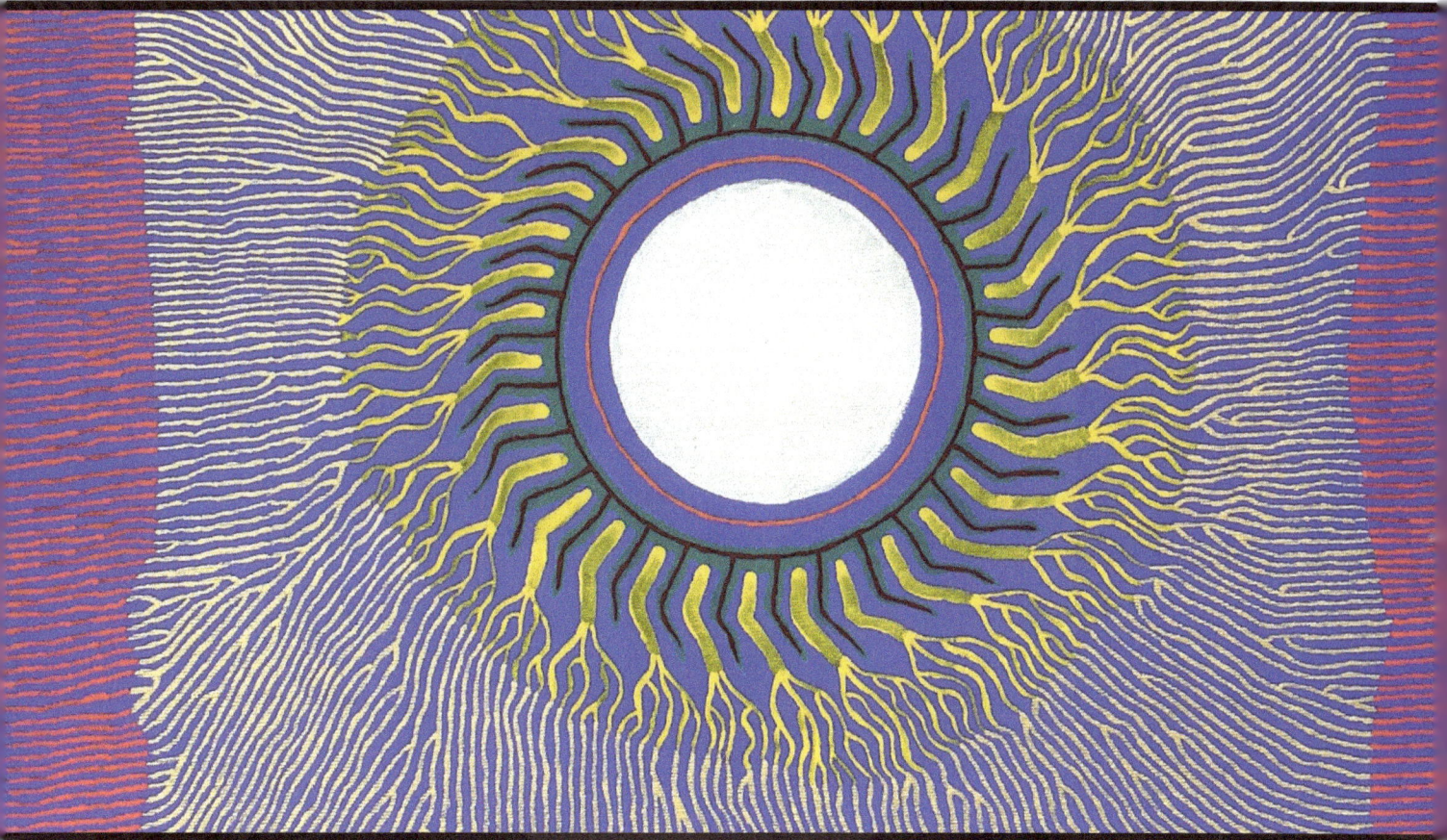

Calling for action on the related traumas of suicide and over-incarceration

Author:	Pat Dudgeon	Published:	January, 2017

Efforts to stop the over-incarceration of Aboriginal and Torres Strait Islander people need to be informed by the same principles that should inform suicide prevention work, according to Professor Pat Dudgeon, a Bardi woman and a leading psychologist.

These principles include respect for human rights, community control and empowerment, holistic understandings of health that incorporate spirituality, culture and healing, and a focus on sustainable, strength-based capacity building.

Dudgeon, Indigenous National Mental Health Commissioner and leader of the **Aboriginal and Torres Strait Islander Suicide Prevention Evaluation Project** (ATSISPEP), made these recommendations in a keynote address to the Northern Territory Tony Fitzgerald Human Rights Awards in Darwin, on Larrikia Country.

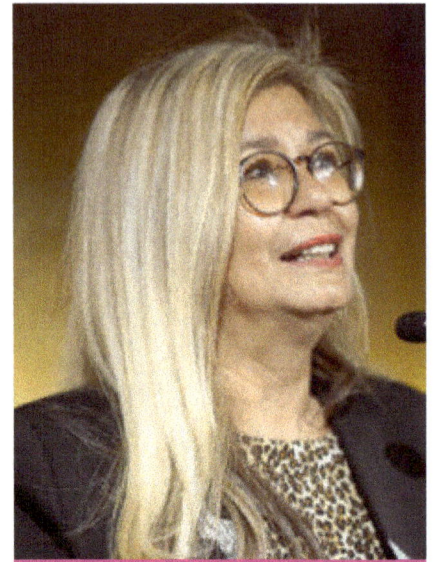

Professor Pat Dudgeon

Her speech came on the same day that the Australian Human Rights Commission's **Social Justice and Native Title Report 2016** was released, urging the Australian Government, "as a matter of urgency", to support the development of justice targets, Justice Reinvestment initiatives and other evidence-based state and territory legislative, administrative and service delivery initiatives to reduce Indigenous incarceration rates.

An edited version of the speech follows below.

Pat Dudgeon writes:

Although I live and work in beautiful Noongar country in Perth, my people are from the Kimberley on the north coast of Western Australia. I was born and raised in beautiful Larrikia country, here in Darwin, so I feel that I have a special connection here as well.

I am especially delighted to be here to honour those who have worked towards human rights. As an Indigenous woman, I have a strong commitment towards social justice and have worked towards this all my life.

We live in a fair minded and civil society – Australia is a progressive society and, certainly over my lifetime, there have been massive changes for the better. But for my people and me, the struggle for social justice and recognition will go beyond our lifetimes.

I commend those who are committed to making positive social changes. I also pay respects and acknowledge those whose human rights we work for. They are not passive victims but desire their own self-determination and come to the table with great strengths and enrich our shared society.

With this in mind, I would like to do two things in the words that follow. I will briefly acknowledge those who have gone before us and share a project that I am part of in my work.

This year, there was a memorial function for the late Rob Riley, to mark the 20th year anniversary of his death. Rob Riley's life and times symbolised the injustices that were perpetrated upon Australia's Indigenous people. He suffered the pain of being stolen from his family as a baby; he was institutionalised and grew up in a racist society. He was a child victim of the Stolen Generations and was taken from his mother as a baby in 1955 and placed in Sister Kate's Children's Home.

Rob Riley was a significant political activist and leader of Aboriginal Australia. I understand that he and Tony Fitzgerald were colleagues and admired each other. He influenced politics and policy in unprecedented ways and he was a voice representing Indigenous diversity at many levels. He was respected across all areas, from the remote outback, urban centres, to the halls of power in Canberra.

He held many important official positions such as the director of the Aboriginal Legal Service Western Australia; he was a key figure in the Royal Commission into Black Deaths in Custody, and instigated the Inquiry into the Stolen Generations, and held key positions such as advisor to the office of the Commonwealth Minister for Aboriginal Affairs. The influence of his activism includes most of the major struggles of Aboriginal politics since the 1970s to his death in 1996.

Worn down by endless struggles for equality with changing governments, both at state and federal levels, who failed to deliver on promises, and beset by his own personal demons as a consequence of his institutionalisation, he took his life 20 years ago.

He left too early but he left a legacy for us. He said:

"*Aboriginal people have great strengths including creativity, endurance, humour, compassion and spirituality. These characteristics of Aboriginal people have enabled their survival through the period of dispossession and oppression... This has helped us (Aboriginal peoples) through the worst of times.*

They will go on sustaining us until, with your understanding and support and commitment, we are ready and able to enjoy with all Australians, the best of times.

Finally, I say to you, two thoughts that I keep in the back of my mind when the struggle along the road to social justice and equity gets a bit tough:

You can't be wrong if you're right, and,

You don't stop fighting for justice simply because those around you don't like it. Just keep on fighting.

Although I propose this from an Indigenous perspective - it is a truth for all the marginalised, different and oppressed groups who make up our society. We have struggles and we have great riches to share with each other.

I work in Indigenous suicide prevention. We have just finished the national Aboriginal and Torres Strait Islander Suicide Prevention Evaluation Project Report, **Solutions that work: what the evidence and our people tell us**, that was launched in Parliament House in Canberra.

This signified the end of two years work – some of this included holding roundtables around the country and speaking with Aboriginal and Torres Strait Islander people about what they thought the solutions needed to be.

The summary of this work told us that:

- Poverty, disadvantage, unemployment, racism, lack of housing/overcrowding, transgenerational trauma and

issues around incarceration contribute to Aboriginal and Torres Strait Islander suicides.

- What they told us also reminded us of the history of colonisation and how it has contributed to the present situation.

- All the roundtables and the literature and program reviews emphasised the importance of culture and identity, the need for local leadership in determining problems and finding the solutions.

- The people who contributed to the report were concerned that many programs and services were not culturally relevant. Self-determination was needed.

Our recommendations included:

Community control and empowerment: projects should be grounded in community, owned by the community, based on community needs and accountable to the community.

Holistic: based on Aboriginal and Torres Strait Islander definitions of health incorporating spirituality, culture and healing.

Sustainable, strength based and capacity building: projects must be sustainable, both in terms of building community capacity and in terms of not being 'one off'; they must endure until the community is empowered.

Partnerships: projects should work in genuine partnerships with local Aboriginal and Torres Strait Islander stakeholders and other providers to support and enhance existing local measures not duplicate or compete with them.

Safe cultural delivery: projects should be delivered in a safe manner.

Innovation and evaluation: projects need to build on learnings, try new and innovative approaches, share learnings, and improve the evidence base.

There are similarities with our work in suicide prevention and with the youth and incarceration in the Northern Territory - particularly the Royal Commission into Youth Detention.

Both have attracted much media attention. Both suicide and youth incarceration are the tips of icebergs of larger suffering and issues and the demand for greater changes to be made.

There needs to be upstream population health approaches that empower and increase resilience, so that youth are not becoming incarcerated or taking their lives.

But these long-term investments and immediate actions need to take place simultaneously.

At the hard end – in immediate intervention – things need to be done differently. For suicide prevention, this requires recognition of cultural differences and working in partnership with communities. This can make programs and services much more effective with better outcomes.

With youth incarceration, there are different views about what has happened and what needs to happen in the future. But from the information we have, from the event of establishing a Royal Commission to investigate the situation, we know that something is broken and it needs to be fixed.

When I saw the media images of youths being restrained, it had a great impact on me.

I know the situation is not simple, but I know that if we treat people like monsters – then they will become monsters. Yet, the greatest cost is to us as a society: we become monstrous ourselves.

So, we need to challenge ourselves and the way we do things, the way we see things.

This is about human rights and how we uphold and practise this in every part of our society and at every level - from policy, practices in programs and services and in our everyday lives - the attitudes we have and the behaviours we do.

We have to ask ourselves: what kind of world do we want our children and grand children to live in?

I know that I want to live in a world where each person is valued, and where the inherent dignity of all members of the human family is the foundation of freedom, justice and peace in the world.

This means – as we heard in our community consultations for the ATSISPEP report – that we need to do much more to "keep out of prison those who should not be there".

Our report has given governments and communities clear advice on the ways forward to tackle the related traumas of suicide and over-incarceration. It is time for action.

Professor Pat Dudgeon, from the Bardi people of the Kimberley, a psychologist and academic at the University of Western Australia, chairs the ATSISPEP project.

Malcolm Turnbull, I hope you have your listening ears on

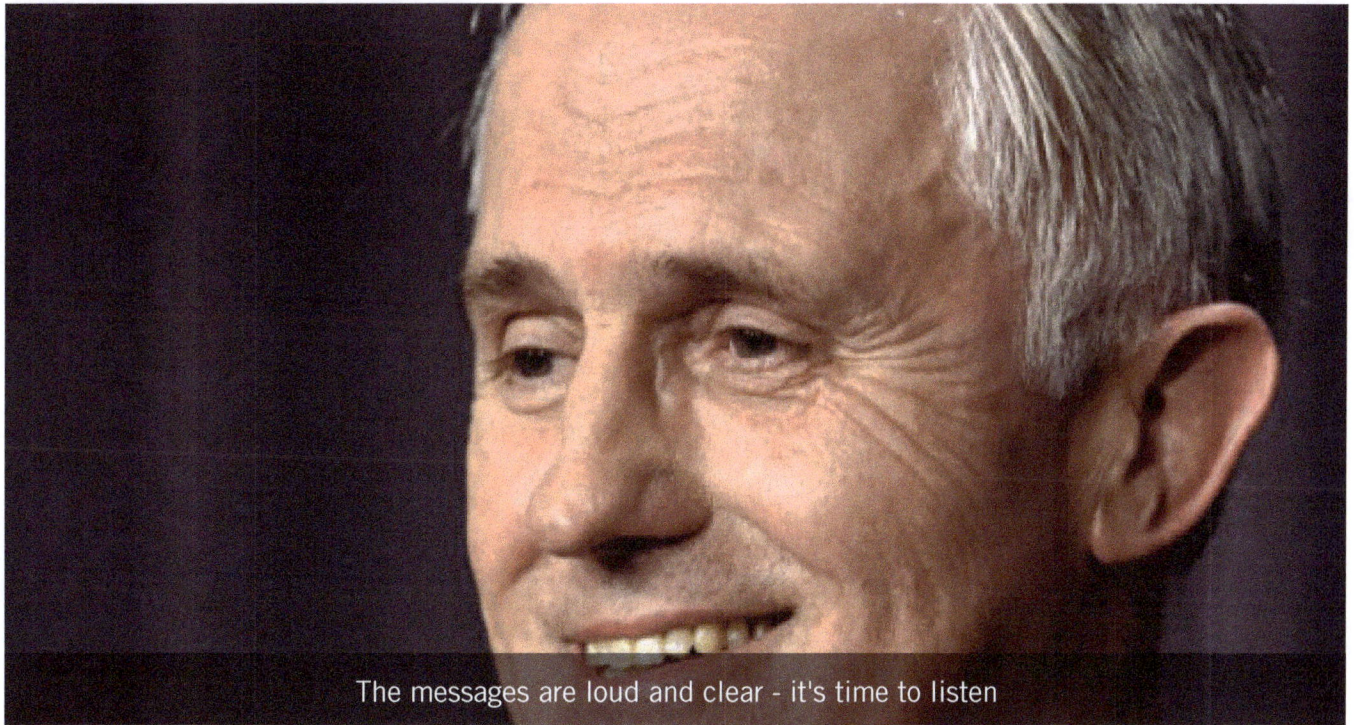

The messages are loud and clear - it's time to listen

Author:	Summer May Finlay	Published:	October 19, 2016

My mum has always said, there is a difference between hearing and listening.

Hearing is the physical act of being able to hear, and listening is the part where you pay attention to what is being said.

The Commonwealth Government has clearly not been "listening" to the Aboriginal and Torres Strait Islander sector and their allies on justice and over-incarceration.

Funding and the recent cuts, unmet need, prevention, justice targets, support for people with Foetal Alcohol Spectrum Disorder (FASD) and Aboriginal and Torres Strait Islander led solutions were the focus of recommendations in a recent Senate inquiry into Aboriginal and Torres Strait Islander experience of law and enforcement and justice services. None of these recommendations is anything that hasn't been said before.

At least one of the recommendations in the report has been part of almost every Aboriginal and Torres Strait Islander incarceration media release from the non-Government sector. The themes have also been a part of multiple Senate Inquiry submissions and most of these themes were also included in the recent Redfern Statement.

Cheryl Axleby, co-chair of the National Aboriginal and Torres Strait Islander Legal Services, agrees: "In the last generation we've had numerous seminal reports which have emphasised repeatedly that the legal assistance sector is not resourced adequately and therefore cannot provide equitable access to justice for our peoples. Despite this, many of those report recommendations remain unimplemented and, as a result, our people are stripped of natural justice."

In the Social Justice Report 2001, the Social Justice Commissioner Dr William Jonas AM raised the issue of Aboriginal and Torres Strait Islander justice issues including mandatory sentencing, the need for diversionary programs and education of Aboriginal and Torres Strait Islander juveniles of their legal rights. In 2014, the United Nations Committee against Torture's concluding observations on the fourth and fifth periodic reports of Australia also raised concerns that mandatory sentencing disproportionately affects Aboriginal and Torres Strait Islander people.

Justice reinvestment , a diversionary program, was also the focus of recommendations from the latest Senate inquiry. Justice Reinvestment is not new. Currently Justice Reinvestment is being explored in two towns in New South Wales, with a research project in Cowra and a trial in Bourke that is supported by Just Reinvest.

In 2013, a Senate Inquiry supported the approach. A Family Violence Prevention Legal Services (FVPLS) submission to the Senate Standing Committee on Legal and Constitutional Affairs was based on the significant value of Justice Reinvestment in reducing Aboriginal and Torres Strait Islander incarceration. A Parliamentary inquiry into the harmful use of alcohol in Aboriginal and Torres Strait Islander communities released in 2015 also recommended investing in Justice reinvestment.

Justice targets for Aboriginal and Torres Strait Islander incarceration are also not a new concept. National Congress of Australia's First Peoples 2013 Justice Policy called for justice targets to be included in Closing the Gap on Indigenous Disadvantage Framework. The 2014 Social Justice and Native Title Report called for Aboriginal and Torres Strait Islander justice targets. Change the Record, a collaboration of Aboriginal and Torres Strait Islander and mainstream organisations, also supports Justice targets.

Many organisations have highlighted the funding cuts affecting the sector since the Coalition Government took office in 2013. In that year, the National Association of Community Legal Services raised the issue of proposed funding cuts to Aboriginal and Torres Strait Islander Legal Services, FVPLSs and Legal Aid Commissions – despite the unmet need and the impact this would have on Aboriginal and Torres Strait Islander people.

In March 2015, a coalition of 26 organisations, including National Aboriginal and Torres Strait Islander Legal Services, FVPLSs and National Congress of Australia's First Peoples, wrote an open letter to the then Prime Minister Tony Abbott, saying the "cuts to legal services will have disastrous impact on Aboriginal and Torres Strait Islander communities".

FASD is also an issue that has been raised before. The 2014 Inquiry into the harmful use of alcohol in Aboriginal and Torres Strait Islander communities raised the need for greater investment in prevention and also support for people with FASD coming in contact with the legal system.

In 2015, Amnesty International in the "A brighter tomorrow: Keeping Indigenous kids in the community and out of detention in Australia" report highlighted the issue of young people with FASD coming in contact with the justice system and the additional preventative resources needed to support people with FASD.

Change the Record has been calling for Aboriginal and Torres Strait Islander led solutions since its inception in 2015. The Redfern Statement called for Aboriginal-led solutions and also called for all funding cuts to Aboriginal and Torres Strait Islander legal services to be reversed. Self-determination is a key principle of the United Nation Declaration on the Rights of Indigenous Peoples, of which Australia is a signatory.

Not listening to the sector and implementing the recommendations has an impact on Aboriginal and Torres Strait Islander people.

Cheryl Axleby said: "The downstream costs of failing to invest in the legal assistance sector are many. But perhaps the biggest cost is life. In the past three months alone, close to ten Aboriginal and Torres Strait Islander women, men and children have lost their lives in custody. Reports in of themselves can't save lives but implementing the recommendations can."

National Aboriginal and Torres Strait Islander Legal Services, FVPLS and Change the Record and the National Association of Community Legal Centres all welcome the recommendations from the Senate inquiry into Aboriginal and Torres Strait Islander experience of law and enforcement and justice services recommendations.

But of course they do – it's what they have been saying for years.

It's time now for the Government to listen and act.

Malcolm Turnbull, do you have your listening ears on?

List of Recommendations

The committee recommends that the Commonwealth Government adequately support legal assistance services, and that specifically funding should focus on:

- community legal education for Aboriginal and Torres Strait Islander people;

- outreach workers to assist Aboriginal and Torres Strait Islander people; and

- interpreters for Aboriginal and Torres Strait Islander people in both civil and criminal matters to ensure that they receive effective legal assistance.

The committee recommends that the Commonwealth Government take all necessary steps in the development and implementation of a plan for the collection of consistent national data on all aspects of Indigenous incarceration placed on the agenda for the next meeting of the Council of Australian Governments Law, Crime and Community Safety Council.

The committee recommends that the Commonwealth Government, prior to the next Council of Australian Governments meeting, explicitly state the measures it is putting in place to assist states and territories to develop, implement and meet Indigenous justice targets.

The committee recommends that the Department of Health prepare a communication plan for those working in areas such as the criminal justice field, to accompany the release of the National Fetal Alcohol Spectrum Disorders (FASD) Diagnostic Tool.

The committee recommends that the Commonwealth Government, through the Council of Australian Governments, work with states and territories, to develop and implement guidelines for the appropriate management of offenders diagnosed with Fetal Alcohol Spectrum Disorders.

The committee recommends that the Commonwealth Government continue to fund initiatives which promote the National Health and Medical Research Council's guidelines that for women who are pregnant, planning a pregnancy or breastfeeding, not drinking alcohol is the safest option.

The committee recommends that the Commonwealth Government contribute to the development of justice reinvestment trials at sites in each state and territory.

The committee recommends that much greater attention is given to Aboriginal led, managed and implemented justice reinvestment programs such as the Bourke Project and Yirriman, and that the Commonwealth Government support Aboriginal led justice reinvestment projects.

The committee recommends that the Commonwealth Government work with the states and territories in supporting programs which strengthen families and communities through a focus on early intervention and support.

The committee recommends that administrative responsibility for Family Violence Prevention Legal Services be returned to the Attorney-General's Department.

The committee recommends that the Council of Australian Governments task the Council of Australian Governments Law, Crime and Community Safety Council to review state laws such as mandatory sentencing which have a disproportionate effect on Indigenous Australians in order to quantify the effects and report to the Council of Australian Governments.

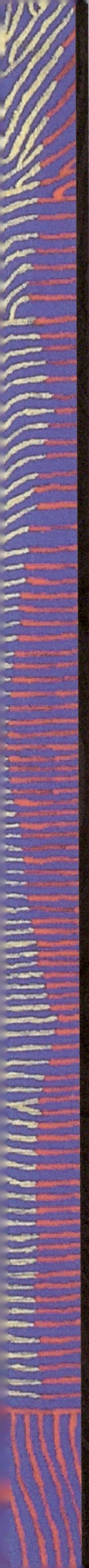

#JustJustice

Tackling the over-incarceration
of Aboriginal and Torres Strait
Islander peoples

#JUSTJUSTICE

"Malcolm Turnbull,
do you have your
listening ears on?"

Summer May Finlay

13. The #JustJustice story

" *The success of the crowdfunding was an example of the power of connective action and of an engaged, collaborative network*

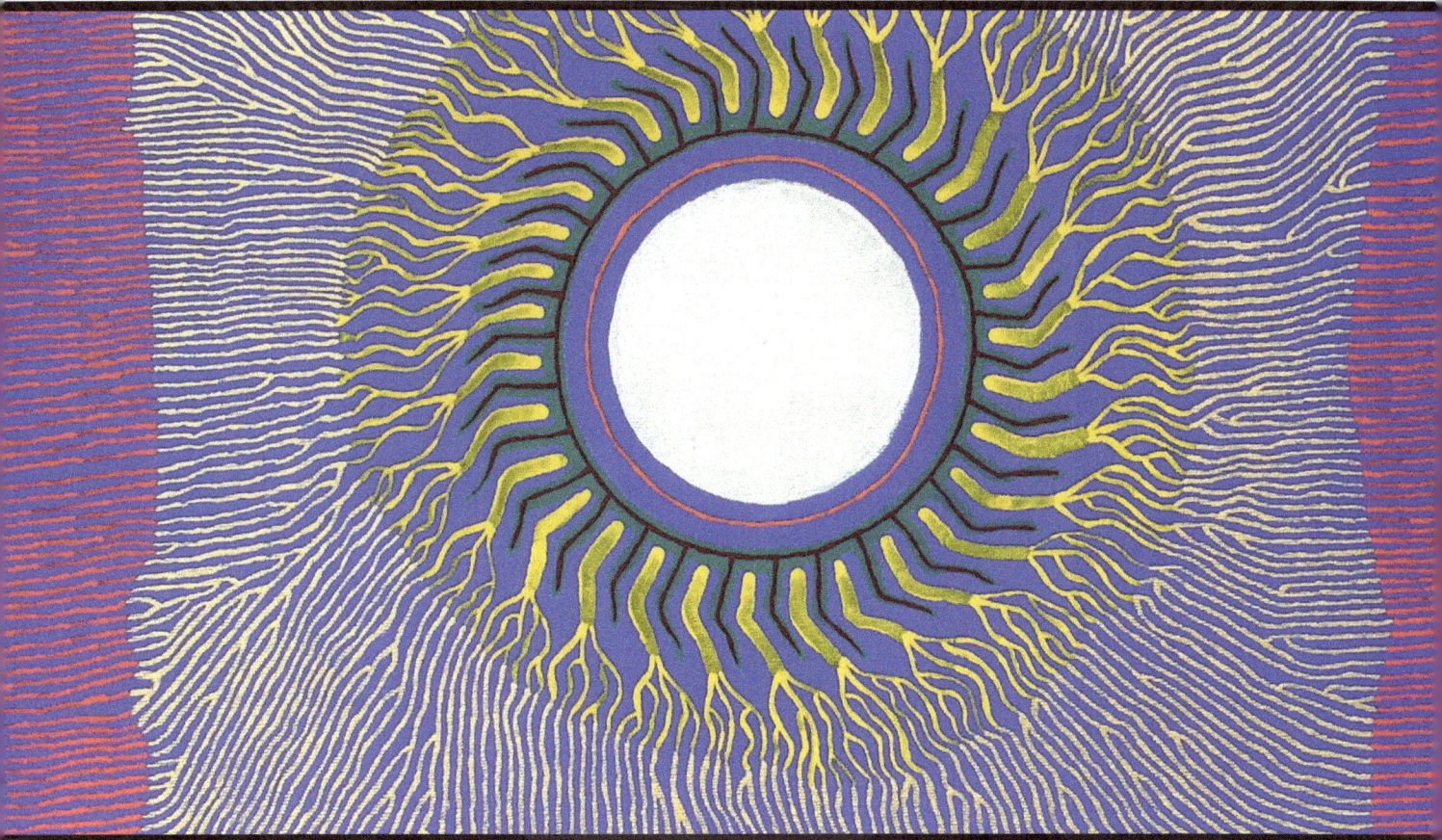

Thanks for helping to make some #JustJustice – wrapping up the crowdfunding campaign

Author:	Melissa Sweet		Published:	July 16, 2015

In coming months, Croakey hopes to bring you stories from Aboriginal and Torres Strait Islander people from across the country about the impacts of over-incarceration – upon individuals, families, and communities – and about related issues.

#JUSTJUSTICE

We also will be sharing stories from communities that highlight effective, culturally appropriate solutions to help reverse the increasing rates of imprisonment.

And we hope to put the spotlight on government policies and practices that are contributing to the over-incarceration of Aboriginal and Torres Strait Islander peoples.

All this will be possible thanks to the generosity of more than 300 contributors to the #JustJustice crowdfunding campaign, which concluded successfully at the Pozible platform on 7 June (their names are listed below and on the #JustJustice homepage).

In the days leading up to the campaign deadline, the #JustJustice team members (Summer May Finlay, Marie McInerney, Mitchell Ward and myself) were not hopeful about our prospects. Just three days out from deadline, we had 108 supporters and needed to raise $10,000 to reach our target.

We consoled ourselves with the thought that just by doing the crowdfunding campaign, this was helping to put the spotlight on over-incarceration as a critical health concern for Aboriginal and Torres Strait Islander people. It was terrific, for example, seeing GP Dr Edwin Kruys engage with the campaign by interviewing Summer May Finlay and writing about it for his blog, Doctor's Bag.

On the final Sunday morning of the campaign, less than 12 hours from deadline, we needed about $6,000 to reach the target – otherwise none of the pledges would be realised. And this was the Sunday of a long weekend.

Luke Pearson, the founder of @IndigenousX, gave some much-needed motivation that morning. His advice was to "go hard" on Twitter as there was "too much on the table to throw away".

As we acted on his advice – and others joined us in creating a Twitter storm – the pledges began to flow in, thick and fast, and the despondency that we had been feeling transformed into exhilaration (as so joyously represented in the "happy dance" that Finlay promised if the campaign reached its mark, not really expecting she would be called to deliver).

In the end, we passed the funding target with a few hours to spare.

The success of the #JustJustice crowdfunding was an example of the power of connective action and of an engaged, collaborative network on Twitter, as many people took it upon themselves to give up time on a long weekend to support the campaign by spreading the word via Twitter, Facebook and their networks.

The campaign hashtag #JustJustice trended number one in Canberra and Brisbane during the day as supporters around the country joined in.

Having hundreds of people joining into support the campaign and say "this issue matters" sent a powerful message and was also empowering in itself.

If you want to know how to help support a crowdfunding campaign, look at some of the tweets at the bottom of this post from some of the generous supporters of #JustJustice.

Warm thanks in particular to Dr Marie Bismark for not only constant tweeting but relieving our anxiety levels greatly on the Sunday afternoon with her promise to cover any funding gap if we couldn't get the campaign over the line.

It was also encouraging to see politicians engaging with the campaign by retweeting, and with some donating. Thanks Senator Sue Lines, Victorian Health Minister Jill Hennessy, federal opposition health spokesman Stephen Jones, Senator Penny Wright, Queensland Health Minister Cameron Dick, and others.

We also enjoyed a few celebrity moments; Sir Michael Marmot, one of the global leaders for action on the social determinants of health, retweeted #JustJustice, and we also appreciated the RTs and support of cartoonist First Dog on the Moon, Van Badham and Todd Sampson.

Thanks also to Dr Mark Lock, Darren Parker, Anne Messenger and others who wrote for Croakey during crowdfunding campaign, as well as to Professor Tom Calma, Mick Gooda, Dr Marshall Watson and others who contributed their time and expertise. We also are grateful to those who have since come forward, volunteering their services to help the campaign.

We would particularly like to acknowledge Jesuit Social Services and Frank Meany as the campaign's two premium sponsors. It would not have happened without their support.

Statement from Jesuit Social Services

Jesuit Social Services is proud to support the #JustJustice project and investigate solutions to the over-incarceration of Aboriginal and Torres Strait Islander people. As Mick Gooda has said, this issue is a public health catastrophe. Jesuit Social Services has nearly 40 years of experience working with people in and exiting the prison system and we know of the significant discrimination and disadvantage experienced by many Aboriginal people that too often drives contact with the justice system. We know also of the strength in Aboriginal communities that supports people's reintegration after prison.

We are committed to working alongside, and in partnerships with Aboriginal controlled organisations and Aboriginal community leaders to strive for social change and improved outcomes for the people we work with. On an organisational level, Aboriginal staff members of Jesuit Social Services have recently convened an Aboriginal Advisory Group to consolidate our knowledge of working with Aboriginal program participants and communities, and to lead our reconciliation process and cultural education.

We were moved to support #JustJustice because we believe there is scope for significant and prolonged change. We hope that the solutions-focused work completed by health, policy and criminal justice experts as well as researchers and journalists will serve to influence those in power, like politicians, policy makers and educators.

Thanks also to the other premium sponsor, Frank Meany, who will be known to many Croakey readers for his work with One Vision.

We would also like to acknowledge the Change the Record campaign now underway. Follow them on Twitter : @Change_Record.

We encourage #JustJustice supporters and Croakey readers to take the Change the Record pledge here.

The Change the Record campaign pledge says:

" *The rates at which Aboriginal and Torres Strait Islander people are experiencing violence and being put in prison far exceeds that of non-Indigenous Australians. And we have reached a crisis point.*

I want to be part of an Australia where Aboriginal and Torres Strait Islander communities and families are safer and stronger. I want to change the record.

We need to:

• Close the gap in rates of imprisonment by 2040; and

• Cut the disproportionate rates of violence to at least close the gap by 2040 with priority strategies for women and children,

I call on all levels of government to:

• Invest in early intervention, prevention and diversion strategies, which address the root causes of violence and imprisonment; and

• Work in partnership with Aboriginal and Torres Strait Islander people, communities, services and their representatives, to develop and implement solutions.

Warm thanks to all those who donated to the campaign

Jessica Adams; Kodie Alderton; Kristin Alford; Meegan Argent; Ruth Armstrong; Scott Avery; Bunty Avieson. Andrew.

Wendy Bacon; Pippa Bailey; David Bain; Phillip Baker; Virginia Barbour; Lesley Barclay; Richard Barnes; Justin Barrie; Anthony Baxter; Katy Bell; Sophie Benjamin; Donna Benjamin; Tess Bennett; Marie Bismark: Belinda Bos; Catherine Bouris; Frank Bowden; Cath Bowtell; Deborah Brian; Edwina Brown.

Lorraine Callow; Jane Cameron; Don Cameron; Elissa Campbell; John Carney; Bren Carruthers; Stacy Carter; Janice Catherall; Jonathan Champ; Megan Chapman; Simon Chapman; Rick Chen; Richard Chirgwin; Nicholas Chu; Curtis Cifuentes; Julian Cleary; Mikaella Clements; Monica Clements; Nicole Cloonan; Nicholas Coghlan; Karen Coombs; David Corbet; Kulja Coulston; Colin Cowell; Alan Crabbe; Anthony Cran; Gemma Crawford; Dan Crawford; George Crisp.

Kaaren Dahl; Paul Davis; Tom Dawkins; Johan de Wit; Maddy Dell; Deejbah; Jennifer Doggett; Rebecca Dominquez; Elissa Doxey; Evelyn Doyle; Sue Ducker; Barb Dunford.

Alison Edwards; M. Edwards; Bruce Enting.

Alison Fairleigh; Rhonda Finlay; Summer May Finlay; Jack Fisher; Hannah Fitch-Rabbitt; Tal Fitzpatrick; Malcolm Forbes; Louise Francis; Bronwyn Fredericks; Amy Free; Mary Freer; Gavin Frost.

Ben Gallan; Wendy Garthon; Lynore Geia; Julie Gibson; Fiona Gillies; Thomas Gorman; Jannine Graham; Kirra Greaves; Catherine Greenhill; Joanna Gregg; James Griffiths; Carmel Grimmett; Nicholas Gruen.

Rod Hagen; Mukesh Haikerwal; Amanda Hand; Karen Harbutt; Tony Harewood; Ash Harper; Mark Harris; Ros Hart; Ros Harvey; Karen Hauser; Katrina Hawke; Marita Hefler; Jill Hennessy; Carl Heslop; Noel Hodda; Caroline Homer; Fiona Horn; Michelle Hostrup; Amy Hourigan; Leigh Hughes; Bradley Hughes; Nerida Hyett.

Rebecca Ivers.

Melanie James; Bonnie James; Eliza Jane Berlage; Jesuit Social Services; Louise Johansson; Mindy Johnson; Claire Jones; Just Judith.

Thomas Kane; Celia Karpfen; Fiona Katauskas; John Kelly; John Kelly; Jack Kerosene; Garth Kidd; Paul Kidd; Amy Knibbs; Edwin Kruys.

Joshua La Macchia; Shihui Lai; Rob Lake; Kay Lam Macleod; Eleni Lambropoulos; Collette Lancaster-Lockwood; Kathy Landvogt; Bronwyn Lapham; Helen Lawrence; Natalie Leader; Hen Learner; Kim Leevers; Chris Lemoh; Debra Lewis; Nicole Lindsay; Sue Lines; Mark Lock; Yvonne Luxford.

Sean M Elliott; Daniel Machuca; Imogene Malcolm; Miska Mandic; Melinda Mann-Yasso; Liza Marsh; Fiona Martin; Rosalie Martin; Bonita Mason; Chris Mayes; Amy Maynard; Jo McCarthy; Edward McCauley; Ruth McCausland; Danny McCormick; David McDonald; Lea McInerney; Joanne McMahon; Mandy McNulty; Barbara Meaker; Frank Meany; MEDAXS; Jasmine Melit; Kris Melmouth; Claire Merquita; Sue Miers; Julie Milland; John Millard; Janine Mohamed; Brett Montgomery; Brenda Moon; Wes Mountain; Sarah Mumml; Matthew; Susie Munro; Nicole Murphy; Melissa Murray.

Danielle Nagle; Jack Nairn; Christy Newman; Peter Noble; Kerrie Noonan.

Mike O'Connor; Isabelle Oderberg; Kristine Olaris; Kat Olesen; Dee O'Loughlin; Firstdog Onthemoon; Lesley Parker; Ruth Parslow; Gregory Paul Miller; Michele Payne.

Hannah Quinn.

Freya Rachel; Black Rainbow; Greg Randolph; Val Ranson; Daniel Reeders; Martin Rees; Clare Renner; Mel Riordan; Geoffrey Roberts; Penny Robinson; Lucie Robson; Juan Rodriguez; Lisa Rooke; Emma Rooksby; Morgan Rose; Ben Ross; Matt Rush; Lesley Russell; Lucie Rychetnik. @redheadedition.

John Salmond; Eliza Sarlos; E Saunders; Brad Sayer; Kristy Schirmer; Nicholas Schmidt; Bronwen Scott; Sara Scrutton;

Andi Sebastian; Karen Seita; Joyce Seitzinger; Tim Senior; Caroline Shepherd; Margaret Simons; Liana Skewes; Cobi Smith; Brian Smith; Matthew Smith; Warwick Smith; Sharron Smyth; Paul Snelling; Michael Stanley; Pippa Stearn; Bronwyn Stell; Ruth Stewart; Stockler family; Jeff Sundstrom; Christene Sweet; Jan Sweet; John Sweet.

David Taylor; Jane Thomas; Dr Mel Thomson; Nina Tinning.

Kylie Valentine; Luke van der Beeke; Beau Vass, Jaklene Vukasinovic.

Fiona Walls; Lucie Walters; Andrew Weatherall; Kimberlee Weatherall; Calli Weitenberg; Simon Weller; Garda White; Becky White; David Wickenden; Bethany Wilksch; Paul Williams; Eden Winnacott; Sharyn Wise; Senator Penny Wright; Mary Wyatt.

Zuleyka Zevallos; Rebecca Zosel; Anthony Zwi.

Our sincere thanks to the other 44 donors who chose to remain anonymous.

If you donated but your name is not mentioned above, it may be because your pledge was not realised (due to problems with the credit card, Pay Pal etc) or because you asked to be anonymous. If you believe you should be listed here, please get in touch with @croakeyblog.

Launching #JustJustice: Mick Gooda calls for action on a "public health catastrophe"

Author:	Mick Gooda	Published:	April 09, 2015

The over-incarceration of Aboriginal and Torres Strait Islander Peoples is a "public health catastrophe", and Mick Gooda, the Aboriginal and Torres Strait Islander Social Justice Commissioner, plans to make it a priority issue for the remainder of his term.

At Croakey we are delighted that Mick Gooda is supporting our new crowdfunding campaign – #JustJustice – which aims to investigate and profile solutions to over-incarceration.

Gooda was a keynote speaker at a conference 'Prison Health – From the Inside Out', that kicked off yesterday in Geraldton, Western Australia, as featured in this ABC news report.

Sandy Davies, chairman of the Geraldton Regional Aboriginal Medical Service, hopes the conference will identify alternatives to imprisonment for minor offences, and also lead to more effective strategies for improving prisoners' health.

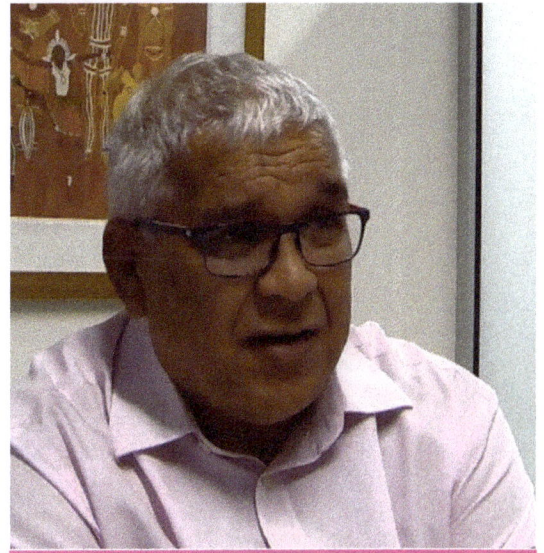

Mick Gooda - talking #JustJustice

The conference continues today – follow the discussion on Twitter at #PrisonHealth and #JustJustice. Also follow live conference tweeting from @DameyonBonson and @WePublicHealth – who this week is Croakey moderator and journalist Marie McInerney.

Mick Gooda writes:

Calling for leadership and action

Tackling the over-incarceration of Aboriginal and Torres Strait Islander peoples will require leadership and action at multiple levels.

We need to shift the dominant narrative, which suggests that "lock them up" policies produce safer communities.

This is not true. The evidence from around the world tells us that putting people in jail for minor crimes does not create safer communities. But it does create a cycle of incarceration that is tearing apart families and communities.

The mental health impacts of over-incarceration are devastating, affecting the social and emotional wellbeing of children, families and communities well into the future.

I am supporting the #JustJustice campaign because we need to encourage a public debate that is focused on ensuring effective, evidence-based solutions to over-incarceration.

Over-incarceration is not only a public health catastrophe; it is also a terrible waste of taxpayers' money – imprisonment is not only ineffective, it's terribly expensive.

Health sector can help

The health sector has an important role to play in this debate; much of the evidence developed by health researchers could help create a fairer criminal justice system.

For example we know from the health sector that having interpreters who are familiar with the health system can make a real difference for Aboriginal and Torres Strait Islander patients.

Similarly, interpreters who understand the criminal justice system can make a real difference. There are countless stories of people ending up in jail without understanding what's just happened to them. If people don't understand the charges they're facing, how can they instruct their lawyers and get a proper defence?

We should also be looking at alternatives to imprisonment for unpaid fines.

Police services could also be learning from work in the health sector to improve the cultural competence of health professionals. We need to be talking with the police services around Australia about issues like unconscious bias, and my sense is that the time is right for these conversations.

Police need to be encouraged to exercise their discretion in the right way; because it is at that first contact point, the one between police and our mob, where the justice system is at its most flexible, as such, how they manage that first contact can often dictate how the rest of the system reacts.

For instance, deciding whether to issue cautions or what charges to lay means they are in positions to stop the cycle of incarceration from starting.

Justice targets matter

At a national level, we need to have justice targets as part of the Closing the Gap agenda. We know that targets focus peoples' attention and efforts.

We would like the Prime Minister to be talking about Justice Targets on the first sitting day of every Parliament, as he does now with other Closing the Gap Targets.

I will be working with the National Justice Coalition to progress justice targets. I hope the Government upholds its 2013 election promise to do the same.

Reducing the over-incarceration of Aboriginal and Torres Strait Islander peoples is one of the most important issues on my agenda for the remaining two years of my appointment.

I encourage the health sector engage in this issue of national importance. A fairer justice system will help to improve the health and social and emotional wellbeing of Aboriginal and Torres Strait Islander peoples. This is a crucial issue for children, for women, for men, for families, for communities.

I encourage Croakey readers and the wider health system to support the #JustJustice series, and to engage with addressing this critical public health issue.

Mick Gooda was the Aboriginal and Torres Strait Islander Social Justice Commissioner at the time this article was published. He is now Royal Commissioner for the Royal Commission into the Child Protection and Youth Detention Systems of the Northern Territory.

List of contributing authors

Michelle Adams
Louis Andrews
Wayne Applebee
Ruth Armstrong
Anna Arstein-Kerslake
Scott Avery
Ethan Blue
Dameyon Bonson
Antoinette Braybrook
Kelly Briggs
Liana Buchanan
Jack Bulman
Madeleine Calleja
Tom Calma
Julian Cleary
Clinton
Paul Collis
Amy Coopes
Adele Cox

Michaela Crowe
Eddie Cubillo
Pat Dudgeon
Shane Duffy
Paul Dutton
Julie Edwards
Elizabeth Elliott
Gina Fairley
Summer May Finlay
Brendan Fletcher
Bronwyn Fredericks
Gerry Georgatos
Mick Gooda
Piers Gooding
Christina Grant
Sam Harkus
Andrew Jackomos
Debbie Kilroy
Robyn Layton

Marlene Longbottom
Ray Lovett
Heather McCormack
Marie McInerney
Bernadette McSherry
Amy McQuire
Anne Messenger
Michael Moore
Roxanne Moore
Kathleen Musulin
Holly Northam
Anna Olsen
Patrick O'Sullivan
Tiffany Overall
Darren Parker
Kirstie Parker
Sharon Payne
Luke Pearson
Yvette Roe

Rosemary Roe
Lynda Ryder
Eugene Schofield-Georgeson
Tim Senior
Bill Shorten
Phyllis Simmons
Mark Skulley
Antony Stockdale
Melissa Sweet
Sharman Stone
Dayna Veraguth
Clinton Walker
Julie Walker
Mitchell Ward
Richard Weston
Megan Williams
Jason Wing
Karen Wyld

List of contributing organisations

This list includes organisations that have contributed articles to #JustJustice, as well as organisations that are signatories to statements published as part of the series.

Aboriginal Medical Services Alliance NT

Aboriginal Peak Organisations Northern Territory

Amnesty International Australia

ANTaR

Australian Council of Social Service

Australian Lawyers Alliance

Australian Medical Association

Black Rainbow

Change the Record Coalition

Close the Gap Steering Committee

Family Matters

Family Violence Prevention Legal Services

First Peoples Disability Network

Geraldton Regional Aboriginal Medical Service

Healing Foundation

Human Rights Law Centre

Indigenous Allied Health Australia

IndigenousX Pty Ltd

Jesuit Social Services

Law Council

Lowitja Institute

Menzies School of Health Research

National Aboriginal and Torres Strait Islander Legal Services

National Aboriginal Community Controlled Health Organisations

National Association of Community Legal Centres

National Congress of Australia's First Peoples,

National Health Leadership Forum

Northern and Central Land Councils

Oxfam Australia

Public Health Association of Australia

Queensland Association of Independent Legal Service Inc

Reconciliation Australia

Save the Children

Secretariat for National Aboriginal and Islander Child Care

Sisters Inside

The Conversation

Uniting Church in Australia, Queensland Synod

Victorian Aboriginal Community Controlled Health organisation

Behind the scenes, with #JustJustice

Australia's failure to provide a culturally safe and fair justice system for Aboriginal and Torres Strait Islander people is bound up with many other colonial legacies that contribute to health inequities.

The health sector, enmeshed in these legacies, has a moral and ethical responsibility to engage with addressing these injustices. The sector also has the power to help reframe public and policy debate towards fairer policies and better outcomes for Aboriginal and Torres Strait Island people.

The #JustJustice project has sought to contribute to this reframing of debate and to prod the health sector to engage more proactively.

This is in keeping with the journalistic mission of Croakey.org, an independent, low-budget social journalism project for health that seeks to work with community in putting the spotlight on under-served issues.

Over-incarceration certainly fits that remit. Despite many, many reports and inquiries over more than a century, governments have yet to take the necessary across-the-board action responding to the wealth of recommendations that have been put forward, by Royal Commissions, inquiries, reports, research and communities.

The #JustJustice project can be seen through many lenses, including as an example of using connective networks to power public interest journalism. It represents innovation in both the funding and the doing of journalism; #JustJustice has been funded by community, and undertaken by working with community.

It also represents the development of journalism as a collaborative, transdisciplinary process – the #JustJustice team has brought together people with diverse knowledges and skills, including cultural knowledge, Aboriginal and Torres Strait Islander health, journalism, communications, public health, community development, and graphic design.

#JustJustice was funded on Sunday, 7 June, 2015 – after a nail-biting race to the crowdfunding finish line.

Just three days out from crowdfunding deadline, we had 108 supporters and needed to raise $10,000 to reach our target (otherwise the campaign would not realise any of the pledges).

> *The #JustJustice project can be seen through many lenses, including as an example of using connective networks to power public interest journalism*

On that final day, a Sunday on a long-weekend, the hashtag #JustJustice trended number one in Canberra and Brisbane during the day as supporters around the country joined in.

Thanks to the generosity of 339 donors we finally made it over. A special shout-out to the two premium donors, Frank Meany of One Vision and the Jesuit Social Services, who each contributed $5,000. Without those generous donations, we would not have reached our fund-raising target.

(While 338 donors helped get us over the crowdfunding line, with one landing after the crowdfunding campaign had finished, not all pledges were realised. However, we acknowledge the 339 tally, recognising that even the pledges which were not realised were useful in getting us over the line, and we acknowledge all donors here.)

But it wasn't only the money that was donated. It was the support as people shared our crowdfunding callouts, and sent out the #JustJustice stories via social media. It was also the support that people gave by sharing their often very personal stories during the #JustJustice series.

#JustJustice thus also represents journalism as a process as well as outcomes. Just as important as this book and the articles published at Croakey.org has been the development of relationships and connections for change.

Individuals and organisations across sectors, spheres, and all walks of life connected with the #JustJustice hashtag. #JustJustice also found supporters amongst politicians of all stripes, including some who donated to the crowdfunding campaign at Pozible. We also enjoyed a few celebrity moments; Sir Michael Marmot, one of the global leaders for action on the social determinants of health, retweeted #JustJustice.

Decolonising journalism

The reason that #JustJustice took a different approach to much other mainstream media coverage of over-incarceration is that it was informed by a decolonising methodology for journalism practice.

This meant that it has sought to:

- Provide a useful service for Aboriginal and Torres Strait Islander peoples and communities.

- Recognise the role of colonisation in contributing to incarceration rates and acknowledge how this history plays out in the present.

- Take a strengths-based approach.

- Ensure priority representation of and respect for Aboriginal and Torres Strait Islander peoples, and their expertise, knowledges, cultures and experiences.

- Examine white privilege, particularly within this context.

- Follow proper process. This project recognises the importance of respect and relationships, and puts emphasis on how the project is done, as one of the outcomes.

How to measure the impact of #JustJustice?

It is too early to know the full impact of the project; hopefully some of the stories that have been planted will continue to grow. We hope a research project may explore these matters further someday.

In the meantime, some interim measures are:

- #JustJustice was a collaborative, productive project that produced more than 90 articles from more than 70 contributors.

- We maintained a high-profile, active social media engagement for more than 18 months. On Twitter, there were almost 5,000 participants at the #JustJustice hashtag from April 2015 to November 2016, and there were more than 118.5 million Twitter impressions (see below for more details). The #JustJustice hashtag was supported at different times by the curated rotated accounts, @IndigenousX and @WePublicHealth. The #JustJustice memes designed by Mitchell Ward were widely shared.

- #JustJustice reached out beyond the articles, Periscope broadcasts and social media discussions. We took #JustJustice to conference presentations and media interviews (see timeline for more details). We gave away #JustJustice Twitter tips (get yours here).

- After the successful launch of the first edition of the #JustJustice book, Western Sydney University provided a $5,000 grant to enable a second edition, and further dissemination strategies.

Nonetheless, we remain acutely conscious that #JustJustice is a drop in the ocean, compared to what is needed to shift policy, practice and debate.

Significantly, just a few days after the launch of the #JustJustice crowdfunding campaign in 2015, a massive $52.5 million police and justice complex was officially opened in Carnarvon

We have sought to contribute to a conversation, working alongside organisational-based campaigns like Change the Record. But so much more needs to be said and done.

We hope that those who have supported, contributed to and read #JustJustice will continue to take the issues forward. Governments need to know that over-incarceration is an injustice that people care deeply about.

Our stories

For the team members, our #JustJustice stories begin in different places. Below, we share something of our individual and collective #JustJustice journeys.

Melissa Sweet, a non-Indigenous public health journalist, Croakey publisher and editor

My #JustJustice journey began when travelling in Western Australia in 2013 and 2014 as part of research for my PhD, *"Acknowledgement": A social journalism research project relating to the history of lock hospitals and other forms of medical incarceration of Aboriginal and Torres Strait Islander people.* As I interviewed people about the history of the lock hospitals of Bernier and Dorre Island via Carnarvon, and other forms of medical incarceration of Aboriginal and Torres Strait Islander people, I would ask, *Why does this history matter? How does it relate to the present?* Inevitably our conversations would end up canvassing the contemporary issues of over-incarceration and the contribution of hostile, unsupportive and inadequate policies and services.

When I returned from WA in late 2014, I was planning to commission a series of articles for Croakey on the health aspects of over-incarceration. Instead, an idea for a more ambitious project arose out of a chance discussion with Professor Tom Calma AO and Summer May Finlay at the Public Health Association of Australia end-of-year celebrations in 2014. We then discussed this idea further with Mr Mick Gooda, who was then the Aboriginal and Torres Strait Islander Social Justice Commissioner, and other Aboriginal health and social justice leaders. Mr Gooda launched the crowdfunding campaign on 9 April 2015. For the 18 months since then, it has been a privilege and a pleasure to work with the #JustJustice team and also the many others who have contributed to the series. A milestone for the team and the project was when Dr Megan Williams joined us in August 2015, bringing her deep research and community experience to the project.

Significantly, just a few days after the launch of the #JustJustice crowdfunding campaign in 2015, a massive $52.5 million police and justice complex was officially opened in Carnarvon. The

Gwoonwardu Mia Cultural Centre, which stood just over the road from this complex, closed down due to a funding shortfall during the course of the #JustJustice project. The opening of one centre, and the closing of another during the term of this project is profoundly and painfully symbolic.

Summer May Finlay, Aboriginal and Torres Strait Public Health practitioner and occasional writer

Social justice was something I have always been passionate about. One of the first poems I ever performed at a drama eisteddfod while in primary school was Oodgeroo Noonuccal's No More Boomerang, Her poetry called to me. The injustice of what our mob has gone through since invasion resonated. I think that's when I became an advocate for our mob.

In my early 20's I went back to university because I wanted to make a difference for our people. While I was at university I worked as a youth and children's worker for the city of Sydney and was based in Redfern and Woolloomooloo. Here I saw how the justice system treated some of the most under privileged young people and it made me so mad. I believe all kids deserve the opportunity to be the best they can be regardless of their situation. I had gone back to university to make a difference and my experiences reinforced that drive.

It was because of my passion for our mob and my experiences that when Melissa mentioned she had been chatting to Tom Calma about running a series on the solutions to the over-incarceration of Aboriginal and Torres Strait Islander people, I knew I wanted to be involved. At that time, I could never have imagined that we would have been able to do as much as we have done.

This project has taught me so many things. That Australians can be such generous people with both their time, support and money. I learnt that crowd funding is hard work, and posting my happy dance on YouTube meant I would never be able to live it down! I have learnt that to grab people's attention, media doesn't need to be sensationalist. That strength-based approaches which privilege Aboriginal and Torres Strait Islander voices is something people want to read. And I have learnt that a small collective, such as the #JustJustice crew, can create something which has the capacity to make a difference for our mob.

Dr Megan Williams, Aboriginal justice health researcher

Some of my earliest memories visiting family in hospital and prison left an indelible mark, as did my early 1990s work in needle and syringe exchanges. People would get out of prison and come to the needle exchange, not to get injecting equipment but to be somewhere 'safe'. We had a

garden and arts projects and made thousands of condom packs for 2-metre Condoman to distribute in nightclubs. My boss saw what a poor job I did of accompanying Condoman, and instead sent me to a much more suitable course on research and evaluation.

Not long after, my gorgeous cousin took his own life in a low-security correctional centre, one in which I had provided blood-borne virus education. Having been in that landscape played on my mind, as did unanswered questions – how could a person in State 'care' kill themselves when a Royal Commission made recommendations for prevention? Why was a person with a range of health issues criminalised to the point of death?

I decided to refine my 'trade' as a researcher through a PhD at the intersection of justice and Aboriginal health. Being a sensitive human I made a rule – my methodology is of 'solution-focussed stories only'. Out of deep respect for Aboriginal and Torres Strait Islander peoples, I sought to highlight their many efforts that seemed so poorly recognised.

> Now 90 stories have been made accessible

Now 90 stories have been made accessible by #JustJustice. They show in detail how Aboriginal and Torres Strait Islander people provide solutions at multiple levels, and in multiple ways – among individuals, in services, in communities and in making system improvements.

I believe Elders when they say we all have a need and the capacity to grow, and to never give up on anyone. While underlying inequalities drive incarceration rates, it is obvious many other cultures are also suffering – from high suicide rates, obesity and poverty, as well as the effects of climate change. The beauty of the solutions identified by Aboriginal and Torres Strait Islander people through #JustJustice is their universal value – that they are beneficial for everyone.

Marie McInerney, non-Indigenous freelance journalist and editor, Croakey editor

As a freelance journalist with a focus on social justice issues, I was thrilled to be invited to join Melissa, Summer and Mitchell, and later Meg, on the #JustJustice team. In an earlier job, I had edited an edition of the VCOSS magazine Insight on Crime and Justice issues, with a growing sense of outrage at the structural inequities and injustices at work in our system, particularly for Aboriginal and Torres Strait Islander people.

Thanks to the generosity of the Geraldton Regional Aboriginal Medical Service (GRAMS), I was able to attend its Prison Health: From the Inside Out conference in Geraldton that coincided with the launch of #JustJustice. It was packed with insights, but a number stood out. Mick Gooda saying we likely would not have needed to be there had the recommendations of the Royal Commission into

Aboriginal Deaths in Custody been implemented. Academic Harry Blagg saying the most significant policing impact of the NT Intervention was a 250 per cent increase in the rate of arrests for driving offences, which often led to stints in prison. How one health worker in Roebourne working with Aboriginal people exiting prison had a caseload of 300. And the distress of a delegate from a remote community fearing it was about to be shut down by the WA Government.

As important was what I have learnt (am learning) as a journalist in the methodology of #JustJustice – of the power of privileging community voices, how a strengths-based approach shifts the ground (and mindset) in reporting, and the freedom that comes from having my non-Indigenous assumptions and approaches challenged by working closer with Aboriginal and Torres Strait Islander people, particularly with Summer and Meg.

I recently worked on another project involving injustice for Indigenous people, which required generating media interest. "What does it tell us that we don't already know?" was a common question. In many ways and with many voices,

#JustJustice tells us what needs to be done. As the Northern Territory Royal Commission has heard, it's time it got done.

Mitchell Ward, non-Indigenous designer and artist; Croakey web developer

My roles included making logos, Internet memes, and YouTube clips, and designing the #JustJustice book, amongst other things. It was an honour to work with Paul Dutton, who created the art work for the cover that informed the whole book's design. I also worked with Melissa in doing interviews and Periscope broadcasts in WA. Being involved in this project has made me more aware of my own privilege as a white man, and the huge disparity that exists in Australia, with too much money going into policing and prisons, rather than communities. To me, nothing says this more powerfully than the opening of a huge police and justice centre in Carnarvon, as Melissa mentions above, at the same time as the closure of the wonderful resource that was the Gwoonwardu Mia cultural centre. It's been fantastic working on this book hearing from so many people, and the depth of the talent and commitment among communities is inspiring.

Twitter analytics

Symplur analytics from 5 April 2015 to 5 November 2016 show there were 4,899 participants and 118,573,468 Twitter impressions for #JustJustice.

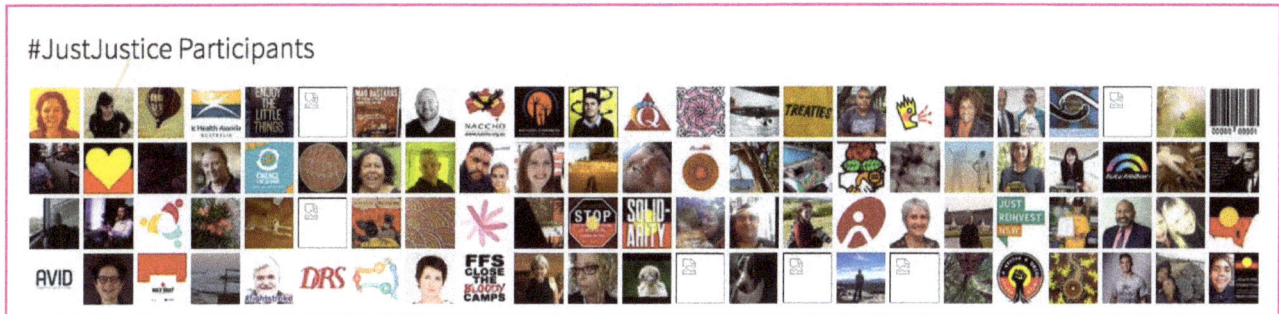

#JustJustice Participants

The Twitter analytics are here.

The #JustJustice Influencers

Top 10 by Mentions	Top 10 by Tweets	Top 10 by Impressions
@croakeyblog 12,940	@croakeyblog 3,781	@croakeyblog 52,092,077
@ontopicaus 10,899	@ontopicaus 3,753	@nacchoaustralia 6,274,289
@mariemcinerney 6,223	@mariemcinerney 788	@ontopicaus 6,162,516
@megbastard 2,942	@indigenousphaa 462	@indigenousx 4,262,043
@wepublichealth 1,918	@bluefishblue292 450	@congressmob 3,062,741
@nacchoaustralia 1,298	@wepublichealth 431	@wepublichealth 3,062,386
@croakeynews 1,244	@megbastard 430	@dameyonbonson 1,553,650
@indigenousx 1,068	@dameyonbonson 394	@wakaflocka 1,548,937
@rocklilydesign 936	@nacchoaustralia 384	@mariemcinerney 1,361,011
@change_record 884	@congressmob 383	@timsenior 1,343,714

The Numbers

118,573,468 Impressions
32,413 Tweets
4,899 Participants
2 Avg Tweets/Hour
7 Avg Tweets/Participant

The Twitter transcript is here.

Acknowledgement of Croakey funders

We acknowledge and thank the members of the Croakey funding consortium convened by the Public Health Association of Australia, including:

Public Health Association of Australia, Alzheimer's Australia, Australian Health Promotion Association, Australian Injury Prevention Network, Australian Healthcare and Hospitals Association, Centre for Primary Health Care and Equity UNSW, Palliative Care Australia, Public Health Advocacy Institute of WA and the McCusker Centre for Action on Alcohol and Youth, Health Services Research Association of Australia and New Zealand, Ragg Ahmed, The George Institute for Global Health, and VicHealth.

The #JustJustice timeline

2014

December 2014: An idea hatches. Discussion between Professor Tom Calma AO, Melissa Sweet and Summer May Finlay regarding possible Aboriginal and Torres Strait Islander justice series.

2015

February 2015: #JustJustice team forms with Summer May Finlay, Melissa Sweet, Marie McInerney, and Mitchell Ward.

8-9 April 2015: Marie McInerney attends Geraldton Aboriginal Medical Service (GRAMS)'s two-day conference 'Prison Health: From the Inside Out".

9 April 2015: Mick Gooda, Aboriginal and Torres Strait Islander Social Justice Commissioner, launches #JustJustice at Croakey, and the crowdfunding campaign begins on Pozible.

10 April 2015: Blog article, Critical Classroom "Please support the #JustJustice public health campaign" http://www.criticalclassroom.com/please-support-the-justjustice-public-health-campaign/

10 April 2015: Media article, Crikey.com "Change the narrative to stop Aboriginal incarceration" – by Melissa Sweet. https://www.crikey.com.au/2015/04/10/change-the-narrative-to-stop-aboriginal-incarceration/

13 April 2015: Radio interview 2SER – Melissa Sweet. http://www.2ser.com/groove-therapy/item/14669-reclaimaustralia-vs-sosblakaustralia-isis-hackers-meerkat-vs-periscope

14 April 2015: Online medical article, MJA Insight "Compounding problems" by Dr Ruth Armstrong (mentions #JustJustice).

22 April 2015: Radio interview, Koori Radio interviews Summer May Finlay.

May 2015: Medical magazine, Medical Observer column – by Melissa Sweet.

2 May 2015: Newspaper article "Barnett's closure plans upset remote communities" The Saturday Paper – by Marie McInerney.

6 May 2015: Blog article, "Doctor's Bag" "Aboriginal over-incarceration: After more than 200 years, let's try our approach" Dr Edwin Kruys interviews Summer May Finlay. https://doctorsbag.net/2015/05/06/aboriginal-over-incarceration-after-more-than-200-years-lets-try-our-approach/

May 2015: Newsletter - In Touch – Public Health Association of Australia. Article about #JustJustice crowdfunding campaign.

May 2015: #IHMayDay2015 - #JustJustice was a topic facilitated by Summer May Finlay.

7 June 2015: Final day for Pozible crowdfunding campaign. Funding target is reached with a few hours to spare.

13 July 2015: Radio interview. 2SER interviews Summer May Finlay. http://www.2ser.com/terms-a-conditions/item/16684-how-to-report-constitutional-recognition-aboriginal-media

August 2015: Dr Megan Williams joins #JustJustice team.

September 2015: #JustJustice presented at Mayo Clinic Healthcare and Social Media Summit – Summer May Finlay http://event.icebergevents.com.au/mayoinoz2015/speakers/summer-may-finlay

September-October 2015: #JustJustice Periscopes and interviews conducted in Western Australia by Melissa Sweet.

December 2015: Marie McInerney attends Cowra Shire Council meeting which declares unanimous support to pursue a Justice Reinvestment pilot, after a three year research project in the town by National Centre for Indigenous Studies at the Australian National University.

2016

16 February 2016: #JustJustice introduced by Dr Megan Williams at the Queensland Corrections Symposium held by the Griffith Criminology Institute, Brisbane.

March 2016: Radio interview, Amy McGuire on 89.9 For the Best Country Let's Talk interviews Summer May Finlay http://www.989fm.com.au/podcasts/lets-talk/summer-may-finlay/

May 2016: Summer May Finlay presents #JustJustice at the Inaugural Aboriginal and Torres Strait Islander Suicide Prevention Conference, Alice Springs.

May 2016: Radio interview, Professor Larissa Behrendt on ABC Radio's Speaking Out interviews Summer May Finlay http://www.abc.net.au/radio/programs/speakingout/speaking-out/7394658

May 2016: #IHMayDay2016 - #JustJustice was a topic facilitated by Summer May Finlay.

September 2016: Paul Dutton finalises art work, "Mother Earth" for the cover of #JustJustice.

September 2016: Summer May Finlay presents #JustJustice at Public Health Association of Australia conference, Alice Springs.

October 2016: The inaugural Closing the Prison Gap: Cultural Resilience Conference is held in northern NSW. Dr Megan Williams presents at the conference, and reports on it for #JustJustice.

October 2016: Summer May Finlay discussed #JustJustice as part of the New News panel, called "Not just news to us", Melbourne.

24 October 2016: Dr Megan Williams discusses #JustJustice at Western Sydney University's Songlines Aboriginal Research Symposium.

27 October 2016: Sydney's Queer Provocations series holds panel discussion on 'Manifesting a World Without Prisons'; Dr Megan Williams introduces #JustJustice.

16 November 2016: NACCHO Aboriginal Health News insert in The Koori Mail. Full-page spread on #JustJustice – by Dr Megan Williams.

27 November 2016: Professor Tom Calma AO launches #JustJustice book at Gleebooks, Sydney.

December 2016: Following the successful launch of the first edition of the #JustJustice book, Western Sydney University makes a $5,000 grant to enable a second edition and dissemination strategies.

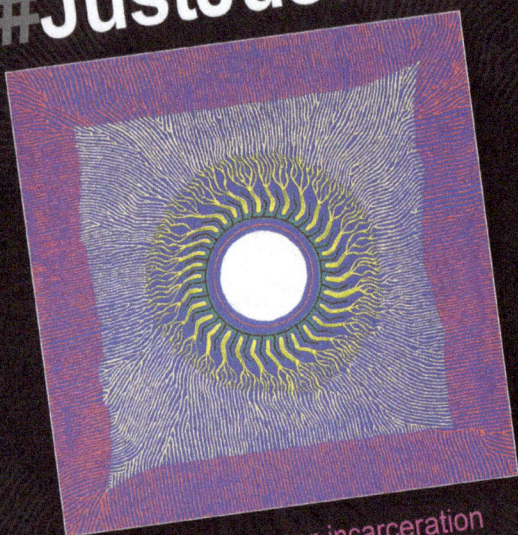

#JustJustice

Tackling the over-incarceration of Aboriginal and Torres Strait Islander peoples

#JUSTJUSTICE

"...it is now time for politicians and policy makers to join us to address this national crisis."

Professor Tom Calma AO

www.ingramcontent.com/pod-product-compliance
Lightning Source LLC
Chambersburg PA
CBHW061011030426
42336CB00028B/3452